ESSENTIAL MANAGEMENT OF OBSTETRIC EMERGENCIES

CLINICAL
EMERGENCY
CARE
SERIES

ESSENTIAL MANAGEMENT OF OBSTETRIC EMERGENCIES

THOMAS F BASKETT

MB BCh BAO (The Queen's University of Belfast)
FRCS(C), FRCS(Ed), FRCOG, FACOG, DHMSA

Professor, Department of Obstetrics and Gynaecology
Dalhousie University, Halifax, Nova Scotia, Canada

Fourth Edition

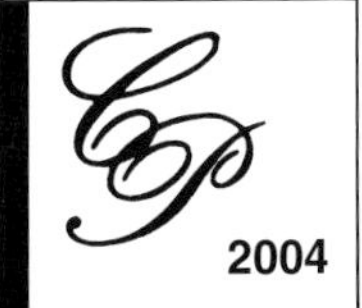

2004

Published by: Clinical Press Limited, Redland Green Farm, Redland Green, Redland, Bristol BS6 7HF

British Library Cataloguing in Publication Data

Baskett, Thomas F.
Essential management of obstetric emergencies.
1. Obstetrics. Emergency treatment.
I. Title II. Series
618.2025

ISBN 1 85457 048X

First edition 1985 John Wiley & Sons Ltd
Second edition 1991 Clinical Press Ltd.
Third edition 1999 Clinical Press Ltd.
Fourth edition 2004 Clinical Press Ltd

Typeset and printed by: Allens Printers Ltd.

Preface to fourth edition

Time moves on and it is now 20 years since I took pen in hand (I still use a pen) to write what I thought would be the first and only edition of this book. After another 20 years of labour ward experience, my own interest and the encouragement of others has been enough to warrant bringing this book up to date.

Despite advances in medical knowledge, pharmaceuticals and technology there has been little or no improvement in maternal and perinatal mortality in the developing world in the past 30 years. Even in developed countries, where maternal and perinatal mortality rates are low, preventable factors are to be found in one-third to one-half of all cases. Severe morbidity occurs at 20-30 times the rate of mortality and can lead to permanent disability. Most of the preventable factors are due to the omission of basic clinical principles, rather than a lack of high technology.

All chapters have been completely revised and the references and bibliography brought up to date. As in the last edition I recommend that readers consult the *Pregnancy and Childbirth Module of the Cochrane Data Base of Systematic Reviews* for recent advances. I have added two new chapters: Vaginal Delivery after Caesarean Section and Emergency Obstetric Hysterectomy as I feel these topics are of sufficient importance to warrant their own brief, self-contained chapters.

While this book covers specialist personnel and facilities in well developed obstetric units, it is also aimed at those with minimal specialist training, both nurses and doctors, who work in areas with limited resources. These are the people who sustain maternity services under difficult clinical, and sometimes medico-legally challenging conditions: they have my admiration.

As always I am grateful to my wife Yvette who has kept me on track and typed the revised manuscript.

T.F. Baskett

Preface to third edition

Since the earlier editions of this book the era of evidence-based medicine has become firmly established in the specialty of obstetrics. Appropriately, we are now encouraged to base clinical decisions on the best evidence available, especially that from randomised controlled trials. Much progress has been made in this area with the *Pregnancy and Childbirth Module of the Cochrane Data Base of Systematic Reviews*. The value of the Cochrane data base is such that it is recommended for chronic use to provide up-to-date information on all areas in this book. As such, though it does not appear in the suggested reading of each individual chapter, it is so intended.

However, there are many aspects of obstetrical emergencies for which randomised controlled trials have not been carried out, and indeed never will – imagine trying to randomise two methods of management of acute uterine inversion. There are, therefore, a few remaining areas in which the elders can still use the phrase, "In my experience....", with some degree of influence. Thus, some management continues to be based on the best experience available and remains, to a degree, *secundum artem*.

The entire book has been revised. I have omitted the chapter on Venous Thromboembolism as I think it belongs better in a text on medical disorders in pregnancy. I have added two new chapters on Trauma in Pregnancy and Emergency Uterine Relaxation as I feel these are areas of clinical relevance. Otherwise, I have retained the guiding philosophy outlined in the prefaces to the first and second editions.

Once again I am indebted to my wife Yvette who, in addition to her duties as a nurse, has typed the entire manuscript.

T.F. Baskett

Preface to second edition

In the six years since the first edition, the social and clinical aspects of obstetrics continue to evolve. Each chapter has been revised, many extensively. However, I have retained the same format and practical clinical approach to the problems presented. I have added a new chapter on the role of major vessel ligation and embolization in obstetric haemorrhage. This covers an area in which the place of each of these techniques has been clarified in recent years.

The sophisticated medical technology and knowledge associated with intensive care has a critical but small role in the management of obstetric emergencies. I continue to be impressed by the fact that many obstetric emergencies are preventable or easily treated at an early stage by the application of long-established and straightforward clinical principles. It is inevitable that hospitals providing obstetric care will have to deal with emergencies, many of which are predictable. The medical and nursing personnel involved must therefore be prepared to forestall or deal with emergencies when they are readily manageable. It is in this context that I hope this book may be of help.

I am grateful to Mr David Kingham of Clinical Press for the opportunity to produce a second edition of this work. The response to the first edition from doctors and nurses working in the clinical arena has been gratifying and enough to justify the time and effort involved. I can also confirm that there is much truth in the cynical aphorism that the main stimulus for writing a book is 'in the hope of learning something about the subject'.

T. F. Baskett

Preface to first edition

Most writings approach obstetric care from the viewpoint of the large well-equipped hospital. In fact, most obstetric emergencies originate outside the hospital and in many parts of the world have to be dealt with, at least initially, in nursing stations or smaller hospitals. While this book carries the management through to the level of care available in the large teaching hospital, I have tried also to outline the appropriate treatment when limited facilities are all that are available. This book is therefore directed at those who may be involved with obstetric emergencies at all levels of care: nurses, family practitioners, and obstetricians in training. Rather than provide only a list of management, I have tried to outline the pathophysiology so that the clinical presentation and rationale for the advised treatment are understood. Having done this, I have been somewhat dogmatic in the sections on management as a positive and decisive course of action is needed when dealing with any emergency. I have not provided an exhaustive list of references but named a few relevant articles for readers who seek a wider view of the topic.

I have mixed feelings towards my brother Peter's role in this book. As Wiley's adviser in emergency medicine, he asked me to produce this volume as the first in a series, each of which will cover a different area of emergency care. He therefore involved me in a year's hard work, but on the other hand I have learned much and benefited greatly from his enthusiasm and guidance. The publishers have also earned my gratitude for their unobtrusive and helpful direction.

Much of my own experience with obstetric emergencies was gained during a 10-year period as a consultant in obstetrics and gynaecology to a remote area of the Canadian north. It is to the people of this area that I dedicate this book.

T.F. Baskett

Contents

CHAPTER 1

Maternal and perinatal mortality

Maternal and perinatal mortality rates indirectly reflect the socio-economic and health service standards of a country. Unfortunately, in developing countries the statistics are often unavailable or inaccurate, whereas in developed countries definitions are not standardised, so that comparisons may be meaningless. It is not intended to cover the causes of maternal and perinatal mortality in detail, but to outline trends and highlight the main threats to the mother and baby.

MATERNAL MORTALITY

DEFINITIONS

'The beginning of wisdom is the definition of terms.' (Socrates)

In recent years attempts have been made to standardise the definition of maternal death. The most widely accepted is that endorsed by both the World Health Organisation and the International Federation of Gynaecologists and Obstetricians: 'The death of a woman while pregnant or within 42 days of termination of pregnancy, irrespective of the duration and the site of pregnancy, from any cause related to or aggravated by the pregnancy or its management but not from accidental or incidental causes.' In the United Kingdom and the United States deaths up to one year after delivery are reviewed. The maternal mortality rate is expressed as the number of direct and indirect obstetric deaths per 100,000 live births or maternities. Maternities include both live and stillbirths. Maternal deaths are classified as follows:

Direct obstetric deaths are 'deaths resulting from obstetric complications of the pregnant state (pregnancy, labour, and puerperium), from interventions, omissions, incorrect treatment or from a chain of events resulting from any of the above.' For example: abortion, ectopic pregnancy, hypertensive diseases of pregnancy, antepartum and post partum haemorrhage, and puerperal sepsis.

Indirect obstetric deaths are 'deaths resulting from previous existing disease, or disease that developed during pregnancy and which was not due to direct obstetric causes, but which was aggravated by the physiological effects of pregnancy.' For example: anaemia, cardiac disease, and diabetes.

Coincidental deaths are 'from accidental or incidental unrelated causes which happen to occur in pregnancy or the puerperium'. For example: motor vehicle accident, homicide, malignancy, and unrelated infectious diseases.

There is evidence that extending the review beyond 42 days in the puerperium will significantly increase the detection of maternal deaths.[1,2] For example in the latest United Kingdom report (1997-1999), by extending the review from 42 days to one year, there were an additional 107 (28%) late maternal deaths. Of these 7 per cent were direct, 36 per cent indirect and 57 percent coincidental.

Of all women dying in pregnancy and the puerperium approximately 40 percent are direct, 30 per cent indirect, and 30 percent coincidental deaths, although this will vary widely between developed and undeveloped countries.

Many national statistics report only direct obstetric deaths and it is estimated that even countries with well-developed reporting systems will miss 20-55 percent of maternal deaths.[3]

MAIN CAUSES OF MATERNAL DEATH

Probably the most complete and accurate statistics of maternal mortality come from the reports on confidential enquiries into maternal deaths in the United Kingdom. This report has been produced every three years since 1952. For the most recent triennial report (1997-99) there were a total of 242 direct and indirect deaths. The leading causes of direct maternal death were:

1. Thromboembolism
2. Hypertensive disorders of pregnancy
3. Sepsis
4. Ectopic pregnancy
5. Amniotic fluid embolism
6. Haemorrhage

In the United States, from 1991-97, the main causes of direct deaths were hypertenisve disorders, thromboembolism, amniotic fluid embolism, sepsis, ectopic pregnancy and haemorrhage.[4] In Australia, for the triennium 1994-96, direct maternal deaths were due to thromboembolism, amniotic fluid embolism, hypertensive disorders, ectopic pregnancy, sepsis and haemorrhage.[5]

The difference in safety of child bearing between developed and developing countries is starkly illustrated by the following figures: There are more than 500,000 maternal deaths in the world each year (one per minute). Of these 99 per cent occur in developing countries. In some developing countries the maternal death rate exceeds 1000 per 100,000 maternities compared to 5-20 per 100,000 in developed countries. In developing countries the main causes of maternal death are haemorrhage, sepsis, eclampsia, obstructed labour and its sequelae, illegal abortion and anaemia. In addition many women succumb to general medical and infectious diseases aggravated by pregnancy.[6,7] These factors are often related to women reproducing too young, too old and too often.

The underlying causes of maternal mortality are often associated with three factors known as the **"Three Delays"**.

- Delay in seeking care: the decision by the patient and/or the initial provider to seek care.
- Delay in reaching care: usually based on lack of transportation and sometimes lack of money.
- Delay in receiving care: they reach the local health centre or hospital but that institutuion does not have adequate personnel, equipment or drugs to provide the appropriate care.

The delays are often a mixture of socio-cultural, socio-economic and health system factors. These can apply in both developed and developing countries – although more pronounced in the latter.

The recommended response to this is for the local community/health centres to provide six basic emergency obstetrical functions – known as emergency obstetric care (Em OC). These are:

- Oxytocics
- Antibiotics
- Magnesium sulphate
- Manual/electrical suction evacuation for incomplete/septic abortion
- Manual removal of placenta
- Vacuum extraction for obstructed labour

The more major referral centres should be able to provide EmOC and, in addition, facilites for blood transfusion, laparotomy and caesarean section.

Because maternal deaths are rare in developed countries it has been suggested that a more accurate measure of the standard of maternal care is to study 'near-miss' cases, which may be defined as those women requiring critical care.[8] For every maternal death there may be 20-25 women who require intensive care.[9,10]

PERINATAL MORTALITY

A stillbirth is caused by factors in the antenatal or intrapartum course of pregnancy. A neonatal death may be due to similar factors, in addition to the availability and quality of neonatal care. When maternal death rates fall the perinatal mortality rate becomes a better marker of the standard of obstetric care.

DEFINITIONS

Perinatal mortality definitions have been even more variable than those of maternal mortality, so that comparisons between countries and even regions of the same country are fraught with statistical pitfalls. Many of these are based on legal definitions. Others are defined by gestational age which is often uncertain.

The following definitions are suggested by the World Health Organization and the International Federation of Gynaecologists and Obstetricians and should be used:

Stillbirth rate: The number of stillbirths weighing ≥500g per 1000 total births.

Early neonatal mortality rate: The death of a liveborn baby ≥500 g within 7 days of birth per 1000 live births.

Late neonatal mortality rate: The death of a liveborn baby ≥500g within 28 days of birth per 1000 live births.

Postnatal mortality rate: The number of deaths >28 days and up to one year per 1000 live births.

Perinatal mortality is the sum of all stillbirths and neonatal deaths, and has two accepted definitions:

Standard perinatal mortality rate: The number of stillbirths and early neonatal deaths ≥1000 g per 1000 total births. This is the definition recommended for international comparison.

Extended perinatal mortality rate: The number of stillbirths and late neonatal deaths ≥500g per 1000 total births. This is a more sensitive indicator of the standard of obstetric care and should be used whenever possible.

MAIN CAUSES OF PERINATAL DEATH

LOW BIRTH WEIGHT

This is the most common factor involved in perinatal death, although there may be many different antecedents:

1. Spontaneous preterm rupture of the membranes and/or preterm labour.
2. Intrauterine growth restriction.
3. Induced labour because of antenatal complications such as hypertensive disease, antepartum haemorrhage, blood group incompatibilities, etc. These and other antenatal complications may, of course, also lead to spontaneous premature labour and intrauterine growth restriction.

The main causes of death among the low birth weight are, extreme immaturity, respiratory distress syndrome, intraventricular haemorrhage and sepsis.

INTRAUTERINE ASPHYXIA

This is still a major cause of perinatal death, particularly stillbirth. In many cases there are clinical factors leading to failure of placental oxygen transfer. These may be acute (abruptio placentae, cord prolapse) or more insidious (hypertensive disease, prolonged pregnancy). Death may occur before labour or the hypoxia may only become manifest during the stress of labour when the uterine contractions cause a reduction in intervillous space blood flow. If the baby does not die *in utero*, fatal hyaline membrane disease and/or intraventricular haemorrhage secondary to the hypoxia may occur early in the postnatal period.

UNEXPLAINED

In several cases of stillbirth there are no clinical antecedents and autopsy shows only non-specific changes of hypoxia but no other fetal or placental pathology. Such 'unexplained' cases form an increasingly large (40-65 per cent) proportion of all stillbirths.

CONGENITAL ANOMALIES

As other causes are reduced, this group produces about 15-25 per cent of all perinatal deaths – particularly those in the neonatal period. The frequency of the different types of abnormalities varies in different countries, but the most common are: central nervous system, cardiac, chromosomal, and multiple system anomalies. As comprehensive programmes of antenatal screening and early pregnancy termination for congenital anomalies are established, this cause of perinatal mortality may be reduced.

FACTORS ASSOCIATED WITH MATERNAL AND PERINATAL MORTALITY

Age: There is an increased risk of maternal and perinatal death at the extremes of reproductive age. The teenage mother has a slightly increased risk and the woman over 35 years a much greater risk than the ideal 20-30 age group.[4]

Parity: The risk is slightly increased in the first pregnancy and greatly increased in fifth and subsequent pregnancies,[4,11] although this effect is ameliorated with good obstetric care.

Socio-economic: In all countries those at the lower end of the socio-economic scale have a greater risk of death in pregnancy. The possible reasons are many: poor education, poor nutrition, poor housing and sanitation, less likely to seek or, in countries where this is required, be able to afford obstetric care.

Smoking: Women who smoke have a slightly higher perinatal mortality. This seems to be due to both the adverse effects of smoking and the fact that there are more smokers in low socio-economic groups.

Geography: In some countries this is an important factor. It is impossible to provide sophisticated maternity care to patients living in remote areas. Although it has been shown in the Canadian north and other countries, that with careful application of resources the risks can be reduced.[12-14] In many instances poor socio-economic conditions and higher age and parity are linked to geographic isolation.

Obstetric care: All studies show a very significant relationship between a lack of antenatal care and higher maternal and perinatal mortality. This is one of the biggest factors and has an important bearing on all the other associated factors. For example, the unmarried teenage primigravida's increased risk can be eliminated if she seeks and receives good obstetric care.

REDUCTION OF MATERNAL AND PERINATAL MORTALITY

The reduction in maternal mortality rates in developed countries has been impressive. Indeed,it is a reflection of the degree of improvement that maternal deaths, once expressed per 1000 births, are now so rare they are expressed per 100,000 births. In developed countries the direct obstetric death rate is 5-10 per 100,000 maternities. This represents an eightfold improvement in the last 30 years and a 50-60 fold improvement in the last 60 years.

Perinatal mortality rates have also dropped, but not so precipitously. Over the past 50 years there has been a four-to-fivefold decrease in perinatal deaths, with an accelerated reduction over the past 20 years.

In developed countries the standard perinatal mortality rate should be below 10 per 1000 total births.

The main reasons for this improvement are:

- Better education and socio-economic conditions
- Better nutrition and general health
- Lower age and parity
- The increased provision and utilisation of obstetric services and hospital delivery
- Safer anaesthesia
- Blood transfusion
- Antibiotics
- Maternal and perinatal death reviews

Further improvements in maternal and perinatal mortality can be expected with emphasis on the following:

1. In developing countries the maternal and perinatal mortality rates are so appallingly high that even the provision of very basic maternity services and emergency obstetric care (EmOC) will produce great improvement. However, even in countries with freely available sophisticated medical services the irreducible minimum of mortality has not been reached,as demonstrated by the fact that 40-50 per cent of all maternal, and 25-50 per cent of all perinatal deaths, are due to ideally preventable factors.

   The biggest gains are not going to be made by advances in sophisticated medical technology but by the efficient and equitable application of currently existing knowledge and techniques. Improvement in education and the elimination of illiteracy are major factors. All studies and reviews of this subject have shown that improved education and status of women in their community are the main factors associated with a fall in maternal and perinatal mortality.

   The organisation of local resources and regionalisation of care suitable for the socio-economic and geographic conditions are the main factors. Careful selection and referral of high risk pregnancies to the appropriate level of perinatal care is important.
2. Continued improvement of socio-economic conditions should bring a concomitant increase in the standard of general health, nutrition, housing, and education.
3. A careful and critical review of all maternal and perinatal deaths is essential, no matter how small the hospital. These reviews should be carried out as a fact-finding, rather than a fault-finding, exercise. This is a most important principle. A careful review will often pinpoint avoidable factors that may be prevented in future cases. In assigning a death as preventable under ideal circumstances, most

reviews will single out one or more of three potentially avoidable factors: medical management, medical facilities, and patient actions. The educational value of such reviews is considerable. At a regional and national level proper data collection and analysis will identify the main causes of death and guide relocation of resources or concentration of effort.

4. Adequate training of personnel destined to look after pregnant women, along with continuing education and support. There is much to said for each maternity unit adopting clear guidelines for the common conditions that threaten maternal health, such as: hypertension, eclampsia, haemorrhage and sepsis. Appropriately, such guidelines are being produced by national and regional societies.

REFERENCES

1. Report on Confidential Enquiries into Maternal Deaths in the United Kingdom. Why Mother Die 1997-1999. London: RCOG Press, 2001.
2. Rochat RW, Rubin GL, Selik R. Changing the definition of maternal mortality: a new look at the post partum interval. Lancet 1982;2:831.
3. Schuitemakern N, Roosmalen JV, Dekker G et al. Underreporting of maternal mortality in the Netherlands. Obstet Gynecol 1997;90:78-82.
4. Berg CJ, Chang J, Callaghan WM, Whitehead SJ. Pregnancy-related mortality in the United States, 1991-1997. Obstet Gynecol 2003;101:289-96.
5. Report on Maternal Deaths in Australia, 1994-96. Canberra: National Health and Medical Research Council, 2001.
6. Liskin LS. Maternal morbidity in developing countries: a review and comments. Int J Gynecol Obstet 1992;37:77-87.
7. Donnay F. Maternal survival in developing countries: what has been done, what can be achieved in the next decade. Int J Gynecol Obstet 2000;70:89-97.
8. Drife JO. Maternal 'near-miss' reports? BMJ 1993;307:1087-8.
9. Bewley S, Kreighton S. "Near-miss' obstetric inquiry. J Obstet Gynaecol 1997;17:26-9.
10. Baskett TF, Sternadel J. Maternal intensive care and near-miss mortality in obstetrics. Br J Obstet Gynaecol 1998;105:
11. Baskett TF. Grand multiparity –a continuing threat. Can Med Assoc J 1977;116:1001-4.
12. Baskett TF. Obstetric care in the central Canadian Arctic. BMJ 1978;2:1001-4.
13. Larsen JV, Muller EJ. Obstetric care in a rural population. S Afr Med J 1978;54:1137-40.
14. Elkady AA, Saleh S, Gadaila S, Fortney J, Bayumi H. Obstetric deaths in Menoufia Governorate, Egypt. Br J Obstet Gynaecol 1989;96:9-14.

BIBLIOGRAPHY

American College of Obstetricians and Gynecologists. Committee Opinion No.167. Perinatal and infant mortality statistics. Washington DC: ACOG, 1995.

Anderson AMN, Wohlfahrt J, Christens P, Olsen J, Melbye M. Maternal age and fetal loss: population based register linkage study. BMJ 2000;320:1708-12.

Bastion H, Keirse MJNC, Lancaster PAL. Perinatal death associated with planned home birth in Australia: population based study. BMJ 1998:317:384-8.

Fathalla MF. Reproductive health: a global overview. Early Hum Dev 1992;29:35-42.

Granja AC, Zacarias E, Bergström S. Violent deaths: the hidden face of maternal mortality. Br J Obstet Gynaecol 2002;109:5-8.

Harper M, Parsons L. Maternal deaths due to homicide and other injuries in North Carolina: 1992-94. Obstet Gynecol 1997;90:920-3.

Hoyert DL, Danel I, Tully P. Matenal mortality, United States and Canada, 1982-1997. Birth 2000;17:4-11.

Krishna UR, Coyaji BJ, Rao KB, Raghavan KS. Safe Motherhood. Bangalore: Federation of Obstetrics and Gynaecological Societies of India ,1995.

Lee KS, Khoshuood B, Chen L, Wall SN, Cromie WJ, Mittendorf RL. Infant mortality from congenital malformations in the United States, 1970-1997. Obstet Gynecol 2001;98:620-7.

Liljestrand J. Reducing perinatal and maternal mortality in the world: the major challenges. Br J Obstet Gynaecol 1999;106:877-80.

Maclean AB, Neilson JP (ed). Maternal Mortality and Morbidity. London:RCOG Press, 2002.

Metha S. Contraception and women's health. Int J Gynecol Obstet (suppl)1995;48:165-71.

Nagaya K, Fetters MD, Ishikawa M et al. Causes of maternal mortality in Japan. JAMA 2000;283:2661-7.

Naidu S, Moodley J, Adhikari M, Ramsaroop R, Morar N, Dunmoye OO. Clinico-pathological study of causes of perinatal mortality in a developing country. J Obstet Gynaecol 2001;21:443-7.

Nkata M. Maternal deaths in teenage mothers. J Obstet Gynaecol 1997;17:344-5.

Rao KB, Maternal mortality in a teaching hospital in Southern India. Obstet Gynecol 1975;46:397-400.

Sach BP, Fretts RC, Garden R et al. The impact of extreme prematurity and congenital anomalies on the interpretation of international comparisons of infant mortality. Obstet Gynecol 1995;85:941-6.

Vandecruys HIB, Pattinson RC, MacDonald AP, Mantel GD. Severe acute maternal morbidity and mortality in the Pretoria Academic Complex: changing patterns over 4 years. Eur J Obstet Gynecol Reprod Biol 2002;102:6-10.

Westergaard HB, Langhoff Roos J, Larsen S et al. Intrapartum death of non malformed fetuses in Denmark and Sweden in 1991: a perinatal audit. Acta Obstet Gynecol Scand 1997;76:959-63.

Wilcox A, Skjaerven R, Buekens P. Birth weight and perinatal mortality. A comparison of the United States and Norway. JAMA 1995:273:709-11.

CHAPTER 2

Antenatal care

Good antenatal care is the cornerstone of management aimed at reducing maternal and perinatal mortality and morbidity. The main principles will be outlined here:

AIMS OF ANTENATAL CARE

1. **Complete medical examination:** This may be the first opportunity in several years for a thorough general medical assessment of the woman. It should always be remembered that the physiological stresses imposed by pregnancy may unmask latent disease: e.g. rheumatic heart disease, gestational diabetes. The course of a medical disease may be worsened by pregnancy or the disease itself may jeopardise the developing fetus.
2. **Obstetric examination:** The pelvic examination in early pregnancy has the following aims:
   - To confirm the diagnosis of pregnancy
   - To assess the uterine size and confirm gestational age
   - To rule out concomitant gynaecological disease
   - To take appropriate cytology and bacteriology specimens
3. **Early detection of pregnancy complications:**
   - Pre-eclampsia
   - Rhesus and other isoimmunisation
   - Multiple pregnancy
   - Malpresentations
   - Anaemia
   - Intrauterine growth restriction
4. **Education:** Advice regarding nutrition, breast feeding, smoking, alcohol, drugs, exercise, and intercourse can be incorporated into antenatal classes.
5. **Engender confidence toward pregnancy, labour and motherhood:** Much of this is provided by those directly looking after the women but good antenatal and postnatal classes can be of great help.
6. **Risk assessment and appropriate plan for antenatal care and delivery.**

HISTORY AND EXAMINATION

FIRST VISIT

Menstrual History

This is a crucial part of the history as it is the most likely source of the correct gestational age. This calculation is done by Naegele's rule, which is based on the mythical normal woman who has a 28 day cycle and ovulates two weeks before the start of her next menstrual period – ie. on day 14. The rule is to add seven days to the first day of the last menstrual period and count back three months to reach the expected date of confinement (EDC). The features to note are:

- First day of last menstrual period:

If not specifically asked, many women will give the date of the end of the period as their last menstrual period. In the case of a seven-day period this would alter the calculation of the expected date of confinement by seven days.

- Normality of last menstrual period:

An implantation bleed may occur at about the time of the expected period (i.e. about 10-14 days after ovulation). This is almost always much lighter and shorter than a normal period. If an implantation bleed is mistaken for a true period, the gestational age calculation would be behind by about four weeks.

- Cycle duration and regularity:

The calculation of gestational age by Naegele's rule is based on a 28-day cycle. Women with a variable cycle, particularly oligomenorrhoea, will require an adjustment to this calculation.

- Cycle interruption:

A calculation adjustment is needed in those women who have not re-established regular cycles after pregnancy, lactation or the contraceptive pill.

Family History

The family history may reveal factors that increase the likelihood of maternal complications or fetal abnormalities:

- Twins
- Diabetes mellitus
- Hypertension
- Hereditary disease

Past Medical History

Past or current medical disorders and associated medications may threaten the mother and fetus, for example:

- Diabetes mellitus
- Epilepsy
- Rheumatic fever
- Renal disease

Past Surgical History

- General surgical procedures
- Gynaecological procedures
  - Myomectomy scar may increase the risk of uterine rupture.
  - Conisation of cervix and therapeutic abortion may increase the risk of cervical incompetence and premature labour.

Past Obstetric History

Like history in general, many complications of pregnancy have a tendency to recur. It is for this reason that the previous obstetric history holds a wealth of valuable relevant information:

- Antenatal complications, e.g. pre-eclampsia, premature labour, iso-immunisation
- Induction of labour and indication
- Assisted vaginal delivery
- Caesarean section – indications, type of section, and complications
- Third stage complications – post partum haemorrhage and/or manual removal of placenta
- Neonatal outcome, e.g. intrauterine growth restriction, macrosomia, congenital anomaly, perinatal death or morbidity.

On the other hand, one or more totally normal pregnancies is the best prognostic factor for a successful outcome in subsequent pregnancies.

Examination

- Height and weight
- General medical examination
- Pelvic examination

SUBSEQUENT VISITS

Traditionally the frequency of antenatal visits has been every four weeks until 28 weeks gestation, every two weeks until 36 weeks and then every week until delivery. However, this may be reduced for many normal women (especially multipara) and will depend on local experience, facilities, and guidelines.[1] In complicated pregnancies more frequent visits will be necessary.

Examination

- Weight
- Blood pressure
- Presence or absence of oedema
- Measure symphysis – fundal height
- Fetal lie, presentation, and relationship of the presenting part to the pelvic brim
- Quickening
- Fetal heart auscultation

SCREENING TESTS

First Visit

- Complete blood count – this is done mainly to detect common iron deficiency anaemia, but also to pick up the rare blood dyscrasia such as leukaemia or thrombocytopenia
- Blood group and antibody screen
- Sickle cell haemoglobinopathy screen in appropriate populations
- Serological test for syphilis
- Human immunodeficiency virus (HIV) testing. If feasible this should be offered to all pregnant women along with appropriate counselling. When positive, treatment of the mother can reduce mother-to-fetus transmission.
- Hepatitis B testing will lead to appropriate management and immunisation of the infant to reduce the risk of mother-to-infant tranmission.
- Rubella immunity detection
- Urine for protein and sugar
- Mid-stream urine for culture: it is worth seeking asymptomatic bacteriuria as its eradication will greatly reduce the incidence of pyelonephritis in later pregnancy
- Cervical cytology, if not done within the past year
- Cervical culture for chlamydia and gonorrhoea: this will depend on local experience, though in most places the prevalence is high enough to warrant such a screen.

Subsequent Visits

- Haemoglobin at 28-30 weeks: more often if anaemia is common in the local population
- If Rhesus negative, check antibody at 28 weeks and give prophylactic Rh (D) immune globulin
- If Rhesus positive, check for atypical antibodies at 28 weeks

- Blood sugar screen at 26-28 weeks for gestational diabetes. This will be done earlier in patients at high risk for this condition
- Urine for protein and sugar at each visit
- Universal or selective third trimester vaginal culture screen for Group B streptococcus.
- Maternal serum biochemical screening and ultrasound markers for fetal anomaly may be used in some regions (see later).

The above represents an acceptable outline of antenatal care. Most regions will have a standard antenatal form on which to record such data. Obviously factors such as prevalence of diseases, availability of medical services and geographic realities will influence the details of antenatal care in any particular area.

ANTEPARTUM FETAL ASSESSMENT

In developed countries, maternal mortality has fallen so low that over the last 30 years the focus of antenatal care has increasingly centred on the fetus. Despite the fact that the last 30 years has seen an explosion of tests and technical equipment to aid antepartum fetal assessment, it should be remembered that the important principles of antenatal care remain unchanged. Those working in areas without the equipment to perform sophisticated tests of fetal evaluation should not feel that they cannot provide safe and adequate antenatal care. On the contrary, the main error in antenatal care that puts both the mother and fetus at risk, is the omission of the sound clinical principles laid down decades ago. The plethora of tests now available for fetal assessment can be confusing. They are often overused and misinterpreted.

In broad terms fetal assessment is aimed at evaluating four aspects of fetal development and health:

1. Gestational age and maturity
2. Fetal growth
3. Fetal well-being (oxygenation)
4. Fetal anomaly

GESTATIONAL AGE AND MATURITY

Menstrual History

As outlined above, a carefully taken menstrual history is the most important single guide to gestational age.

Coital History

In patients with limited coital opportunities, the date of conception may be narrowed down or even pinpointed precisely.

Quickening

The time the patient is first aware of fetal movement is a rough guide only. Most primigravidae will experience quickening between 18 and 20 weeks and most multiparae between 16 and 18 weeks. Even these limits are quite variable.

Auscultation of Fetal Heart

If the fetal heart can be heard using an ordinary fetal stethoscope the patient is likely to be at least 20 weeks' gestation. This will vary depending on the patient's obesity and the skill of the observer.

Uterine Size

This is only of value if the uterine size is assessed with bimanual examination in the first four months. Even then the accuracy may be diminished by obesity, uterine retroversion, a tense patient, and an unskilled observer. It must be stressed that even in early pregnancy the abdominal assessment of uterine size is quite inaccurate. For example, an 8-10 week size, anteverted uterus may be palpable just above the pubic symphysis, whereas a 14 week size, retroverted uterus may not.

Pregnancy Test

The standard urine pregnancy test is usually positive by five weeks' amenorrhoea. This may help in that one can assume that on the date of a positive pregnancy test the patient was at least five weeks' gestation. The newer immune assays for hCG allow even earlier detection.

Ultrasound

This technique has revolutionised the assessment of gestational age and, indeed, antepartum fetal assessment in general. Unfortunately it is frequently misused and misinterpreted. In the first three months the crown-rump length may help pinpoint gestational age to ±7 days. If done in the early second trimester (16-20 weeks) this is accurate to within 7-10 days. In the third trimester the accuracy falls to 3 weeks. This level of accuracy is based on the normal range of biometry for fetuses of a given gestational age. If there is any technical error in the measurement then the range of accuracy falls even more. Thus, if gestational age is in doubt, the optimum time for ultrasound is during the first 20 weeks. In the third trimester ultrasound is of limited help in assessing gestational age.

Amniocentesis

It is not within the scope of this book to go into the details of this test. It is used less often than in the past but may still be indicated when consideration is being given to induction of labour or elective caesarean section, and assurance of fetal pulmonary maturity is required. This investigation, which measures fetal pulmonary surfactant, either as the lecithin:sphingomyelin ratio or the phosphatidyl glycerol content, is concerned with functional maturity rather than gestational age.

X-ray

With the advent of ultrasound and amniocentesis, radiological signs of gestational age are rarely, if ever, sought. They are retained here largely for historical interest. The most consistent and practical signs are the appearance of the ossification centres of the fetal knee. The distal femoral epiphysis appears at 36 weeks' gestation and the proximal tibial epiphysis at 38-40 weeks. On the other hand the absence of these epiphyses does not indicate lack of maturity, as many full-term fetuses will have neither.

The importance of accurate assessment of gestational age in the subsequent management of high risk pregnancy is stressed. The first person to see the patient has the best chance to get an accurate menstrual history and early bimanual uterine assessment and thus is in the best position to pinpoint gestational age. This should be carefully recorded on the antenatal form. When a reliable ultrasound service is available, an early pregnancy review, including gestational age, is helpful.[2]

FETAL GROWTH

In theory, fetal growth may be excessive (e.g. macrosomia with maternal diabetes) or reduced (intrauterine growth restriction). In clinical practice we are mainly concerned with intrauterine growth restriction (IUGR) because of the association with increased perinatal asphyxia and neonatal morbidity and mortality. Deviation from the normal growth pattern has to be quite marked or it will escape clinical detection. This is underlined by the fact that about half of those infants with IUGR are not detected before birth. On the other hand diligent clinical efforts to seek IUGR in the antenatal period will lead to over diagnosis in about 50 per cent of cases.

Estimation of Fetal Growth

Clinical

1. Look for any **antecedent cause:** e.g. chronic hypertension or renal disease. About half of the cases have no obvious cause or associated factors.
2. **Maternal weight gain** may indirectly reflect utero-placental function and fetal nourishment. Poor weight gain, therefore, should increase suspicion, although IUGR often occurs with normal weight gain.
3. **Uterine measurement.** This is usually done by measuring the symphysis-fundal height. In the latter half of the pregnancy this measurement, in centimetres, usually corresponds to the number of weeks gestation.[3,4] This is by no means an absolute rule and the main value of this method is the serial trend. Provided it is done carefully, this is one of the best clinical screening methods for fetal growth, although it has not been proven to improve perinatal outcome. Some clinics combine this with measurement of abdominal girth.
4. **Abdominal palpation** seeking an impression of fetal size and the amount of amniotic fluid (which is often reduced in severe IUGR).

Ultrasound

A number of ultrasonic measurements have been correlated with fetal growth. These include the biparietal diameter (BPD), abdominal circumference and femur length. It is important to remember that the normal range of these measurements at a given gestational age, plus the range of technical error, mean that 2-3 weeks between measurements is required before one can pronounce on the adequacy or inadequacy of growth. With intrauterine growth restriction (IUGR), there is usually preferential redistribution of blood within the fetus to the brain and heart. Thus, the head measurements may continue to grow normally in the presence of significant IUGR. The abdominal circumference, however, is more sensitive to the early changes of IUGR as it measures an area of the fetus reflecting the loss of fat and liver glycogen stores that occur earlier in fetal malnutrition. Thus, when seeking ultrasound confirmation of IUGR, both the BPD and abdominal circumference are necessary. The other end result of the redistribution of blood within the fetus is reduced renal perfusion leading to a decrease in fetal urine production and thence to oligohydramnios. Various measures of amniotic fluid volume are used, including the single deepest pocket of fluid and four-quadrant pocket assessment – the sum of which gives the amniotic fluid index. Although oligohydramnios is a very important sign of IUGR, it tends to be a late manifestation.

More advanced ultrasound techniques involving Doppler studies of blood flow in the umbilical cord and within the fetus, along with assessment of fetal urine production, may produce earlier and more precise detection of IUGR. Indeed, Doppler umbilical artery waveform in cases of IUGR is one of the few antepartum tests that has been shown to improve perinatal outcome.

FETAL WELL-BEING

The term 'well-being' is usually taken to mean the absence of fetal asphyxia, so that tests of fetal well-being are aimed at assessing the adequacy of utero-placental perfusion and fetal oxygenation. The following methods of assessment are available:

Clinical Assessment

This entails careful antenatal appraisal seeking factors known to be associated with an increased risk of fetal asphyxia and selecting these patients for more detailed fetal assessment. For example: hypertensive disorders, antepartum bleeding, suspected IUGR, prolonged pregnancy, etc.

Biophysical Assessment

1. **Fetal movement counting** by the mother is an attractive and readily available method of fetal assessment. The rationale is based on the finding that many babies suffering chronic and progressive asphyxia *in utero* move less and less before death. There are many approaches to maternal fetal movement counting, with one of the most practical being the Cardiff 'count-to-ten' method. While this test is not infallible, it has the merit of a simple screening method and is available to all.[5]
2. **Fetal heart assessment** is one of the most commonly used biophysical tests:

a) The **non-stress test** or **cardiotocography** is based on the finding that when the normal fetus moves the fetal heart rate accelerates. This test is simple to do but requires a fetal heart monitor. It is possible to modify the test and, using auscultation alone, apply the same principles without a fetal heart monitor.[6]

b) The **contraction stress test** and the **oxytocin challenge test** also require a fetal monitor. They evaluate the fetal heart response to either Braxton Hicks or oxytocin-induced contractions. These are time consuming (45-90 min) and have largely been supplanted by the other biophysical tests.[7]

3. The **fetal biophysical profile** has been developed in an attempt to provide more comprehensive fetal assessment. Using the fetal heart monitor and real time ultrasound five fetal biophysical variables are assessed: the non-stress test, fetal movement, fetal tone, fetal breathing movements, and amniotic fluid volume. This method requires more sophisticated equipment but has a higher predictive ability than single tests of fetal assessment.[8]

If one has limited resources the triad of fetal movement counting, non-stress test and amniotic fluid volume assessment is a reasonable compromise, with the more comprehensive tests reserved for difficult cases.

Biochemical Assessment

Over the last three decades many hormones (e.g. oestriol) and enzymes have been measured in maternal blood and urine in an attempt to find a relationship with feto-placental function. Many of these had a general correlation with fetal outcome but were too variable to be of much help with individual cases and they have been replaced by the biophysical tests.

FETAL ANOMALY

Anything abnormal that a fetus can do is more likely to be done by an abnormal fetus. Thus if one remembers that **abnormal babies do abnormal things** it serves as a reminder to consider fetal anomalies in the following situations:

History

- Past history of fetal anomaly
- Family history of fetal anomaly
- Advanced maternal and, to a lesser extent, paternal age
- Diabetes mellitus (higher incidence of all abnormalities, especially major CNS anomalies)
- Drugs and high alcohol intake

Clinical

- Abnormal amniotic fluid volume—both polyhydramnios (e.g. major CNS and upper GI tract anomalies) and oligohydramnios (e.g. obstructive uropathy) have a strong association with fetal anomalies.

- Abnormal fetal growth – many abnormal fetuses exhibit either growth restriction (e.g. chromosomal anomalies) or, less likely, certain types of abnormaly large anomalies.
- Malpresentations – abnormal fetuses more often lie in abnormal positions.
- Twins – the chance of one or other twin being abnormal is greater than with a singleton pregnancy.
- Complications of pregnancy such as bleeding, premature labour, and premature rupture of the membranes are more common with an abnormal fetus.
- The abnormal fetus is more likely to produce abnormal results in response to tests of fetal well-being.

When the possibility of fetal anomaly is raised by the above findings, the following tests may be appropriate:

1. **Genetic amniocentesis:** This may be necessary to clarify the findings of abnormal results involving maternal serum biochemical screening and ultrasound markers for fetal anomaly.
2. **Chorionic villus sampling (CVS):** It was hoped that this procedure, carried out in the first trimester, might replace second trimester amniocentesis in selected cases. However, the procedure-related risks of CVS are greater than those of amniocentesis. In addition, the results of karyotyping from placental tissue are fraught with ambiguity related to placental mosaicism and maternal overgrowth.
3. **Cordocentesis:** This may be used in special centres for carefully selected fetuses, especially the small for gestational age fetus, with suspected chromosomal abnormalities and for haematological disorders.
4. **Ultrasound:** With the advances in ultrasound technology the definition of fetal anatomy has made rapid strides so that in skilled hands many fetal structural anomalies can be diagnosed.
5. **X-ray:** This may still help with skeletal anomalies but has been largely supplanted by ultrasound.

ROUTINE OBSTETRIC ULTRASOUND

Arguments can be advanced in favour of universal ultrasound in early pregnancy. These include, precise estimation of gestational age, screening for multiple pregnancy, baseline measurement against which subsequent fetal growth can be followed, screening for markers of fetal abnormalities, and the detection of structural fetal anomalies. Skilled routine ultrasound can reduce the induction rate for prolonged pregnancy and will increase the detection of fetal anomalies, allowing the option of second trimester termination. Apart from converting perinatal loss due to anomalies to second trimester termination, routine ultrasound has not been shown to reduce perinatal mortality. In addition, the equipment, trained personnel and expense necessary to provide this service to a high standard in all pregnancies is not available in many areas. Other than screening and detection of fetal anomalies the cost effectiveness remains unproven and the potential for additional expensive, inappropriate and possibly harmful testing and intervention exists. Thus, the debate on the advisability, or otherwise, of routine ultrasound screening in pregnancy continues. However, in many regions with appropriate facilities, routine ultrasound assessment of early pregnancy has been incorporated into normal antenatal care.

SCREENING FOR FETAL ANOMALY

In recent years it has been established that maternal serum screening of certain biochemical markers (alpha-fetoprotein, PAPP-A oestriol, hCG) at 16 weeks gestation can, in association with maternal age, increase the identification of fetal chromosomal abnormalities (Down's syndrome, trisomy 18). In addition to the use of ultrasound to screen for major structural anomalies at 18-20 weeks gestation, there are more subtle features such as nuchal transluency and choroid plexus cysts that can be identified in the first trimester and are also markers for an increased risk of aneuploidy. Thus, in some regions combined serum screening, along with first and second trimester ultrasound screening is offered to all pregnant women. Implementation of such screening programmes requires sophisticated coordination of personnel and facilities including: information and counselling services, laboratory and ultrasound.

The whole field of antepartum fetal assessment is large and developing rapidly. It is beyond the scope of this book to cover it in detail, so that the above account represents an outline only. The interested student is referred to suggested reading at the end of this chapter and encouraged to consult the Cochrane Database.

PREGNANCY RISK ASSESSMENT

It has long been known that patients with certain complications in pregnancy require different levels of care to achieve the best outcome. Factors in the past obstetric performance, medical history or complications arising in pregnancy will increase the risk of maternal and perinatal mortality and morbidity. Such pregnancies are therefore designated 'high risk'. In the 1970s attempts were made to quantitate the degree of risk using various scoring systems. Factors known to increase the risk to mother and/or fetus are identified and the degree of risk apportioned by assigning a score to each factor. The cumulated score from all factors operating in a given pregnancy is added and represents the total risk score. The total score is correlated with perinatal outcome and from this analysis pregnancies can be grouped as high or low risk. Many risk-scoring forms have been developed, but are often long and cumbersome to complete. This type of risk assessment will only be used in clinical practice if it is simple and easily incorporated into normal antenatal care. Examples of these have been applied to large populations and found to correlate well with perinatal outcome.[9,10]

Most studies using pregnancy risk assessment have focused on perinatal outcome, and have shown that about 70 per cent of the perinatal mortality and morbidity comes from 25 per cent of pregnancies with identifiable antepartum risk factors. The addition of intrapartum risk assessment can improve the predictability of outcome, although not all studies support this.[11] Of the factors that cause an increased risk of perinatal mortality and morbidity about one-third are identifiable at the first visit from the past obstetric history and medical examination, one-third develop during pregnancy, and one-third arise during labour.

The main purpose of risk assessment is as a guide to rational planning for suitable pregnancy care, including the need for consultation and appropriate place of delivery. This may be particularly helpful in geographic areas with variable levels of care. Some of the main intrapartum factors that increase risk-premature labour, premature rupture of the membranes, prolonged first stage of labour, and meconium staining – can be identified early enough to allow transfer of the patient to an appropriate hospital.[12]

This risk approach has been criticised, with the valid observation that applying population data to individuals has limitations and women labelled ‘high risk’ can be put under extra stress and subjected to unnecessary additional testing and intervention.[13] Furthermore, the term ‘risk factor’ has also been condemned as being merely a ‘risk marker’, associated with an outcome rather than its cause.

Risk assessment is really the practical application of clinical common sense and its limitations should be realised. Medicine deals with probabilities and to a degree risk scoring helps predict and quantitate those probabilities. It must be stressed, however, that in individual cases risk scoring can be quite misleading: either falsely reassuring or falsely alarming. Thus, blind adherence to the predictive value of an individual score is clearly not indicated. The main value of a risk-scoring form is that it facilitates a disciplined and systematic review of the factors influencing each pregnancy. This, allied to clinical appraisal, can aid the overall pregnancy risk assessment and help define the appropriate level of care.

REFERENCES

1. Jewell D, Sharp D, Sanders J, Peters TJ. A randomised controlled trial of flexibility in routine antenatal care. Br J Obstet Gynaecol 2000;107:1241-7.
2. Crowther CA, Kornman L, O'Callaghan S, George K, Furness M, Willson K. Is an ultrasound assessment of gestational age at the first antenatal visit of value? A randomised clinical trail. Br J Obstet Gynaecol 1999;106:1273-9.
3. Belizan JM, Villar J, Nardin JC, et al. Diagnosis of intrauterine growth retardation by a simple clinical method: measurement of uterine height. Am J Obstet Gynecol 1978; 131: 643-6.
4. Gardosi J, Francis A. Controlled trial of fundal height measurement plotted on customised antenatal growth charts. Br J Obstet Gynaecol 1999;106:309-17.
5. Pearson JF, Weaver JB. Fetal activity and fetal well-being: an evaluation. BMJ 1976; 1:1305-7.
6. Baskett TF, Boyce DA, Lohre MA, Manning FA. Simplified antepartum fetal heart assessment. Br J Obstet Gynaecol 1981;88:395-7.
7. Baskett T F, Sandy E A. The oxytocin challenge test and antepartum fetal assessment. Br J Obstet Gynaecol 1977;84:39-43.
8. Manning FA, Morrison I, Harman CR, Lange IR, Menticoglou S. Fetal assessment based on biophysical profile scoring: experience in 19,221 referred high-risk pregnancies. Am J Obstet Gynecol 1987;157: 880-4.
9. Coopland AT, Peddle LJ, Baskett TF. A simplified antepartum high-risk scoring form: statistical analysis of 5,459 cases. Can Med Assoc J 1977;116:999-1001.
10. Morrison I, Olsen J. Perinatal mortality and antepartum risk scoring. Obstet Gynecol 1979;53:362-6.
11. Morrison I, Carter L, McNamara S. A simplified intrapartum numerical scoring system: the prediction of high-risk in labor. Am J Obstet Gynecol 1980;138:175-80.
12. Webster MA, Linder-Pelz S, Martins J. et al. Obstetric high-risk screening and prediction of neonatal morbidity. Aust NZ J Obstet Gynaecol 1988;28:6-11.
13. A, Chard T. The effectiveness of current antenatal care. In:Studd J (ed). Progress in Obstetrics and Gynaecology. Edinburgh: Churchill Livingstone. 1996;12:3-18.

BIBLIOGRAPHY

Adair CE, Kowalsky L, Quon H et al. Risk factors for early-onset group B streptococcal disease in neonates: a population – based case – control study. Can Med Assoc 2003;169:198-203.

American College of Obstetricians and Gynecologists. Practice Bulletin No.9. Antepartum fetal surveillance. Washington DC. ACOG,1999. (Obstet Gynecol 1999;94. No 4.)

Baskett T F. The fetal biophysical profile. In :Progress in Obstetrics and Gynaecology. Studd J (ed.). Edinburgh:Churchill Livingstone. 1989; 7:145-59.

Baskett T F, Liston R M. Fetal movement monitoring: clinical application. Clin Perinatol 1989;16: 613-25.

Baskett TF, Nagele F. Naegele's Rule: a reappraisal. Br J Obstet Gynaecol 2000;107:1433-5.

Bucher HC, Schmidt JG. Does routine ultrasound scanning improve outcome in pregnancy? meta-analysis of various outcome measures. BMJ 1993;307:13-7.

Coeverden de Groot HA. Provision of a community perinatal service in a developing country. Aust NZ J Obstet Gynaecol 1993;33:225-9.

Cuckle H. Biochemical and ultrasound screening for Down's syndrome: rivals or partners? Ultrasound Obstet Gynecol 1996:7:236-8.

Divon MY, Feber A. Evidence – based antepartum fetal testing. Prenat Neonat Med 2000;5:3-8.

Dornan JC, Harper SA, Bailie CAL. Prenatal screening. Br J Obstet Gynaecol 1998;105:573-5.

Hogberg U, Larsson N. Early dating by ultrasound and perinatal outcome: a cohort study. Acta Obstet Gynecol Scand 1997;76:907-12.

Jones-Pereyra, J. Emphasis on preventative perinatology: a suitable alternative for developing countries. Semin Perinatol 1988;12:381-8.

Koong D, Evans S, Mayes C et al. A scoring system for the prediction of successful delivery in low-risk birthing units. Obstet Gynecol 1997;89:654-9.

McIntosh GC, Olshan Af , Baird PA. Maternal age and the risk of birth defects in offspring. Epidemiology 1995;6:282-8.

Resnik R. Intrauterine growth restriction. Obstet Gynecol 2002;99:490-6.

Roberts T, Henderson J, Mugford M, Bricker L, Neilson J, Garcia J. Antenatal ultrasound screening for fetal abnormalities: a systematic review of studies of cost and cost effectiveness. Br J Obstet Gynaecol 2002;109:44-56.

Royal College of Obstetricians and Gynaecologists. Guideline No.31. The investigation and management of the small-for-gestational-age fetus. London: RCOG, 2002

Society of Obstetricians and Gynaecologists of Canada. Clinical Practice Guideline No.90. Antenatal fetal assessment. J Soc Obstet Gynaecol Can 2000;22:456-62.

Urbaniak SJ, (ed). Consensus conference on Anti-D prophylaxis. Br J Obstet Gynaecol 1998;105(suppl): 1-44.

Work BA. Screening general obstetric populations for risk assessment. Clin Perinatol 1994;21:699-705.

CHAPTER 3

Miscarriage

The legal and clinical definitions of miscarriage vary in different countries. Many will accept the following as a working definition: a fetus weighing less than 500g, or less than 20 weeks gestation if the weight is unrecorded. (In fact the fetus weighs about 400g at 20 weeks, and 500g at 22 weeks).

Approximately 20 per cent of all women will have spotting or bleeding in early pregnancy. The incidence of pregnancy loss from clinically diagnosed miscarriage is about 15 per cent. Many miscarriages occur before pregnancy diagnosis and may be regarded by the woman as a normal or 'delayed heavy' period. In a recent study, up to 22 per cent of pregnancies detected by sensitive hCG assay aborted spontaneously before clinical detection. The total pregnancy loss after implantation, including clinically diagnosed pregnancies, was 31 per cent.[1]
Other miscarriages that are called 'spontaneous' may in fact be initiated by illegal means. In many parts of the world miscarriage is a leading cause of maternal death.[2]

It is not proposed to cover medically induced abortion in this text.

PATHOPHYSIOLOGY

The underlying mechanism usually involves haemorrhage into the decidua basalis leading to necrosis of the implantation site and complete or partial detachment of the conceptus. The detached conceptus acts as a foreign body, stimulating uterine contractions, dilatation of the cervix and complete or partial expulsion of the products of conception. In very early miscarriage the process often leads to complete expulsion of the products of conception. From 6 to 14 weeks some placental tissue is often retained.

About 75 per cent of all spontaneous miscarriages occur before 10 weeks' gestation. In approximately half of the cases of first trimester miscarriage the gestational sac is empty, representing early death of the 'blighted ovum'. In 50-60 per cent of spontaneous miscarriages there is a chromosomal abnormality of the conceptus. Thus, early miscarriage is nature's way of expelling abnormal zygotes. This may occur very early in gestation, so that the pregnancy is undiagnosed, or later in the first trimester when the abnormal zygote has degenerated so much as to present as a blighted ovum or anembryonic pregnancy.

Second trimester miscarriage is much less common (1-2 per cent), the fetus is usually normal and the process is more like a miniature labour.

TYPES OF MISCARRIAGE

1. Threatened
2. Inevitable
3. Incomplete
4. Complete
5. Missed
6. Septic

Recurrent or habitual miscarriage (three or more consecutive spontaneous miscarriages) warrants a full investigation of potential correctable causes. This is outside the scope of this book.

THREATENED MISCARRIAGE

Threatened miscarriage is diagnosed when pregnancy has been confirmed and there is light bleeding coming through a closed cervix. The uterus should be of appropriate size and consistency for the gestational age. Thus in all respects, other than bleeding and perhaps mild crampy hypogastric pain, the pregnancy seems normal.

It is not uncommon for women to bleed around the time of the first missed period as the trophoblast is implanting. This 'implantation bleed' may mimic threatened miscarriage. It is usually light and settles quickly. It is also prudent to consider the differential diagnosis of ectopic pregnancy.

Approximately half of those women with threatened miscarriage who seek medical advice will eventually lose the pregnancy. If the bleeding is red and light the prognosis for continuation of the pregnancy is quite good. If there is recurrent or continued dark brown loss the pregnancy will often end in miscarriage.

The standard urine pregnancy test is of limited value in these cases. The test is based on detection of human chorionic gonadotrophin (hCG) secreted by the chorionic villi, which may continue after the embryo is dead. Thus, a positive test may be registered with incomplete and missed/delayed miscarriages.

MANAGEMENT

1. Bed rest, until the bleeding has ceased, is the traditional treatment. This need not be in hospital and in very few cases will it alter the eventual outcome. Along with the advice to abstain from coitus, the main value of this treatment is that the woman feels she has done her best to avert the pregnancy loss that will ensue in half the cases. After the bleeding has settled the woman gradually resumes full activity.
2. If no ultrasound facilities are available the above management is appropriate and time will clarify whether the woman will abort or the pregnancy continue. If available, ultrasound can help diagnose the eventual outcome sooner so that appropriate treatment can be initiated without delay (see later). In general, if the fetus is seen to be viable on ultrasound the outlook for continuation of the pregnancy is optimistic but not assured.

INEVITABLE AND INCOMPLETE MISCARRIAGE

Miscarriage is inevitable when the products of conception have become detached and nothing can prevent their eventual expulsion. The miscarriage is incomplete when part of the products of conception have been expelled but portions remain *in utero*. The management of both these types of miscarriage is the same.

CLINICAL FEATURES

1. **Bleeding** is usually heavier than a period, often associated with the passage of clots, and can be profuse and life threatening.
2. **Pain** is usually described as like either period or labour pains and is due to uterine contractions trying to expel the remaining products. The pain can be relatively mild or very severe.
3. **Cervical dilatation.** This is not always obvious or to the extent of accepting one finger. However the cervix is usually patulous.
4. The **uterus** should be smaller and firmer than expected for the gestational age.

MANAGEMENT

1. Treatment of hypovolaemic shock with intravenous crystalloid or colloid and blood transfusion may be required.
2. Evacuation of the uterus is the curative treatment:

- General anaesthesia is often given for this procedure. But if circumstances dictate, paracervical block, augmented by inhalation or intravenous narcotic analgesia, is usually adequate.
- An intravenous oxytocin infusion during the procedure may contract the uterus, reducing the chances of uterine perforation and cutting down blood loss.
- In later abortions it may be possible to push the finger through the cervix and loosen the products, facilitating their evacuation.
- The anterior lip of the cervix is grasped with ring forceps and gentle traction used to straighten the uterus. A tenaculum is unnecessary and serves only to tear and cause troublesome bleeding from the vascular and friable pregnant cervix. Using a second pair of ring forceps the uterine cavity is explored. These are gently advanced through the cervix until the fundus is reached, the ends opened, rotated 90°, closed and removed. This is repeated until the larger pieces of tissue are all removed.
- This is followed by **gentle** curettage with the broadest ended, suction curette that can be inserted through the cervix. An empty uterus is confirmed by the 'gritty' feeling of the curette on the uterine wall. It is important not to curette too vigorously because of the risk of causing intrauterine scarring and adhesions (Asherman's syndrome)

3. The technique outlined above is the traditional and more formal operative approach to evacuation of the uterus. Increasingly, in selected patients with inevitable/incomplete miscarriage, evacuation is undertaken in the outpatient or emergency department setting without admission to hospital. There are a variety of simple portable suction devices to facilitate this procedure under a combination of paracervical block, inhalation analgesia and intravenous sedation. This is much more cost-effective and involves the least hospital exposure for the patient.
4. All tissue removed should be sent for pathological assessment to confirm intrauterine pregnancy and pick up the rare case of trophoblastic disease that presents in this manner.
5. All patients must have their blood group checked and, if Rh negative without antibodies, be given Rh immune globulin to protect against isoimmunisation.

In an area where evacuation of the uterus is not possible because of lack of facilities, a different approach is needed:

- Give an intravenous infusion of 30 units oxytocin in 1000 ml crystalloid. This should help reduce the bleeding until the patient can be transferred to an appropriate facility and may aid spontaneous expulsion of the products.

- Pass a vaginal speculum and if products are seen protruding through the cervix, grasp and remove them with ring forceps.

On rare occasions a patient may be seen with bleeding, severe cramping pain and appear profoundly shocked with pallor, hypotension, and bradycardia. Speculum examination reveals products in the cervical os. This represents a form of vasovagal shock with strong uterine contractions trying to force the products of conception through the cervix. This responds rapidly to pulling the products through the cervix with ring forceps. This requires no anaesthesia and produces a dramatic and gratifying improvement in the patient's condition.

PERFORATION OF THE UTERUS DURING CURETTAGE

It is often said that a blunt curette is less liable to perforate the uterus than a sharp curette. It is not the sharpness of the curetting edge that is the danger but the width of the instrument, and more particularly the skill of the operator at the other end of the curette! A sharp curette used gently is safer than a blunt curette used roughly. If available, suction curettage is preferable.

If perforation does occur the following guidelines should serve:

1. If the products have been completely evacuated just observe the patient and, if stable, no active treatment is required. The event should be carefully documented.
2. If the patient continues to bleed vaginally, or if there are signs of intraperitoneal bleeding, or if the products have not been completely evacuated, do a laparoscopy. This should allow completion of the curettage under direct vision. If the perforation is not bleeding, no more need be done. If a small perforation is bleeding those with the skills may be able to suture this via laparascope. If not, a laparotomy should be performed to suture the laceration which, if extensive and lateral, may even require hysterectomy.

COMPLETE MISCARRIAGE

Complete spontaneous expulsion of the products of conception is most likely to occur before 6 weeks and after 12 weeks' gestation. The history, and examination of the tissue passed, allied to the clinical findings of a firm uterus, minimal bleeding and a patulous cervix support the diagnosis of complete miscarriage. If ultrasound is available and confirms that the uterus is empty, evacuation is not necessary.

MISSED/DELAYED MISCARRIAGE

In this variety of miscarriage the embryo dies but the uterus fails to respond in the normal manner and the products of conception are retained. There is bleeding into the chorio-decidual space and ultimately the embryo and placental tissue are partially absorbed and incorporated into a mass of organised blood clot known as a **carneous mole**. If the fetus dies in the early second trimester the amniotic fluid is usually absorbed and the fetus may be partially absorbed or mummified. The placenta shrinks and can become quite adherent to the uterine wall.

CLINICAL FEATURES

1. Early symptoms of pregnancy subside.
2. Signs of pregnancy regress: the uterine size remains static and eventually shrinks. The patient loses weight and pregnancy-induced breast changes disappear.
3. There may be a brown discharge, episodes of threatened abortion or no bleeding at all.
4. The standard urinary pregnancy test may remain positive for some time after the death of the embryo.
5. Ultrasound can confirm the diagnosis.

MANAGEMENT

Eventually nature will respond and expel the products of conception, either as a complete or incomplete miscarriage. There are two reasons for avoiding a prolonged wait once the diagnosis has been confirmed. The woman may suffer emotionally knowing the diagnosis and waiting in suspense for spontaneous miscarriage to occur. The other risk is of disseminated intravascular coagulation, which develops in a small proportion of patients six weeks or longer after death of the embryo (see Chapter 8). Some women will opt for non-intervention, at least for a while, and this should be accomodated.

EVACUATION BY DILATATION AND CURETTAGE (D & C)

This can be one of the more dangerous operations in gynaecology. Some of my worst haemorrhagic moments have occurred with these cases. There seem to be all of the disadvantages and none of the advantages of pregnancy. The uterus is friable and prone to perforation, but not so contractile in response to oxytocic drugs. The placental tissue may have become organised and adherent to the uterine wall. Its removal opens sinuses and the adherence may cause strips of myometrium to tear off, worsening the haemorrhage and leading to Asherman's syndrome. If the cervix is firm, closed and uneffaced it may be traumatised by forceful dilatation. In such cases the pre-operative intra-cervical placement of Laminaria or one of its synthetic variants will reduce cervical trauma and aid subsequent evacuation of the uterus.[3]

Safeguards

1. Check the coagulation profile before operation.
2. Blood group and screen
3. Evacuation to be done by an experienced operator.
4. Only attempt D & C if the uterus is less than 10-12 weeks' size.
5. Infuse oxytocin during the D & C.
6. Have facilities available for hysterectomy.

MEDICAL MANAGEMENT OF SPONTANEOUS MISCARRIAGE

Over the past ten years many departments have advocated a more conservative, non-surgical approach to early pregnancy loss.[4-7] They argue that without intervention most women will completely abort the products of conception within a week of diagnosis, without an increase in short or long term morbidity. Others advocate the use of mifepristone followed by misoprostol, or misoprostol alone, especially for inevitable or incomplete miscarriage. Misoprostol is chosen over surgical evacuation for the uterus >12 weeks' size.

This is an area of management that is evolving and will depend on local availability of the medications. Various combinations, routes of administration (oral versus vaginal), dosage and timing are being tested. Local protocols should be established and evaluated. Efficient backup surgical evacuation services must be available.

Thus, depending on the clinical circumstances and facilities, women with early pregnancy loss can be offered the options of waiting, medical, or surgical evacuation of the uterus.

With the increasing use of first trimester ultrasound screening, the diagnosis of missed/delayed miscarriage is being made earlier and more often. Medical management can be offered, and may be more acceptable to this group of women.

THE USE OF ULTRASOUND IN PATIENTS WITH FIRST TRIMESTER BLEEDING

In some areas of the world ultrasound is not readily available and the diagnosis and management of miscarriage must be based on clinical features alone. Indeed, in the majority of cases this is all that is required. If, however, skilled ultrasound is available it can help distinguish those patients with missed, incomplete or complete miscarriage that make up about half of the cases clinically diagnosed as threatened miscarriage. This will either provide reassurance, or else confirm the need for uterine evacuation without delay. Great care is needed in the interpretation of ultrasonic findings in very early pregnancy. If the gestational age is earlier than suspected a misdiagnosis of blighted ovum can easily be made. In doubtful cases it is therefore advisable to repeat the scan in 1-2 weeks before accepting this diagnosis.

In a patient with a miscarriage thought to be complete, ultrasound can help confirm or deny the presence of products of conception. This may avert the need for anaesthesia and evacuation of the uterus, or alternatively, confirm its necessity.

Thus, ultrasound has revolutionised the management of patients with bleeding in early pregnancy. In most instances the diagnosis can be precisely obtained and the appropriate treatment instituted without delay. Hospital admission and unnecessary bed rest at home can be avoided. A more accurate prognosis can be provided and patient anxiety, associated with delay and uncertainty, reduced.

SEPTIC MISCARRIAGE

Sepsis can complicate any type of miscarriage, but most often the incomplete variety. In countries with easy access to medically induced termination of pregnancy the incidence of septic miscarriage is low, suggesting that many cases are the result of illegally attempted abortion. The reported incidence of sepsis with miscarriage therefore varies from 5 to 25 per cent.

Patients who become pregnant with an intrauterine contraceptive device (IUCD) *in situ* are prone to develop sepsis. It is felt that the threads of the device, protruding through the cervix, may act as a 'wick' for ascending infection coupled with a pregnancy. Thus, any patient who becomes pregnant with an IUCD *in situ*, and the threads visible, should have the device removed by traction on the threads.

CLINICAL FEATURES

In addition to the usual features of the underlying miscarriage:

1. Pyrexia-usually >38°C.
2. Uterine tenderness and possibly evidence of pelvic peritonitis. In most cases the infection is contained in the decidua. In others there is metritis, parametritis, and pelvic peritonitis. In less than 5 per cent septic shock supervenes.
3. Offensive vaginal discharge-not in all cases.

4. Seek signs of illegal interference, such as cervical trauma, that may increase the suspicion of uterine perforation.

MANAGEMENT

1. Treatment of any associated hypovolaemic shock with intravenous crystalloid, colloid and blood as required.
2. Appropriate intrauterine and blood cultures should be taken and sent for aerobic and anaerobic cultures.
3. Intravenous antibiotics will be guided to some extent by local knowledge of causative organisms and their sensitivity. A reasonable choice, in the patient who is not seriously ill, is ampicillin 1 g 4-6 hourly and gentamicin 60-80 mg 8 hourly. The antibiotics should be continued long enough to ensure complete resolution of the infection. This will be guided by the clinical response and the subsequent culture reports.
4. Evacuation of the uterus: Removal of the septic focus is the cornerstone of treatment. Once initial stabilisation of the patient has been achieved, and the antibiotics have been infused for 1-2 hours, the uterus should be emptied without further delay. If the uterus is less than 12 weeks' size this is done by curettage, and if greater than 12 weeks' size it is done by oxytocin infusion followed by curettage if necessary. Curettage must be performed very gently as the infected uterus is very susceptible to perforation. In addition, the possibility of prior perforation due to illegal interference must be kept in mind.

   In most patients this treatment is all that is required and once the septic products are removed the patient recovers rapidly and completely.

The emotional sequelae of miscarriage should not be overlooked. It must be remembered that some women view miscarriage in the same light as a stillbirth and need to grieve accordingly. They, or their husband, frequently harbour guilt regarding coitus or some other event that they feel may have been responsible. An opportunity to ventilate these feelings along with follow-up and discussion of future reproductive prognosis is essential. In this context it is always more appropriate to use the word 'miscarriage' with the woman and her relatives. The word 'abortion' still has connotations of deliberate or illegal termination with the lay public, and may add unnecessary hurt at a vulnerable time.

SEPTIC SHOCK

This is a rare, but dreaded, complication of septic miscarriage. It can also occur in obstetric patients with chorioamnionitis, puerperal endomyometritis, and pyelonephritis. With modern obstetric practice and easy access to medically induced termination of pregnancy the incidence has fallen markedly in the past 25 years.

PATHOPHYSIOLOGY

In the majority of cases gram-negative bacteria are responsible: particularly *Escherichia coli,* and species of *Klebsiella, Enterobacter, Proteus, Pseudomonas, and Bacteroides*. Gram-positive bacteria are incriminated less often but staphylococci, streptococci, and the clostridia can cause a similar picture.

The exact mechanisms involved in the pathophysiology of septic shock are not fully understood. It was thought to be a direct action of the endotoxin released from the cell wall of gram-negative bacteria. It is now felt that the endotoxin exerts its effect indirectly by initiating an exaggerated host immune response via a series of complex events involving the complement, kinin, endorphin, coagulation and fibrinolytic systems. Through these systems, and released chemical mediators such as prostaglandins, catecholamines, histamine, cytokines, glucocorticoids, beta-endorphin, and lysosomal enzymes, profound cardiovascular changes occur. Initial vasodilatation and increased capillary permeability are followed by vasoconstriction, impaired myocardial contractility, hypotension, and reduced tissue perfusion leading to hypoxia, metabolic acidosis, and cardiovascular collapse. The reduced tissue perfusion is manifested by oliguria, adult respiratory distress syndrome (shock lung), intractable hypotension, coma, and eventual death.

CLINICAL FEATURES

The signs and symptoms of the associated cause, e.g. septic miscarriage, puerperal endomyometritis, pyelonephritis, etc., will be present.

In the initial stages of vasodilatation the patient may be alert, tachypnoeic, tachycardiac, and hypotensive, but with warm peripheries:the so-called 'warm shock' phase. Later, as vasoconstriction supervenes, the patient becomes less alert remains tachycardiac and hypotensive, but the peripheries are pale and clammy: the so-called 'cold shock' phase.

If, in a patient with septic miscarriage, hypotension develops that seems out of proportion to the blood loss, septic shock should be suspected. A rapid intravenous infusion of 500-1000 ml crystalloid should correct the hypotension if the shock is due to hypovolaemia but not if it is due to sepsis.

The temperature is usually elevated (38-41°C) initially, but as the reduced tissue perfusion upsets the hypothalamic temperature regulating function the patient can become hypothermic or hyperthermic.

The white cell count may be normal or elevated, with the differential showing increased immature granulocytes.

Disseminated intravascular coagulation may develop (see Chapter 8) and in cases with clostridial sepsis there may be extensive haemolysis.

The end organ sequelae of reduced tissue perfusion, with increasing hypoxia and acidosis, are oliguria, adult respiratory distress syndrome, cardiac failure, peripheral circulatory collapse, and coma.

MANAGEMENT

Just as the exact pathophysiology is uncertain so the treatment of septic shock is controversial and still evolving. If at all possible the assistance of intensive care facilities and personnel should be enlisted. The broad principles of treatment will be outlined here:

1. **Investigations:** Depending on the severity of the patient's condition the following investigations may be needed:
   - Cultures and Gram stain of the urine, blood and septic site.
   - Haemoglobin, haematocrit, platelets, white cell count and differential.
   - Coagulation profile.
   - Serum electrolytes, creatinine, and blood urea.
   - Arterial blood gases.
   - Urinalysis.
   - Chest X-ray.
   - Abdominal and pelvic X-ray looking for air under the diaphragm or a foreign body, either of which may indicate uterine perforation. In cases of suspected clostridial sepsis there may be a myometrial gas pattern.

2. **Intravenous antibiotics:** The initial antibiotic combination must cover all likely causative organisms and sensitivities. This, and the availability of antibiotics, will vary in different locations. A suitable routine involves three antibiotics:
   - Penicillin G 5 million units 4 hourly or ampicillin I g 4 hourly.
   - An aminoglycoside: gentamicin or tobramycin 1.0-1.5 mg/kg 8 hourly. Care must be taken due to the potential ototoxicity of the aminoglycosides. In oliguric patients dose adjustment based on drug serum levels is advisable.
   - Metronidazole 500 mg 8 hourly.

   The combination of penicillin and the aminoglycoside will cover most of the probable pathogens except *Bacteroides fragilis* and some species of *Pseudomonas*. The metronidazole will cover the

Bacteroides. Alternatives to metronidazole are clindamycin, cefoxitin, and chloramphenicol. If *Pseudomonas* species are isolated carbenicillin or ticarcillin may be necessary.

3. **Removal of the septic focus:** This is the most important aspect of treatment and may involve:
   - Evacuation of the uterus by D & C or oxytocin, as outlined in the management of septic abortion.
   - Laparotomy if the uterus has been perforated in an illegal abortion. Surgical management will depend on the findings but will often necessitate hysterectomy.
   - Hysterectomy may have to be considered in patients not responding to treatment following curettage, suggesting that the process has progressed to myometrial microabscess formation. It may also be required in patients with severe clostridial infections and extensive myometrial gas formation not responding to other measures.

4. **Maintain circulation and tissue perfusion:** This is best monitored by a combination of central venous pressure (CVP) measurement, urine output, and the patient's mental state. The CVP will allow guided transfusion of appropriate blood, colloid or crystalloid solutions. In the critically ill patient insertion of a Swan-Ganz catheter is necessary.

   The use of **vasoactive and inotropic drugs** is controversial and must be guided by experts. The beta-adrenergic properties of isoproterenol and dopamine may enhance peripheral tissue perfusion. If depressed myocardial function is present inotrophic drugs such as dobutamine or epinephrine are given. If congestive heart failure develops the patient is digitalised. Corticosteroids are advocated by some authorities, but their place is still controversial. They are usually given in doses of 2 g of hydrocortisone intravenously every 4 hours (or equivalent dose of another corticosteroid). Immunomodulation treatment in the form of recombinant human activated protein C has shown promise in trials.

   Metabolic acidosis is corrected with intravenous sodium bicarbonate.

5. **Respiratory support** may be required with oxygen and mechanical ventilation monitored by arterial blood gases.

6. **Disseminated intravascular coagulation** may require specific treatment (see Chapter 8).

REFERENCES

1. Wilcox L J, Weinberg C R, O'Connor J F et al. Incidence of early loss of pregnancy. N Engl J Med 1988;319: 189-94.
2. Laguardia K D, Rotholz M V, Belfort PA. 10-year review of maternal mortality in a municipal hospital in Rio de Janeiro: A cause for concern. Obstet Gynecol 1990;75: 27-32.
3. Johnson N. Intracervical tents: usage and mode of action. Obstet Gynecol Surv 1989;44: 410-20.
4. Henshaw RC. Medical management of miscarriage; non surgical uterine evacuation of incomplete and inevitable spontaneous abortion. BMJ 1993;306:894-5.
5. Luise C, Jermy K, May C, Costello G, Collins WP, Bourne TH. Outcome of expectant management of spontaneous first trimester miscarriage: Observational study. BMJ 2002;324:873-5.
6. Jonge ETM. Randomised clinical trial of medical evacuation and surgical curettage for incomplete miscarriage. BMJ 1995;311:662.
7. Chipchase J, James D. Randomised trial of expectant versus surgical management of spontaneous miscarriage. Br J Obstet Gynaecol 1997;104:840-1.

BIBLIOGRAPHY

Balk RA. Severe sepsis and septic shock. Definitions, epidemiology, and clinical manifestations. Crit Care Clin 2000;16:179-86.

Bradley E, Hamilton-Fairley D. Managing miscarriage in early pregnancy assessment units. Hospital Med 1998;59:451-6.

Creinin MD, Moyer R, Guido R. Misoprostol for medical evacuation of early pregnancy failure. Obstet Gynecol 1997;89:768-72.

Everett C. Incidence and outcome of bleeding before the 20th week of pregnancy: prospective study from general practice. BMJ 1997;315:32-4.

Franche RL. Psychologic and obstetric predictors of couples' grief during pregnancy after miscarriage or perinatal death. Obstet Gynecol 2001;97:597-602.

Hemminki E. Treatment of miscarriage: current practice and rationale. Obstet Gynecol 1998;91:247-53.

Mabie WC, Barton JR, Sibai BM. Septic shock in pregnancy. Obstet Gynecol 1997;90:553-61.

Regan L, Rai R. Epidemiology and the medical causes of miscarriage. Best Prac Res Clin Obstet Gynaecol 2000;14:839-54.

Royal College of Obstetricians and Gynaecologists. Guideline No. 25. The management of early pregnancy loss. London: RCOG, 2000.

Turner MJ, Flannelly G M, Wingfield M et al. The miscarriage clinic: an audit of the first year. Br J Obstet Gynaecol 1991;98: 306-8.

CHAPTER 4

Ectopic pregnancy

The incidence of ectopic pregnancy has increased worldwide during the last 30 years, such that approximately 1-2 per cent of all diagnosed pregnancies are ectopic. The significance of this is underlined by the fact that 5-10 per cent of all maternal deaths are due to this complication.

TYPES

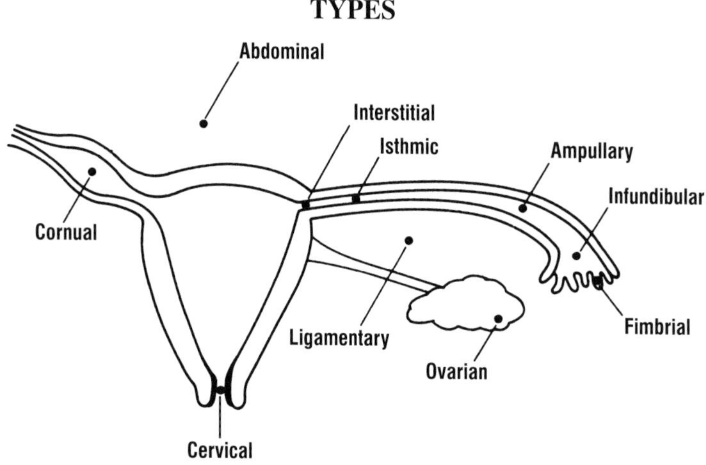

Figure 4.1 Ectopic pregnancy – sites

EXTRAUTERINE

1. **Tubal:** by far the commonest – approximately 97 per cent:
   - Fimbrial 1-2 per cent
   - Ampullary/infundibular 65-70 per cent
   - Isthmic 20-25 per cent
   - Interstitial 1-2 per cent
2. **Ovarian**

3. **Ligamentary**
4. **Abdominal**
   - Primary
   - Secondary

UTERINE (Extremely rare)

1. **Cervical**
2. **Cornual** – in the rudimentary horn of a bicornute uterus which may or may not connect with the uterine cavity.

AETIOLOGY

Anything that impedes or delays the passage of the ovum down the tube can cause ectopic pregnancy.

1. **Congenital abnormalities of the tube**
   (a) Diverticula
   (b) Accessory ostia
   (c) Duplication or partial duplication
2. **Previous tubal inflammatory disease**
   This may be post-operative, post-abortal, puerperal, tuberculous or, most commonly, due to sexually transmitted diseases, especially chlamydia and gonorrhoea. Intratubal and peritubal adhesions can kink and compress the tube. The damage may be more subtle and interfere with normal ciliary and peristaltic tubal function.
3. **Extraneous tubal distortion**
   Uterine fibroids, ovarian and broad ligament cysts may lead to attenuation and narrowing of the tube. Previous abdominal surgery (e.g. appendicectomy) may cause adhesions that distort the tubal anatomy.
4. **Previous tubal surgery**
   (a) Failed tubal ligation: either due to the rare occurrence of a fertilised ovum being trapped distal to the ligature at the time of operation, or later recanalisation allowing passage of sperm but not the fertilised ovum.
   (b) Tubal reanastomosis to reverse sterilisation.
   (c) Infertility surgery, e.g. salpingostomy, salpingolysis, etc.
5. **Contraceptive practice**
   (a) The intrauterine contraceptive device (IUCD), particularly those with progesterone, is associated with an apparent increase in the risk of ectopic pregnancy, with a predilection towards the ovarian site. Some 5 per cent of pregnancies that occur with the IUCD in place are ectopic. This increase is largely relative, as

the IUCD prevents virtually all intrauterine pregnancies but less of the tubal and ovarian type. The other factor implicating the IUCD is its association with an increased incidence of pelvic inflammatory disease.

(b) Progestin only contraceptive pills have been linked with a higher rate of ectopic pregnancy.[1]

6. **Induction of ovulation with gonadotrophins**
   This can be associated with high oestrogen levels which may alter ovum maturation and tubal transportation.[2]
7. **Overdevelopment of the ovum**
   Iffy has shown that in some cases the embryo of an ectopic pregnancy is older than the menstrual history suggests.[3] He feels that the underlying mechanism is one of ovulation dysfunction with late ovulation and inadequate steroid production by the corpus luteum producing a short luteal phase and withdrawal bleeding before the fertilised ovum can implant in the uterus. He suggests that the ovum is forced back up the tube by retrograde menstruation. This could account for the not uncommon finding of a tubal pregnancy and corpus luteum on contralateral sides.
8. **Abnormal embryo**
   An abnormal conceptus may be more likely to implant in the tube.[4]
9. **Reproductive technology**
   Pregnancies achieved with the aid of the new reproductive technologies (e.g. *in vitro* fertilisation) are associated with an increased incidence of ectopic pregnancy.[5]

The main reasons for the rising incidence of ectopic pregnancy are the increase in sexually transmitted diseases, tubal surgery and assisted reproductive technology. Also contributing to this rise is the use of sophisticated diagnostic aids that permit earlier diagnosis and intervention in cases that previously may have been missed and undergone spontaneous resolution.

PATHOLOGY

TUBAL PREGNANCY

Reaction of the tube

The trophoblast invades the tube as it would the uterus. This induces a decidual reaction in the endosalpinx, but this tends to be patchy and cannot contain the invasion of the trophoblast. Thus, erosion of the tubal wall is common and often the trophoblast interposes between the muscularis and serosal layers.

The ampulla is the commonest site and, as this is the widest part of the tube, it is not so liable to early rupture. The isthmus is narrow, less distensible, and prone to early rupture. The interstitial portion of the tube is a rare site and the pregnancy may extend into the uterus and even be expelled by this route. If the tube does rupture in the interstitial area the bleeding can be profuse because of the large vessels involved.

Outcome of Tubal Pregnancy

Absorption or Mummification

Usually the pregnancy dies before six weeks'gestation because of deficient placentation. If very small it may become absorbed in the tube or, after abortion, into the peritoneal cavity. The dead embryo may become mummified, infected or calcified (lithopaedion).

Tubal Abortion

This is a common outcome of ampullary pregnancy. The conceptus is separated from the tubal wall by chorio-decidual haemorrhage producing a **haematosalpinx**. The pregnancy may be extruded into the peritoneal cavity-complete **tubal abortion** – or only partially extruded – **incomplete tubal abortion**. If the pregnancy remains in the haematosalpinx as a **missed tubal abortion** it may become organised like a carneous mole – a tubal mole.

With any of these types blood may collect around the tube as a **peritubal haematocoele** or run down into the pouch of Douglas to form a **pelvic haematocoele**.

Tubal Rupture

The tubal wall may be so distended by the pregnancy sac and so deeply penetrated by the trophoblast that it may rupture. This may be sudden or a gradual erosion and is much less common than tubal abortion.

Intraperitoneal rupture may lead to:

1. Haemoperitoneum.
2. Peritubal haematocoele.
3. Pelvic haematocoele.
4. Secondary abdominal pregnancy-in these rare cases it is likely that the embryo is initially expelled from the tube but the placenta remains in the tube, i.e. a **tubo-abdominal pregnancy**. Eventually the chorionic villi grow out through the opening until the whole placenta is found outside the tube.

Extraperitoneal rupture (between the leaves of the broad ligament) may lead to:
1. Broad ligament haematoma.
2. Ligamentary pregnancy.
3. Secondary intraperitoneal rupture.

OVARIAN PREGNANCY

This is very rare but seems a little more likely in patients with an IUCD. Many apparent cases are in fact extruded tubal pregnancies that have become adherent to the ovary.

Spiegelberg's four criteria must be fulfilled to establish the diagnosis:

1. The tube on the affected side must be normal and separate from the pregnancy sac.
2. The pregnancy sac must occupy the position of the ovary.
3. The sac must be attached to the uterus by the ovarian ligament.
4. Ovarian tissue must be histologically demonstrable in the wall of the pregnancy sac.

CORNUAL PREGNANCY

The ovum implants in the rudimentary horn of a bicornute uterus which may or may not communicate with the rest of the uterine cavity. If it communicates, such a pregnancy may be extruded into the uterine cavity or it may develop until the twelfth to sixteenth week before rupturing, as the area is quite distensible. Excision of the horn is required.

CERVICAL PREGNANCY

This is extremely rare. The ovum implants in the cervical canal. Abortion usually occurs and the bleeding from the non-retractile cervix can be so severe as to warrant hysterectomy. Other measures to achieve haemostasis and preserve the uterus include: tamponade with a Foley catheter bulb, intracervical injection of vasopressin, trans-vaginal uterine artery ligation, angiographic embolisation and hysteroscopic resection.[6-8]

ABDOMINAL PREGNANCY

Primary abdominal pregnancy is extremely rare. External transmigration of the ovum may be a factor in some cases. It may implant anywhere in the peritoneal cavity. Haemorrhage and cessation of the pregnancy in the early weeks is likely but very occasionally it may advance close to term. This may be heralded by spurious uterine contractions. Laparotomy is needed to remove the fetus but the placenta is usually left to absorb as, attempts to remove it cause haemorrhage from areas where it is difficult and dangerous to achieve haemostasis.

CHANGES IN THE UTERUS

These changes are due to the normal uterine response to the hormones of early pregnancy:

1. There may be increased vascularity, enlargement, and softening of the uterus, so that it may mimic a normally pregnant uterus up to 8 weeks' size.
2. There is a decidual reaction in the endometrium but this can be patchy and both proliferative and secretory endometrium may be present at curettage. The Arias-Stella changes with cells of atypical appearance may also be seen, but this is not specific for ectopic pregnancy.

CLINICAL FEATURES

There are no signs or symptoms specific to ectopic pregnancy. The clinical presentation may be acute or chronic with varying degrees of each. Although, with earlier diagnosis, the more extreme clinical presentations are not often seen, the full clinical spectrum will be outlined here:

ACUTE PRESENTATION

This is much less common than the chronic presentation and usually follows tubal rupture but can occur with tubal abortion. It is not uncommon for the acute picture to follow an undiagnosed and untreated chronic picture.

1. There is usually a short period of **amenorrhoea**. In about 25 per cent of cases there is no history of a missed period.
2. **Signs and symptoms of early pregnancy** may or may not be present.
3. Acute onset of **pain** in the iliac fossa or hypogastrium.
4. This pain may be associated with **syncope** and collapse.
5. The pain persists and after lying down may be referred to the **shoulder tip** due to sub-diaphragmatic irritation by free blood in the peritoneal cavity.
6. Hypovolaemic **shock**.
7. **Guarding, tenderness**, and **rebound** over the whole lower abdomen, often maximal in one iliac fossa.

8. If there is a lot of free blood the sign of **shifting dullness** may be elicited.
9. In the classic acute presentation a pelvic examination is hardly necessary to confirm the diagnosis and indeed may precipitate further bleeding. If it is performed, moving the cervix will produce marked **cervical excitation pain**. This is sometimes graphically known as 'yelling tenderness' and can also be elicited with other acute adnexal lesions such as salpingo-oophoritis. Because of the marked tenderness and guarding it is unlikely that any of the pelvic contents will be outlined.

CHRONIC PRESENTATION

1. **Amenorrhoea** and signs and symptoms of early pregnancy, as for the acute picture.
2. **Recurrent lower abdominal pain** is the commonest symptom. This may be due to tubal colic, tubal distension or blood leaking into the peritoneum. Epigastric or shoulder tip pain may occur if there is free intraperitoneal blood.
3. Transient **queasiness** and **syncope**, possibly due to a vasovagal response to blood irritating the peritoneum.
4. Irregular **vaginal bleeding** is common. It is usually quite slight and the colour is often dark brown-likened to prune juice. It is usually due to decidual separation, but may come from the tube. On rare occasions the bleeding is heavy. The passage of recognisable decidual tissue is a late and uncommon sign.
5. A pelvic haematocoele may cause pressure on adjacent pelvic organs leading to **rectal tenesmus, dysuria**, and **urinary retention**.
6. Lower **abdominal guarding and rebound tenderness**, usually most marked on one side. In cases with a pelvic haematocoele the abdominal findings may be quite limited and unimpressive.
7. The pelvic examination may reveal quite variable findings. The most consistent and valuable is marked **cervical excitation pain** and tenderness on palpation of the vaginal vault. The uterus may be palpable and feel softened and slightly enlarged, as in a normal early pregnancy. A **tender adnexal mass** may be palpable. This may be fairly discrete and acutely tender, or quite large and ill-defined if the peritubal clot involves ovary and intestines. In the case of an interstitial or cornual pregnancy tender asymmetrical enlargement of the uterus may be found. A pelvic haematocoele may be felt as a tender boggy mass in the pouch of Douglas. If the tenderness is extreme none of the pelvic contents may be outlined.
8. The patient may have a low grade **pyrexia** and **leucocytosis**.
9. **Cullen's sign** – the umbilical 'black eye' – due to accumulation of blood pigments in and around the umbilical skin is a late and rare sign.

DIFFERENTIAL DIAGNOSIS

The potential list of differential diagnoses is legion. The most important are considered here and can often be distinguished by a careful history and examination.

1. **Complication of intrauterine pregnancy:**
   a) Miscarriage.
   b) Early pregnancy plus uterine fibroid or ovarian tumour,
2. **Conditions causing acute abdominal pain:**
   a) Torsion of ovarian tumour, fallopian tube, or subserous pedunculated fibroid.
   b) Salpingo-oophoritis.
   c) Pelvic pain with an IUCD *in situ*.
   d) Appendicitis.
3. **Conditions causing haemoperitoneum:**
   a) Ruptured corpus luteum. This can be especially confusing when a *corpus luteum persistens* causes a short period of amenorrhoea.
   b) Ruptured follicular cyst.
   c) Ruptured endometriotic cyst.
4. **Conditions simulating a pelvic haematocoele:**
   a) Retroverted gravid uterus.
   b) Pelvic or tubo-ovarian abscess.

DIAGNOSIS

The pre-operative diagnostic accuracy of ectopic pregnancy, based on clinical features alone, is notoriously poor: probably in the region of 50 per cent. In recent years a number of diagnostic aids have helped improve on this accuracy, thereby avoiding delay in needed treatment and reducing unnecessary operation.

Human chorionic gonadotrophin (hCG)

The sensitive enzyme-linked immunosorbent assay can detect hCG in the urine two weeks after conception. Thereafter, with a normal intrauterine pregnancy serum hCG levels will double every two days. The increase will be less or non existent in ectopic pregnancy or spontaneous abortion. When the so-called discriminatory zone of hCG ≥1500 iu/l is reached, a normal intrauterine pregnancy sac should be demonstrable using transvaginal ultrasound.

Serum progesterone

These levels will be low (<20 ng/ml) with early pregnancy failure but take longer to perform, cannot differentiate between ectopic and spontaneous abortion, and do not increase the diagnostic sensitivity.

Ultrasound

The value of ultrasound in the diagnosis of ectopic pregnancy has been enhanced by the greater accuracy provided with the transvaginal probe. The main benefit is if an intrauterine pregnancy can be confirmed, the likelihood of a coexistent extrauterine pregnancy is extremely remote. Caution is needed with interpretation of the scan in the 4-6 week gestational range as it is often impossible to confirm a fetal pole. At this stage, use is made of the 'double sac' sign caused by images cast by the amniotic sac and the space that exists between the decidua vera and decidua capsularis prior to fusion. A misleading single sac can be seen in cases of ectopic pregnancy due to the decidual cast. At seven weeks amenorrhoea the fetal heart should be detectable using transvaginal ultrasound.

In a minority of cases, a viable ectopic pregnancy can be located in an extrauterine position, thereby clinching the diagnosis. In others tubal pregnancy will be suspected if there is an empty uterus, a pseudo single sac, a tubal ring (doughnut sign) and/or fluid in the pouch of Douglas.

Thus, the main dilemma arises in the 4-6 week gestation range (2-4 weeks post-ovulation). At this stage, the hCG is positive, but ultrasound may not be able to confirm a normal intrauterine pregnancy. Therefore, we know the patient is pregnant but do not know whether it is intra- or extrauterine and, if intrauterine, whether it is viable or not. In such cases, if the clinical picture warrants observation, it is reasonable to do serial quantitative hCG estimations. With a normal intrauterine pregnancy, the levels usually double every two days, whereas in ectopic and non-viable intrauterine pregnancies, the levels will plateau or fall. Thus, in selected patients, the diagnosis may be clarified without subjecting the patient to anaesthesia and laparoscopy.

Dilatation and Curettage (D & C)

In cases in which the diagnosis is either an ectopic or non-viable intrauterine pregnancy (missed/inevitable miscarriage), the hCG levels and ultrasound findings may not be able to distinguish between the two. In most cases, the diagnosis is a non-viable intrauterine pregnancy and evacuation of the uterus by D & C is indicated. At the time of D & C, placental tissue may be obvious but, if not, the tissue can be thoroughly washed in saline. Chorionic villi (if present) will float to the surface and when observed against the light or by microscope will show the typical fronds with a feathery border. If these are not present, one should suspect that only decidual tissue is present and consider laparoscopy to rule out ectopic pregnancy.

Culdocentesis

This procedure may help confirm the presence of blood in the pouch of Douglas. Through a speculum, the posterior lip of the cervix is grasped with a tenaculum and drawn up under the symphysis. The lower part of the posterior vaginal fornix is steadied with Allis forceps and an 18 gauge needle, attached to a 10-ml syringe, thrust through the dimple of the vagina between the utero-sacral ligaments into the pouch of Douglas. Only if free, non-clotting blood is aspirated is haemoperitoneum confirmed. This procedure is not painless but can be carried out under local anaesthesia in many patients. Its value is limited by false-positive and false-negative rates of 10-15 per cent. With the availability and accuracy of hCG, ultrasound and laparoscopy, this procedure is rarely used.

Laparoscopy

In cases of doubt the pelvis should be visualised by laparoscopy. This is the most accurate diagnostic aid, although it is possible to miss a very early intact tubal pregnancy. In fact, the false-negative and false-positive rate of diagnosis of ectopic pregnancy at laparoscopy is about 3 per cent.

Those who work in an area where laparoscopy is unavailable should not feel reticent about proceeding to laparotomy if the diagnosis of

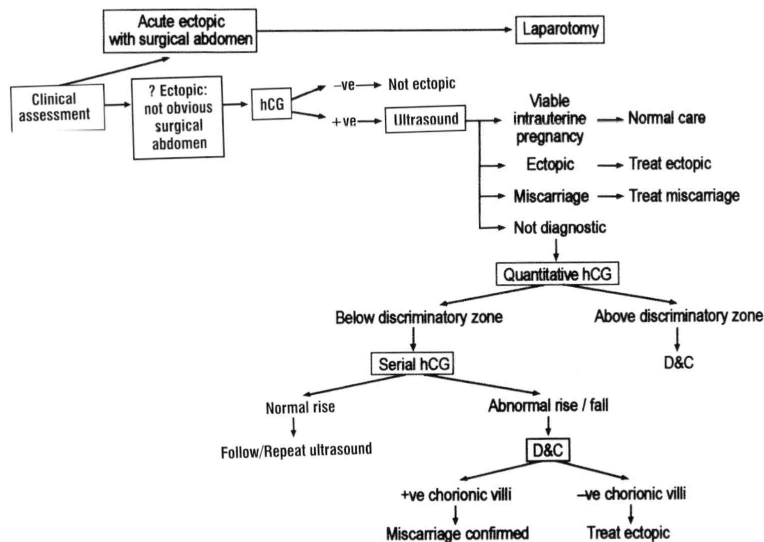

Figure 4.2: Diagnostic evaluation in cases of suspected ectopic pregnancy.

ectopic pregnancy is seriously considered. A small incision can be made for diagnostic purposes, and enlarged if the need for specific surgery is confirmed.

A possible plan for the use of these diagnostic measures in cases of suspected ectopic pregnancy is outlined in Figure 4.2.

Before the more sophisticated and valuable aids of hCG assay, ultrasound, and laparoscopy are enlisted, the diagnosis of ectopic pregnancy must be suspected. Thus, although these tests have revolutionised the diagnostic accuracy, a thorough knowledge of the clinical presentation and its treacherous mimicry is still essential.

MANAGEMENT

In the minority of cases presenting as an acute surgical abdomen with hypovolaemic shock, rapid replacement with intravenous crystalloid, colloid, and blood is indicated (see Chapter 24). It is important to realise that in some cases one will never catch up with the continuing blood loss and that anaesthesia and **laparotomy** must be undertaken before the hypovolaemia is fully corrected. Such cases should be entered rapidly through a lower midline incision. For the inexperienced, and indeed even for the experienced, the apparently endless welling up of blood preventing direct visualisation of the adnexa can be very disconcerting. Time should not be wasted in continued suction and mopping. Grasping the uterus and pulling it upwards should allow one to palpate and see the offending tube. Ring forceps can then be rapidly applied to both medial and lateral sides of the ectopic site to stem the blood loss. The blood and clots are then removed by suction and mopped away to reveal the detailed pathology, and the anaesthetist can begin to catch up replacing the lost blood volume. The initial use of ring forceps is advised so that any structures, inadvertently caught while trying to place the forceps by palpation in a well of blood, are not irrevocably damaged.

Autotransfusion has been used in these acute cases. The blood from the peritoneal cavity is scooped out and filtered through layers of gauze into a jar containing 3.8 per cent sodium citrate and reinfused into the patient. The ratio of blood to citrate solution is 5:1. Such blood will have reduced coagulation factors. This technique has its application in cases with fresh blood in the abdomen, a shocked patient, and no donor blood available.[9,10]

SURGICAL PROCEDURES

Over the past 20 years, opinion has swung in favour of conservative surgery with preservation of the affected tube if at all possible. As a result of improved diagnostic methods, the majority of ectopic pregnancies are diagnosed earlier in gestation and prior to rupture, lending the condition to more conservative surgery than was formerly possible. There appears to be a small advantage for future pregnancy in patients who have undergone the more conservative salpingotomy, compared to those who have salpingectomy, with a similar risk of subsequent ectopic pregnancy (10-15 per cent) in both groups.[11] However, the rate of persistent ectopic is higher with salpingotomy. Indeed, if the contralateral tube is normal, salpingectomy may reduce the chance of subsequent ectopic pregnancy, without reducing the overall chances of another pregnancy.[12]

When feasible, and it usually is, a full pre-operative discussion with the patient should cover the possible findings and surgical options. Depending on the circumstances, and after careful inspection of both adnexa, one of the following operative procedures may be undertaken:

Salpingectomy: This is indicated if the patient does not desire future fertility or if the whole tube is distorted and replaced by the ectopic pregnancy. It has been suggested that this should be accompanied by cornual resection to eliminate the risk, albeit rare, of a subsequent interstitial pregnancy. In fact, cornual resection does not prevent interstitial implantation and may predispose to uterine rupture in a future intrauterine pregnancy. Thus, a simple salpingectomy, excising the tube flush with the uterine wall, is the procedure of choice. Removing the ovary on the same side as the salpingectomy with the theoretical hope that it will improve the chance of future fertilisation is not advised.

Manual Expression: A fimbrial or distal ampullary pregnancy may be amenable to this approach. If the pregnancy has a tenuous hold, and the tubal wall is not eroded, gentle massage may extrude the pregnancy *in toto*-mimicking what happens in a spontaneous tubal abortion. Haemostasis can usually be achieved by compression, coagulation and ligation of discrete bleeding points, or transfixion of the mesosalpinx.

Salpingotomy: This method is appropriate for the most commonly situated ampullary tubal pregnancy. Using needle-tip cautery a longitudinal incision is made over the pregnancy, along the antimesosalpingeal border of the tube. The pregnancy is gently extruded and haemostasis achieved by the same methods as for manual expression. The incision is left open.

Segmental Resection: This approach can be used for pregnancies in the narrow isthmic portion of the tube where salpingotomy is inappropriate. The tube is ligated with non-absorbable suture on either side of the pregnancy, the mesosalpinx below is transfixed and that portion of the tube excised (in the case of laparoscopic surgery, cautery or laser is used). This method has the advantage of simplicity, speed and sure haemostasis. It leaves the patient with the option of future end-to-end reanastomosis after thoughtful discussion and reflection. There are those who advocate primary resection and end-to-end reanastomosis, but this may not be feasible because of the distortion and oedema of the tissues.

With all the conservative surgical methods-manual expression, salpingotomy, and segmental resection-haemostasis will be aided by the pre-operative injection into the mesosalpinx and tube of a solution of either local anaesthetic and adrenaline, 1:100000, or dilute vasopressin, 1:10 solution of pitressin (20 units/ml). Infiltration with 1-3 ml of either of these solutions is usually adequate to diminish the operative bleeding.

Hysterectomy: On rare occasions, this may be indicated for certain forms of ectopic pregnancy, e.g. interstitial, cervical.

Associated Procedures: In individual cases, concomitant salpingolysis, ventrosuspension, or tubal ligation may be appropriate.

Laparoscopic Surgery Versus Laparotomy

An increasing number of reports show that in skilled hands salpingotomy, segmental resection, and salpingectomy can be carried out via laparoscopy in selected cases. This requires extra equipment and skill, and is not appropriate for the occasional laparoscopist. In about 5-10 per cent of cases so performed, repeat operation or medical treatment is required for bleeding or persistent trophoblastic tissue. The main advantage is the reduced post-operative stay and earlier full recovery. For those with the instruments and training laparoscopic surgery can be used for most cases. However, those without the equipment or skill to perform laparoscopic surgery should not feel too badly. A small (7cm) Pfannenstiel incision will often allow the appropriate surgical procedure to be performed safely and rapidly, with minimal difference in postoperative recovery.

Excessive enthusiasm for laparoscopic conservative surgery, particularly by the inexperienced, will be repaid by post-operative bleeding and the need for a second anaesthetic and the laparotomy that should have been done in the first place.

Follow up

Persistent trophoblastic tissue may occur after conservative surgery via both laparoscopy and laparotomy – though less often with the latter route. Therefore, weekly quantitative hCG should be measured, with the expectation of undetectable levels in four weeks. Persistent or rising levels will need either medical treatment with methotrexate or repeat surgery.

Medical Treatment

It is ironic that just over a century after Lawson Tait finally proved the value of surgical management (salpingectomy) for ectopic pregnancy, medical treatment is available in carefully selected cases.

The increasing accuracy of quantitative hCG levels and transvaginal ultrasound have made the early and accurate diagnosis of ectopic pregnancy possible, without recourse to laparoscopy in all cases. Intramuscular methotrexate (50mg/m2 body surface area – about 1 mg/kg body weight) has now been used in several hundred cases with about 90 per cent success. It is only suitable in carefully selected patients, with a small (≤3.0cm), intact tubal pregnancy and low hCGs. Those undertaking medical treatment should establish careful guidelines for follow up and be familiar with the sometimes paradoxical increase in abdominal pain and transient rise in hCG titres that may occur in the first week after treatment.

Injection of the peritubal ectopic site via laparoscopy or ultrasound guidance with hyperosmolar glucose, potassium chloride or methotrexate is, as yet, an unproven technique.

A final point to remember is that all Rh-negative patients with ectopic pregnancy, who are not already isoimmunised, should be protected by Rh immune globulin.

REFERENCES

1. Liukko P, Erkkola R, Laakso L. Ectopic pregnancies during use of low-dose progestins for oral contraception. Contraception 1977;16: 575-80.
2. McBain JC, Evans JH, Pepperell RJ et al. An unexpectedly high rate of ectopic pregnancy following the induction of ovulation with human pituitary and chorionic gonadotrophin. Br J Obstet Gynaecol 1980;87: 5-6.
3. Iffy L. Ectopic pregnancy. In: Principles and Practice of Obstetrics and Perinatology. Iffy L, Kaminetsky HA. (eds). New York; John Wiley & Sons, 1981 pp. 609-33.
4. Poland BJ, Dill FJ, Styblo C. Embryonic development in ectopic human pregnancy. Teratology 1976;14:315-21.
5. Strandel A, Thorburn J, Hamberger L. Risk factors for ectopic pregnancy in assisted reproduction. Fertil Steril 1999;71:282-6.
6. Hurley VA, Beischer NA. Cervical pregnancy: hysterectomy avoided with the use of a large Foley catheter balloon. Aust NZ J Obstet Gynaecol 1988;28:230-2.
7. Ash S, Farrell SA. Hysteroscopic resection of a cervical ectopic pregnancy. Fertil Steril 1996;66:842-4.
8. Vshakov FB, Elchalal V, Aceman PJ et al. Cervical pregnancy: past and future. Obstet Gynecol Surv 1997;52:45-59.
9. AJ, Cuddigan BJ, Wyatt AP. Early experience of intraoperative auto transfusion. J R Soc Med 1988;81:389-91.
10. Obiechina N, Emelife EC, Ezeasor E. The place of autotransfusion in managemnt of ectopic pregnancy – 10 years experience. J Obstet Gynaecol 2001;21:513-5.

11. Bangsgaard N, Lund CO, Otteson B, Nilas L. Improved fertility following conservative treatment of ectopic pregnancy. Br J Obstet Gynaecol 2003;110: 765-70.
12. Royal College of Obstetricians and Gynaecologists. Guideline No.21. The management of tubal pregnancies. London: RCOG,1999.

BIBLIOGRAPHY

Barnhart KT, Gosman G, Ashby R, Sammel M. The medical management of ectopic pregnancy: a meta-analysis comparing 'single dose' and multidose regimens. Obstet Gynecol 2003;101:778-84.

Bouyer J, Job-Spira N, Pouly JL, Coste J, Germain E, Fernandez H. Fetility following radical, conservative-surgical or medical treatment for tubal pregnancy: a population-based study. Br J Obstet Gynaecol 2000;107:714-21.

Carson SA, Buster JE. Ectopic pregnancy. N Engl J Med 1993;329:1174-81.

Clausen I. Conservative versus radical surgery for tubal pregnancy: a review. Acta Obstet Gynecol Scand 1996;75:8-12.

Fylstra DL. Tubal pregnancy: a review of current diagnosis and treatment. Obstet Gynecol Surv 1998;53:320-8.

Gracia CR, Barnhart KT. Diagnosing ectopic pregnancy: decision analysis comparing six strategies. Obstet Gynecol 2001;97:464-70.

Graczykowski JW, Mishell DR. Methotrexate prophylaxis for persistent ectopic pregnancy after conservative treatment by salpingostomy. Obstet Gynecol 1997;89:118-22.

Hobson PT, Bidmead J, Khalid A, Cardozo L, Hill S. Current trends in management of ectopic pregnancy in the United Kingdom. J Obstet Gynaecol 2000;20:74-7.

Kristiansen JD, Clausen I, Nielsen MN et al. Stereomicroscopic demonstration of chorionic villi: differentiation between miscarriage and ectopic pregnancy. Br J Obstet Gynaecol 1993;100:839-41.

Mascarenhas L, Williamson JG, Smith SK. The changing face of ectopic pregnancy. BMJ 1997;315:141.

Olofsson JI, Poromoa IS, Ottander V, Kjellberg L, Damber MG. Clinical and pregnancy outcome following ectopic pregnancy: a prospective study comparing expectancy, surgery and systemic methotrexate treatment. Acta Obstet Gynecol Scand 2001;80:744-9.

Ombelet W, Vandermerwe JV, Van Assche FA. Advanced extrauterine pregnancy: description of 38 cases with literature survey. Obstet Gynecol Surv 1988;43:386-97.

Raziel A, Golan A, Pansky M et al. Ovarian pregnancy: a report of twenty cases in one institution. Am J Obstet Gynecol 1990;163:1182-5.

Shalev E, Yaram I, Bustan M et al. Transvaginal sonography as the ultimate diagnostic tool for the management of ectopic pregnancy: experience with 840 cases. Fertil Steril 1998;69:62-5.

Tulandi T, Sammoutt A. Evidence-based management of ectopic pregnancy. Curr Opin Obstet Gynaecol 2000;12:289-92.

Vermesh M, Graczykowski JW, Sauer MV. Re-evaluation of the role of culdocentesis in the management of ectopic pregnancy. Am J Obstet Gynecol 1990;162:411-3.

Yao M, Tulandi T. Current status of surgical and nonsurgical management of ectopic pregnancy. Fertil Steril 1997;67:421-33.

CHAPTER 5

Acute abdominal pain in pregnancy

Any physician dealing with patients who complain of abdominal pain will benefit from reading the small book *Cope's Early Diagnosis of the Acute Abdomen*.[1] Many of the soundest principles that apply to these patients are laid down in this classic monograph:

- Early diagnosis gives the best prognosis.
- Correct diagnosis leads to correct treatment.
- Try and make a diagnosis at the first examination.
- If one is still in doubt after the first examination, review the history as it is here the answer is most likely to be found.
- Withhold analgesia until you have made a diagnosis and decided upon your initial course of action.
- A patient may have a normal pulse and temperature and still have serious intra-abdominal pathology.
- Severe abdominal pain in a previously well patient, lasting more than six hours, is usually of surgical importance.

In real clinical life, of course, it is common not to be able to make a certain diagnosis at the first examination. The important thing is to try, establish the differential diagnosis, and at least rule out life-threatening conditions that require immediate intervention. As one of my former teachers put it: 'Is she opening sick or watching sick?' One can then start appropriate initial management (e.g. intravenous fluids, cross-match blood, laboratory tests, etc.) and observe the patient closely. Usually the clinical picture will unfold and the diagnosis become clear in a few hours. One of the reasons senior consultants are often the best diagnosticians is because they tend to see the patient at a later stage when the clinical picture has unfolded! As the Chinese proverb says: 'The unlucky doctor treats the beginning of an illness; the fortunate doctor the end.'

In most of the conditions in this chapter surgical treatment is carried out via laparotomy. However, with appropriate facilities and skill, some procedures such as diagnostic,cholecystectomy and appendicectomy are being increasingly done via laparoscopy.

OBSTETRIC CAUSES OF ABDOMINAL PAIN

The most important and common causes: abortion, ectopic pregnancy, abruptio placentae, uterine rupture, and puerperal sepsis are covered in separate chapters. The others will be dealt with here.

PHYSIOLOGICAL

It is not surprising that some of the profound changes associated with pregnancy can cause abdominal pain.

1. Uterine distension in early pregnancy and formation of the lower uterine segment in the later weeks.
2. Distension of the veins in the broad ligament (one need only look at these during caesarean section to appreciate this).
3. Round ligament stretching. This can lead to quite annoying pain for women, especially in the second trimester.

These conditions usually produce relatively mild and unsustained pain, are not associated with other symptoms, and can be differentiated easily on clinical grounds.

INCARCERATED RETROVERTED GRAVID UTERUS

This is a rare complication that occurs when a retroverted pregnant uterus becomes trapped beneath the sacral promontory, usually between 13 and 16 weeks' gestation. As the uterus fills the pelvis the bladder dome is displaced upwards and the bladder base forwards, interfering with bladder emptying and causing urinary retention.

DIAGNOSIS

1. The classic presentation with the patient at 13-16 weeks' gestation giving a clear history of urinary retention and acute hypogastric pain, makes the diagnosis simple.
2. In many cases the presentation is camouflaged. There can be retention with overflow and the patient may complain of frequency rather than retention. The tense bladder may, on examination, be mistaken for the uterus and be an appropriate size for the period of amenorrhoea. Another trap is to misinterpret the swelling for an ovarian tumour.

MANAGEMENT

1. Think of the condition and always catheterise the patient, thereby avoiding the embarrassment and danger of unnecessary laparotomy for an 'ovarian cyst'.
2. Drain the bladder slowly with a Foley catheter. Leave the catheter in place and keep the bladder empty for 24-48 hours. During this time the uterus almost always spontaneously escapes, and once out of the pelvis does not return.
3. Manipulation of the uterus, either with or without general anaesthesia, is very rarely needed.
4. Laparotomy to disimpact the uterus, which may be held down by adhesions requiring surgical division, is described. This is exceedingly rare, but may become more common in pregnancies following *in vitro* fertilisation in patients with extensive adhesions from chronic pelvic inflammatory disease, who in former times would not have achieved pregnancy.

SEVERE PRE-ECLAMPSIA/HELLP SYNDROME

In a minority of cases of severe pre-eclampsia and/or HELLP syndrome (see chapter 7) acute abdominal pain can be the main presenting symptom.

DIAGNOSIS

1. The pain is typically epigastric and right hypochondrial.
2. May be associated with nausea and vomiting.
3. There may be obvious signs of pre-eclampsia: hypertension and proteinuria.
4. In some cases of HELLP syndrome there may be no or mild hypertension only. In such patients, unless the diagnosis is considered and liver function and coagulation tests performed, the case may be labelled cholecystitis and inappropriate treatment given.

MANAGEMENT

1. Appropriate treatment of the severe pre-eclampsia or HELLP syndrome (see chapter 7)
2. In cases with persistent or worsening right hypochondrial pain a subcapsular hepatic haematoma should be considered, and may be confirmed by ultrasound. These patients need to be carefully observed because of the rare progression to rupture and severe intraperitoneal haemorrhage.

ACUTE POLYHYDRAMNIOS

This is a very rare occurrence with sudden and rapid accumulation of amniotic fluid causing uterine distension and acute abdominal pain. It can occur in the second or third trimester.

DIAGNOSIS

1. Sudden and rapid abdominal distension.
2. The uterus is tense and may be tender. There is a fluid thrill and fetal parts are not palpable.
3. Oedema of the legs and lower abdominal wall may develop.
4. The patient can be very distressed with pain, nausea, vomiting, dyspnoea, and orthopnoea.

MANAGEMENT

1. Suspect an associated fetal anomaly and/or multiple pregnancy. Ultrasound is therefore indicated.
2. Amniocentesis and slow release of the excess amniotic fluid is required. Testing of the fluid for fetal pulmonary maturity may be appropriate. If the fetus seems normal, but immature, one can attempt serial amniocentesis to relieve the tension, as the fluid almost always rapidly re-accumulates. Unfortunately this usually fails and the patient delivers prematurely.

NON-OBSTETRIC CAUSES OF ABDOMINAL PAIN

Obviously the pregnant woman is not immune to any of the non-obstetrical conditions that can cause acute abdominal pain. The more important, and particularly those that have a relationship with pregnancy, will be discussed here.

ACUTE APPENDICITIS

The incidence of acute appendicitis in pregnancy is about 1 in 1500 deliveries. The mortality is higher in pregnancy due to delay in diagnosis and the natural reluctance to subject the pregnant woman to laparotomy. Certain changes in pregnancy lead to diagnostic pitfalls as well as reducing the patient's ability to contain the infection. Maternal mortality is highest in the third trimester. Fetal complications are mainly due to associated premature labour. This is less of a problem with early diagnosis and appendicectomy, than with delayed intervention and peritonitis. In uncomplicated appendicitis the fetal loss is 1-2 per cent, rising to 30-40 per cent if peritonitis supervenes.

DIAGNOSIS

The process of acute appendicitis is the same in the pregnant as in the non-pregnant, except that during pregnancy certain factors operate to make the diagnosis more difficult:

1. The symptoms of anorexia, nausea, vomiting, abdominal pain, and urinary frequency are common in the first half of normal pregnancy.
2. In acute appendicitis abdominal pain is a consistent finding, although its character and location may differ. In the early obstructive phase the visceral pain will be epigastric and periumbilical, irrespective of the position of the appendix. As the obstructed lumen of the appendix fills with pus it irritates the overlying parietal peritoneum causing pain and tenderness at the local site. During pregnancy the position of the appendix may change if the caecum is mobile and pushed upwards and laterally by the enlarging uterus (Figure 5.1). Thus the site of the pain, guarding and tenderness may range from low in the right iliac fossa up to the right flank, depending on the stage of pregnancy. The omentum is displaced upwards so that its ability to surround and localise the infected appendix is compromised, facilitating spread of the infection and peritonitis.

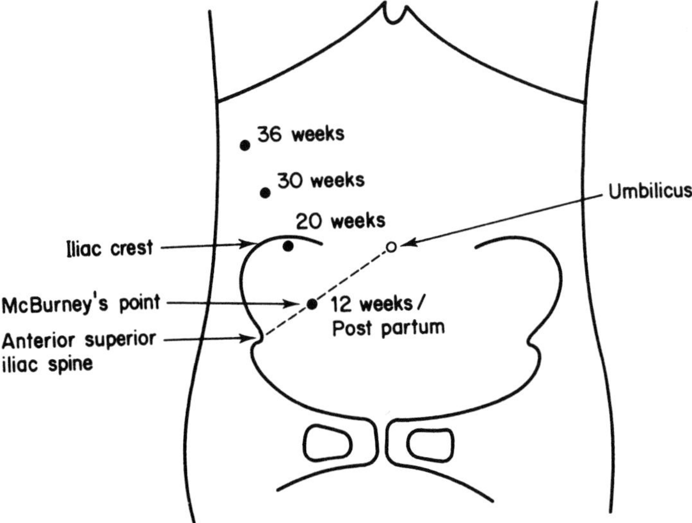

Figure 5.1 Changing position of the appendix during pregnancy.

3. In advanced pregnancy the ability of the distended abdominal wall to display guarding and rigidity is lessened.
4. The displaced, inflamed retrocaecal appendix may overlie the renal pelvis and ureter causing pyuria but usually not bacteriuria. In addition, the retrocaecal appendix not in contact with the parietal peritoneum, may be associated with an absence of point tenderness. For these reasons right-sided pyelonephritis is the disease most commonly confused with appendicitis.
5. The presence or absence of either fever or leucocytosis will neither confirm nor deny the diagnosis.

Thus, careful clinical examination of the patient and her urine, plus an awareness of the vagaries of this condition in pregnancy are the keys to diagnosis. Ultrasound has been used to increase the accuracy of diagnosis in cases of clinical doubt.

MANAGEMENT

1. If the diagnosis is seriously considered laparotomy and appendicectomy should be performed. In early pregnancy diagnostic laparoscopy may be undertaken, as the appendix can be seen in about 75 per cent of cases.
2. Choice of incision: In the first trimester, if there is doubt about the diagnosis, a lower midline or right paramedian incision will allow the flexibility to deal with other gynaecological conditions that may imitate appendicitis. In the second and third trimesters an oblique muscle-splitting incision, of the McBurney type, over the point of maximum tenderness is recommended. The skin incision will be made almost transversely in the skin crease.
3. If the appendix has perforated, or is gangrenous, perioperative antibiotics should be given and the operative site drained.
4. Concomitant caesarean section in late pregnancy is not done except for independent fetal or maternal reasons.

ACUTE PYELONEPHRITIS

This condition occurs in 1-2 per cent of pregnancies. It is commonest in the second and third trimesters. Certain factors predispose the pregnant woman to pyelonephritis by causing stasis in the upper urinary tract:

- As the uterus enlarges to 18 weeks' size, and greater, it can cause ureteric compression at the pelvic brim. This is more marked on the right side due to dextrorotation of the uterus by the sigmoid colon.

- The effect of progesterone leads to dilatation of the ureter and renal pelvis.

DIAGNOSIS

1. Flank pain and chills are the most common presenting symptoms.
2. Pyrexia-ranging from 38 to 41°C.
3. Costo-vertebral tenderness: most often on the right, but may be bilateral or just left sided.
4. Lower urinary tract symptoms of frequency and dysuria may be absent initially.
5. Nausea and vomiting, and tenderness in the right iliac fossa may mimic appendicitis.
6. Urinalysis is essential and should reveal both bacteriuria and pyuria. Urine is then sent for culture and sensitivity.

MANAGEMENT

1. Hydration with intravenous fluids.
2. Intravenous ampicillin 1 gram 4-6 hourly and continue for 48 hours after the symptoms and pyrexia have settled. It may be necessary to add gentamicin because of the increasingly common resistance of *E.Coli* to ampicillin. This is followed by oral antibiotics.
3. If the patient does not get better the antibiotics can be changed on the basis of the urine culture results.
4. Follow-up urine cultures at regular intervals are important as many of these patients get recurrent infection. Asymptomatic bacteriuria found at follow-up should be eradicated with antibiotics. Some patients may require suppressive antibiotics for the remainder of the pregnancy.

URINARY CALCULI

These manifest themselves clinically in about I in 1000 pregnancies.

DIAGNOSIS

1. The patient may present with classical renal or ureteric colic or with more non-specific urinary symptoms such as: flank pain, right iliac fossa pain, haematuria, frequency, and dysuria.
2. Microscopic haematuria.
3. In patients with acute pyelonephritis, in whom the condition does not resolve with appropriate antibiotics, obstruction with urinary calculi should be considered. The same holds for patients with recurrent urinary tract infections.

4. Intravenous pyelography (IVP): In those patients with a firm clinical diagnosis, in whom the pain can be controlled and there is no infection, treatment with hydration and analgesia will usually result in the spontaneous passage of the stone. If this is so then the radiation associated with an IVP can be avoided. If the IVP is needed the radiation can be reduced by doing only one exposure 30 minutes after contrast media injection.
5. Ultrasound may obviate the need for IVP in selected cases.

MANAGEMENT

1. With good hydration and analgesia the vast majority of small calculi (0.5cm) will pass spontaneously. During this time all urine should be strained and any calculi analysed.
2. If this fails and there are continued signs of obstruction, particularly pyelonephritis unresponsive to antibiotics, then the stone will have to be removed or by-passed. This may be achieved by cystoscopy and basket extraction for lower ureteral stones. Other options include internal ureteral stenting, percutaneous nephrostomy and ureterolithotomy. Extracorporeal shock wave lithotripsy is contraindicated in pregnancy.
3. Careful post partum follow-up, when a more extensive and accurate evaluation of the urinary tract can be made, is indicated.

ACUTE CHOLECYSTITIS

More than 90 per cent of cases of acute cholecystitis are associated with gall stones. The pregnant woman is more prone to acute cholecystitis because of altered gall bladder function in pregnancy.

- Gall bladder emptying is slowed and reduced, presumably due to the effect of progesterone on the smooth muscle.
- The equilibrium between cholesterol and bile salts is upset by the increased biliary excretion of cholesterol and a decrease in the bile salt pool. This causes cholesterol saturation and the laying down of cholesterol crystals which may initiate or accelerate stone formation.

DIAGNOSIS

1. The pain is usually constant and initially situated in the epigastrium. It may relent for a few hours and then recur in the right hypochondrium with referral to the scapular region.

2. Anorexia, nausea, and vomiting.
3. Tenderness and rigidity in the right hypochondrium. Murphy's sign may be positive.
4. A distended gall bladder is not often palpable in the pregnant patient.
5. Pyrexia of 38-39°C may be present.
6. Mild, transient jaundice can occur, but if there is a stone in the common bile duct it will be marked and persistent.
7. Ultrasound is often useful in demonstrating gall stones.

MANAGEMENT

1. Intravenous fluids and nasogastric suction.
2. Narcotic analgesia.
3. Intravenous antibiotics if any signs of sepsis.
4. Cholecystectomy is reserved for the small minority of cases that are not controlled by these conservative measures, in whom peritonitis occurs, or if there is unrelieved cystic or common bile duct obstruction.

PELVIC INFLAMMATORY DISEASE

Acute pelvic inflammatory disease (PID) in pregnancy is rare, but can occur. It is widely felt that acute salpingo-oophoritis due to chlamydia and/or gonorrhoea is very unlikely, given the usual pathogenesis via ascending infection. However, the uterine cavity is not obliterated by fusion of the decidua parietalis and capsularis with the products of conception until about 12 weeks gestation. In addition, an infection may occur at the time of fertilisation, in association with threatened abortion or by lymphatic or vascular spread. Of the reported cases, the vast majority occur in the first trimester. Some cases of spontaneous abortion, particularly those associated with sepsis, may be initiated by pelvic inflammatory disease.

DIAGNOSIS

The diagnosis is not easy in many cases because the signs and symptoms of PID are quite variable and the many other causes of abdominal and pelvic pain that occur in pregnancy. Often the diagnosis is made at laparotomy, as suspected appendicitis is the most common differential diagnosis.

1. Lower abdominal/pelvic pain.
2. Variable anorexia, nausea and vomiting.
3. Abdominal signs range from mild tenderness to frank peritonitis.

4. Variable pelvic and adnexal tenderness with cervical excitation pain and adnexal enlargement.
5. Purulent cervicitis is more likely if gonorrhoea is the causative organism.
6. Low-grade pyrexia: 38-39°C.
7. Leucocytosis.

MANAGEMENT

Intravenous antibiotics chosen to cover the commonly involved organisms and taking into the account the developing embryo or fetus. Penicillin, aminoglycoside and erythromycin are commonly used. Even with treatment, pregnancy loss exceeds 50 per cent.

COMPLICATIONS OF UTERINE FIBROIDS

Red Degeneration

The increased uterine growth and vascularity in pregnancy causes many uterine fibroids to substantially increase in size. The increasing oedema in the fibroid can lead to ischaemia and infarction. This can be acutely painful.

DIAGNOSIS

1. This may be aided by prior knowledge of the presence of fibroids.
2. The pain can be acute in its onset and severity.
3. The patient may have anorexia and vomiting.
4. Mild pyrexia and leucocytosis may be present.
5. The tenderness will be localised to the uterus and the fibroid itself, if it is palpable.
6. In some cases ultrasound may help clarify the diagnosis.

MANAGEMENT

Rest and analgesics are all that are required. The pain usually abates in a few days.

Torsion of a pedunculated subserous fibroid may present as an acute surgical abdomen necessitating laparotomy and removal of the infarcted fibroid.

Rupture of a vessel overlying a fibroid is a very rare accident which may occur with the increased vascularity of pregnancy. The presentation is one of intraperitoneal haemorrhage requiring laparotomy.

COMPLICATIONS OF OVARIAN TUMOURS

Ovarian tumours may cause acute pain if they undergo torsion, rupture or bleed. The corpus luteum may also cause pain if it becomes cystic and bleeds. Torsion of adnexal tumours is more common in pregnancy when the changing size of the uterus acts as a rotating force and the intraabdominal relationships are changing. It is more likely to occur in early pregnancy and especially in the puerperium.

DIAGNOSIS

1. The pain is unilateral and often intermittent and colicky initially. Later it becomes constant.
2. Tenderness and rebound on the affected side of the uterus, with signs of peritonitis, mild pyrexia, and leucocytosis developing later.
3. The tender tumour may be palpable, though in later pregnancy this can be impossible to appreciate.
4. Ultrasound should help define the tumour.

MANAGEMENT

Laparotomy and removal of the tumour and any infarcted tissue.

RUPTURE OF THE LIVER, SPLEEN AND INTRA-ABDOMINAL ARTERIAL ANEURYSMS

These are very rare occurrences but have a propensity to happen more often in the pregnant woman.

Hepatic rupture most often occurs in patients with pre-eclampsia and originates as a hepatic haematoma. The patient presents with right upper quadrant pain, with or without nausea and vomiting. In almost all cases this is associated with signs of pre-eclampsia. The diagnosis may be assisted by ultrasound and computerised tomography. When the haematoma ruptures through Glisson's capsule, the presentation is one of generalised abdominal pain associated with intraperitoneal bleeding.

Splenic rupture may occur spontaneously or in response to trauma during pregnancy. Spontaneous rupture is most common in the third trimester and puerperium. The clinical presentation is left upper quadrant and epigastric pain with referral to the neck and left shoulder. This may be followed by signs of intraperitoneal bleeding.

Aneurysms: In decreasing order of frequency, spontaneous rupture of splenic, aortic, renal and ovarian artery aneurysms in pregnancy have been reported.

In all of the above conditions, the initial management is treatment of the hypovolaemia followed by laparotomy and surgical haemostasis.

REFERENCE

1. Silen W. Cope's Early Diagnosis of the Acute Abdomen. 20th ed.New York: Oxford University Press, 2000.

BIBLIOGRAPHY

Acosta AA, Malroy CR, Kaufman RH. Intrauterine pregnancy and co-existent pelvic inflammatory disease. Obstet Gynecol 1971;37:282-5.

Anderson B, Nielson TF. Appendicitis in pregnancy: diagnosis, management and complications. Acta Obstet Gynecol Scand 1999;6:347-51.

Angel JL, O'Brien WF, Finan MA. Acute pyleonephritis in pregnancy. Obstet Gynecol 1990;76:28-31.

Ashkenazy M, Kesler I, Czernobilsky B. Ovarian tumours in pregnancy. Int J Gynaecol Obstet 1988;27:79-81.

Barrett JM, VanHooydrak JE, Boehm EH. Pregnancy-related rupture of arterial aneurysms. Obstet Gynecol Surv 1982;37:557-66.

Blanchard AC, Pastorek JG, Weeks T. Pelvic inflammatory disease during pregnancy. South Med J 1987;80:1363-5.

Butler EL, Cox SM, Eberts EG, Cunningham FG. Symptomatic nephrolithiasis complicating pregnancy. Obstet Gynecol 2000;96:753-6.

Conron RW, Abbruzzi K, Cochrane SO, Sarno AJ, Cochrane PJ. Laparoscopic procedures in pregnancy. Am J Surg 1999;65:259-63.

Davis JL, Mazumder SR, Hobel CJ. Uterine leiomyomas in pregnancy:a prospective study. Obstet Gynecol 1990:75:41-4.

Fegan KS, Calder AA. Surgical emergencies in obstetrics. Contemp Clin Gynecol Obstet 2002;2:333-44.

Firstenberg MS, Malangani MA. Gastrointestinal surgery during pregnancy. Gastroenterol Clin North Am 1998;27:73-88.

Landers D, Carmona R, Crombleholme W et al. Acute cholecystitis in pregnancy. Obstet Gynecol 1987;69:131-3.

Lochman E, Schinfield A, Voss E et al. Pregnancy and laparoscopic surgery. J Am Assoc Gynecol Laparosc 1999;6:347-51.

McColl I. More precision in diagnosing appendicitis. N Engl J Med 1998;338:190-1.

Mourad J, Elliott JP, Erickson L, Lisboa L. Appendicitis in pregnancy. Am J Obstet Gynecol 2000;182:1027-9.

Nair V. Acute abdomen and abdominal pain in pregnancy. Curr Obstet Gynecol 2003;13:14-20.

Neerhof MG, Zelman W, Sullivan T. Hepatic rupture in pregnancy. Obstet Gynecol Surv 1989;44:407-9.

Sajjad Y, Aust TR, Morgan P, Nwosu EC. Rupture of splenic artery aneurysm and literature review. J Obstet Gynaecol 2000;20:633-4.

Sharma K, Tebbutt H. Subcapsular hepatic haematoma following caesarean section. J Obstet Gynaecol 1995;15:109.

Sharp HT. The acute abdomen during pregnancy. Clin Obstet Gynecol 2002;45:405-13.

Sivanesaratnam V. The acute abdomen and the obstetrician. Best Prac Res Clin Obstet Gynaecol 2000;14:89-102.

Smith LG, Moise KJ, Dildy GA et al. Spontaneous rupture of the liver during pregnancy: current therapy. Obstet Gynecol 1991;77:171-5.

Stothers L, Lee LM. Renal colic in pregnancy. J Urol 1992,148:1383-6.

CHAPTER 6

Antepartum haemorrhage

Antepartum haemorrhage is defined as bleeding from the genital tract between 20 weeks' gestation and delivery of the baby. In some countries the range is between 24 weeks and delivery, in keeping with definitions of viability.

CAUSES AND INCIDENCE

Antepartum bleeding occurs in about 2-3 per cent of all pregnancies. The approximate incidence of the various causes of antepartum haemorrhage is:

Placenta praevia	20%
Abruptio placentae	30%
Unclassified	45%
Lower genital tract lesions and others	5%

The lower genital lesions include cervical polyp, cervical carcinoma, vulvo-vaginal varices, and vaginitis. Other rare causes include uterine rupture. These conditions are not discussed here as this chapter will focus on the three main causes of antepartum haemorrhage.

GENERAL MANAGEMENT OF ANTEPARTUM HAEMORRHAGE

When the patient is first seen the cause of the antepartum haemorrhage is usually not obvious. Therefore an initial routine is necessary for all cases:

1. If the patient is seen outside hospital, make a brief clinical assessment (**never** do a pelvic examination), sedate if appropriate and transfer the patient to hospital by the quickest and safest route. The patient should be accompanied and an intravenous drip established.

2. On arrival at hospital the patient should be quickly assessed in case she needs rapid treatment of hypovolaemia. Blood is taken for haemoglobin, haematocrit, coagulation studies, blood type and antibody screen. At least two units of blood should be available in the hospital.
3. Clinical assessment **(excluding** a pelvic examination) may point to the likelihood of either abruptio placentae or placenta praevia as the cause of bleeding (Table 6.1).

Table 6.1 Clinical features of abruptio placentae and placenta praevia

Abruptio Placentae	Placenta Praevia
May be associated with hypertensive disorders, uterine overdistension, trauma	Apparently causeless
Abdominal pain and/or backache	Painless
Uterine tenderness	Uterus not tender
Increased uterine tone	Uterus soft
Usually normal presentation	Malpresentation and/or high presenting part
Fetal heart may be absent	Fetal heart usually normal
Shock and anaemia out of proportion to apparent blood loss	Shock and anaemia correspond to apparent blood loss

4. If the patient is beyond 37 weeks' gestation, or if the bleeding continues unabated, or if the patient is in labour, then pursue **active treatment** (see later).
5. If not, then carry out **expectant treatment** (see later). In practice, however, some cases between 37 and 40 weeks' gestation, with slight bleeding and no clinical signs of abruptio placentae or placenta praevia are initially treated expectantly until placental localisation is obtained.

PLACENTA PRAEVIA

DEFINITIONS AND INCIDENCE

The placenta is situated either partially or wholly in the lower uterine segment.

The **lower uterine segment** is that part of the uterus which passively stretches during labour and takes no active part in expelling the fetus. Anatomically it is the portion of the uterus below the reflection of the utero-vesical peritoneum. In late pregnancy and labour it is that part of the uterus within 3 inches (7 cm) of the internal os. Thus, in practical clinical terms it is the area that can be explored by the examining finger.

TYPES OF PLACENTA PRAEVIA (Figure 6.1)

Type I (lateral or low-lying) – encroaches on the lower uterine segment but not down as far as the internal os.

Type II (marginal) – the lower edge of the placenta extends to the internal os, but does not cover it.

Type III (partial) – when the internal os is dilated it is partially covered by the placenta.

Type IV (complete or central) – the internal os is completely covered by the placenta, even when fully dilated.

Types I and II are called a minor degree and Types III and IV a major degree of placenta praevia. Placenta praevia occurs in about 1 in every 200 deliveries, of which approximately half are major and half minor degrees.

The incidence is increased with high parity, advancing age, previous abortion, smoking and cocaine use, and in those previously delivered by caesarean section. The risk of recurrence is about 5 per cent.

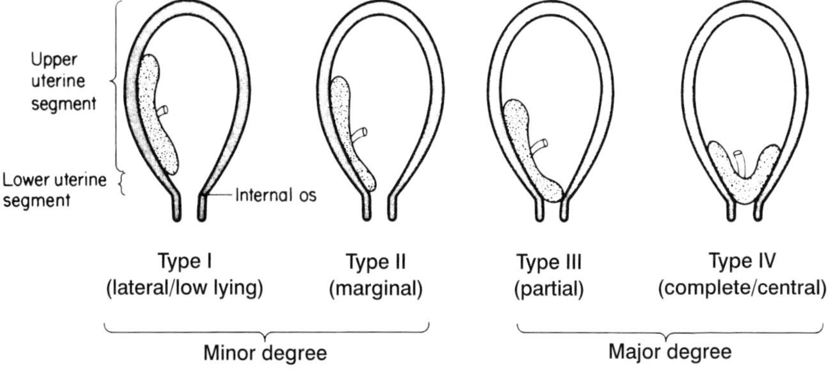

Figure 6.1 Types of placenta praevia.

PATHOPHYSIOLOGY AND CLINICAL FEATURES

- In the later weeks of pregnancy the lower segment of the uterus is formed and stretched. If the placenta is implanted on the lower uterine segment the edge may separate from the uterine wall leading to bleeding. The classic presentation is painless, apparently causeless, and recurrent bleeding in the later weeks of pregnancy.

About 80 per cent of all patients bleed before the onset of labour. In general, major degrees of placenta praevia bleed earlier, more often, and more heavily than minor degrees. However, a complete placenta praevia may, on rare occasions, not bleed until labour starts.

- With the placenta occupying or encroaching upon the lower uterine segment the presenting part is usually high and free and malpresentations are found in about one-third of cases.
- The uterus is soft and not tender.
- The fetal heart is usually present and normal.
- The degree of anaemia and shock corresponds to the apparent blood loss.
- The lower uterine segment does not contract and retract as effectively as the upper uterine segment and as a result post partum haemorrhage is more frequent. In addition the decidual response of the lower uterine segment is poorer and varying degrees of placenta accreta are more likely.
- Abnormalities of the placenta (membranacea, succenturiata, bipartite, etc.) and cord insertion (battledore and velamentous) are more common.

DIAGNOSIS

At term, ultrasound is a very accurate method of placental localisation: <2% false negative or false positive. However, in the early second trimester the lower uterine segment is unformed and only extends 0.5cm from the internal cervical os – the anatomical point from which ultrasound defines placenta praevia. Thus, at this early gestation five per cent of all placentae appear so close to the internal os, as to be judged potentially low-lying. As the lower uterine segment develops in the third trimester, the upper uterine segment and the attached placenta appear to move up and away from the internal os: so-called 'placental migration'. By term only 1 in 200 placentae remain low-lying: the true placenta praevia. Therefore, with the advent of routine second trimester ultrasound, at least five percent of women are earmarked as potential cases of placenta praevia. Transvaginal ultrasound has been shown to be safe and to improve upon the accuracy of transabdominal ultrasound and may help delineate some of these cases. If not, the case should be rescanned at 32 weeks, by which time most will be clearly seen not to be praevia. Those with a major degree of placenta praevia at 32 weeks gestation should be admitted to hospital and delivered at about 37 weeks gestation, unless bleeding or labour necessitates active management before (see below).

Those that remain as a potentially minor degree of praevia should be rescanned at 37-38 weeks, by which time the lower uterine segment is fully formed. In the meantime these women do not need to be admitted to hospital, unless they bleed (see below). An exception would be the rare patient in whom a complete placenta praevia is obvious on ultrasound even in the second trimester. Such patients should be advised against intercourse, travel etc.

MANAGEMENT

All cases that bleed must be admitted to hospital and the principles outlined under general management followed. The first bleed is almost never fatal to either mother or fetus and, with rest, it ceases in almost all cases. This fact forms the basis and rationale for expectant treatment. The first bleed is often called the 'warning bleed', which is a very apt term – a warning to be heeded by both the patient and those who attend her.

EXPECTANT TREATMENT

1. The patient should be kept resting in bed until active bleeding has stopped for three days. In practice, most cases can also be allowed bathroom privileges, as the gymnastic endeavours involved in using a bedpan often exceed those of gently transferring the patient to the bathroom in a wheelchair.
2. Blood is kept available at all times.
3. Seek and treat anaemia. If Rhesus negative, give Rh immune globulin and do a Kleihauer test.
4. When the bleeding has settled, a gentle speculum examination is done to look for lower genital tract lesions. **No** digital examination is performed for fear of disturbing the lower uterine segment and provoking another bleed. Even if a local lesion is found it does not rule out an associated placenta praevia.
5. Ultrasonic localisation of the placenta should be performed. If this is not available the patient should be transferred to a facility where it is.
6. If the ultrasound rules out placenta praevia, there are no features of abruptio placentae, and the bleeding settles, the patient is treated as an unclassified antepartum haemorrhage (see later).
7. If the ultrasound confirms the diagnosis of placenta praevia the patient should remain in hospital. The older texts refer to the bleeding due to placenta praevia as 'inevitable' antepartum haemorrhage. In many ways it is a pity this term has been dropped as it underlines the rationale behind this principle of management. If a patient has a placenta praevia it is virtually inevitable that she will bleed again, if only when she comes into labour. There are those who advocate outpatient management of selected patients with

placenta praevia, e.g. those with a mild bleed that settles, a minor degree of praevia, and who live close to hospital with a telephone and available transportation. There is no solid data upon which to base this decision. However, even minor degrees of placenta praevia can produce a torrential second haemorrhage. In addition, those patients with placenta praevia who bleed before labour have a worse perinatal outcome than those who do not bleed.[1] Thus, in general, even those patients with a minor degree of placenta praevia, who manifest this by bleeding before labour, should be admitted.

8. If less than 34 weeks' gestation consider giving corticosteroids to accelerate fetal pulmonary maturity. At least half of all cases of placenta praevia deliver before 35 weeks.
9. In some patients in the late second and early third trimesters the ultrasound may suggest a minor degree of placenta praevia. The ultrasound can be repeated in about two weeks in the hope that the lower uterine segment may have developed so that the placenta is now seen not to be praevia. The patient can then be treated as an unclassified antepartum haemorrhage.
10. Depending on how long the patient has to be in hospital, tests of fetal growth and well-being may be appropriate.
11. At 37-38 weeks' gestation, or before if indicated, active treatment is instituted.

ACTIVE TREATMENT

This is indicated when the patient reaches 37-38 weeks' gestation, if labour starts, or if there is heavy sustained bleeding. It may also be indicated at earlier gestation in cases, initially treated expectantly, in whom there are repeated bleeds. In most cases with a good ultrasound service the diagnosis of placenta praevia is certain and delivery by planned caesarean section is appropriate.

In a small number of cases where, even with transvaginal ultrasound the findings are equivocal or, ultrasound is not available, the basis of treatment is the double set-up examination. The patient is examined in the operating theatre, with the anaesthetist present, assistants scrubbed and instruments prepared for immediate caesarean section. The fornices are palpated first and if no placenta is felt the examining finger is **gently** pushed through the cervix and the lower uterine segment carefully explored. Placental tissue usually has a gritty consistency that helps distinguish it from clot. Depending on the findings the following options are possible:

1. If no placenta is felt amniotomy is performed and the subsequent labour carefully monitored.

2. If placenta praevia is confirmed the appropriate course is immediate caesarean section. In some cases of Type 1, if there is no bleeding, the cervix is very favourable and the fetal head is settling below the placental edge it is permissible to perform amniotomy and monitor the labour. If there is any doubt, or renewed bleeding, caesarean section should be performed.

Technical aspects of caesarean section for placenta praevia:

- The lower uterine segment may be poorly formed if the delivery is done early in the third trimester or if there is a transverse lie. In such cases a classical caesarean section, or a low vertical incision with the option of extending it into the upper uterine segment, is appropriate. In some patients huge vessels over the lower segment extending into the broad ligament may also make a vertical uterine incision the most prudent. In most cases, however, a low transverse uterine incision can be made.
- If the placenta is placed anteriorly use the hand to quickly separate the edge of the placenta either caudal or lateral, rupture the membranes, deliver the baby, and promptly clamp the cord. This technique is the quickest and should produce less fetal blood loss than directly cutting through the placenta. Ultrasound before the caesarean may help map out the site of the placenta and guide the best direction of the hand to the placental edge.
- Another advantage of the transverse incision is that good exposure of the lower uterine segment is obtained to observe haemostasis. If, despite oxytocics, there is general oozing from the site of placental implantation the whole lower segment can be firmly packed for a few minutes. After this isolated bleeding areas can be oversewn. Another option is the injection of 1-2ml solution of vasopressin (5units in 20ml saline) at multiple subendomyometrial sites of the placental bed.[2] If this fails, and conservation of the uterus is paramount, uterine artery ligation may reduce perfusion enough to achieve haemostasis. Square compression sutures opposing the anterior and posterior walls of the lower uterine segment may help (see chapter 20). If the bleeding cannot be stopped or if there is placenta praevia accreta then caesarean hysterectomy is the definitive treatment (see Chapter 19).
- In cases of known or highly suspected placenta accreta preoperative acute normovolaemic haemodilution may be considered. This entails removing, during one hour preoperatively, about 1000ml maternal blood to a closed – circuit blood storage bag. Concomitantly about three litres of crystalloid are given to maintain a normal pulse and blood pressure. At the time of the surgery the previously withdrawn blood is autotransfused. The acute blood

loss at surgery is therefore of haemodiluted blood and is replaced by the autotransfusion of whole blood.[3,4]

In similar cases, if hospital facilities exist for this purpose, pre-operative vascular catheters can be placed to allow immediate post-caesarean embolisation of the uterine and collateral arteries thereby reducing the need for hysterectomy (see chapter 25).

Nowadays virtually all cases of placenta praevia should be delivered by caesarean section-certainly for fetal reasons and often also for maternal reasons. There are still, however, rare occasions-in certain remote areas or in the case of a dead or pre-viable fetus-where the older techniques of assisted vaginal delivery may be needed. **Braxton Hicks bipolar podalic version** involves pushing two fingers through the cervix and the external hand guiding the breech over the pelvic brim. The two fingers, or ring forceps, grasp a foot and pull it through the membranes and cervix and apply gentle steady traction. The idea is not to pull the fetus forcibly through the cervix but to use the fetal leg and buttocks as a method of placental site tamponade. This is remarkably effective. For cephalic presentations **Willett's scalp forceps**, by putting traction on the fetal head, apply the same tamponade principle. In skilled hands under unusual circumstances both these techniques may have an occasional role.

VASA PRAEVIA

In about 1 per cent of singleton and 5 per cent of multiple pregnancies the umbilical cord inserts into the membranes and the vessels branch out running between the chorion and amnion before joining the placenta. This is called **velamentous insertion of the cord** and is more common with placenta praevia. The vessels running between the membranes are not protected by Wharton's jelly and are therefore vulnerable to compression and rupture. In about 1 in every 5000 pregnancies the vessels in the membranes run across the lower segment and cervix in front of the presenting part-**vasa praevia**. Apart from compression of the vessels during labour causing fetal asphyxia, the vessels may be torn during amniotomy or spontaneous rupture of the membranes leading to fetal exsanguination.

On occasions the wary examiner may feel the vessels in the membranes during a pelvic examination. If bleeding occurs shortly after rupture of the membranes, and particularly if there is fetal tachycardia, this diagnosis should be considered. The definitive diagnosis is achieved by testing for fetal haemoglobin. There are a number of rapid bedside tests based on the resistance of fetal haemoglobin to denaturation by alkali compared to adult haemoglobin. Add a few drops of vaginal blood to 10 ml of 0.1 per cent sodium hydroxide; fetal haemoglobin will remain pink but adult haemoglobin will turn the solution brown within 30 seconds.[5]

If the diagnosis is considered and confirmed by either palpation of the vessels or demonstration of fetal blood the treatment is immediate delivery. In practice the diagnosis is often missed and even when it is considered the fetus can exsanguinate with frightening speed from the onset of detectable bleeding or fetal heart changes. Improvement may come with newer techniques of ultrasound doppler colour flow allowing antenatal diagnosis.[6]

ABRUPTIO PLACENTAE

This is the premature separation of a normally situated placenta. It is sometimes known as 'accidental' haemorrhage to contrast it with the 'inevitable' haemorrhage of placenta praevia. Abruptio placentae occurs in about 1 in 150 deliveries.

AETIOLOGY

The exact mechanism causing abruptio placentae is unknown, but there are a number of associations:

1. Hypertensive disorders.
2. High parity and increased maternal age.
3. Low socio-economic groups, in whom as yet undefined nutritional and other factors may play a role.
4. Prolonged preterm rupture of the membranes.
5. Sudden decompression of an overdistended uterus, e.g. following rupture of the membranes with polyhydramnios and after delivery of a first twin.
6. Trauma, e.g. fall, car accident, amniocentesis-overall an uncommon cause.
7. Circumvallate placenta.
8. Smoking and cocaine use.

TYPES (Figure 6.2)

The bleeding usually passes between the membranes and the uterus to escape through the cervix and appear per vaginam-**revealed haemorrhage**. Much less frequently the blood remains trapped between the placenta and uterus-**concealed haemorrhage**. Not uncommonly a degree of both these types occurs, known as **mixed haemorrhage**.

Cases are also often classified as mild, moderate or severe depending on the blood loss and severity of signs and symptoms.

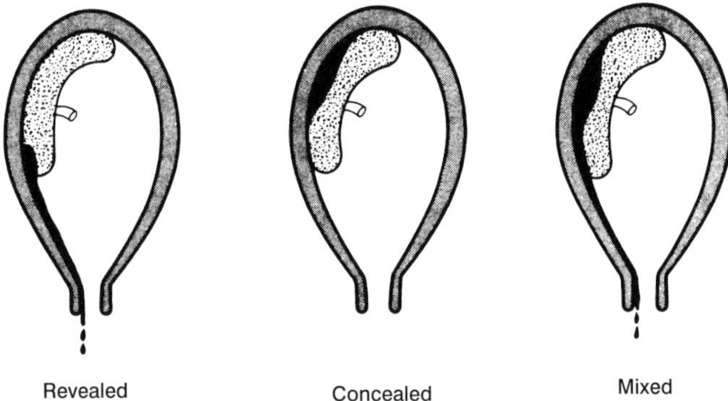

Figure 6.2 Types of abruptio placentae.

PATHOPHYSIOLOGY

Haemorrhage into the decidua basalis with haematoma formation initiates the placental separation. The clot depresses and adheres to the maternal surface of the placenta. When the edge of the placenta separates there is usually little resistance to the blood tracking down between the membranes and uterus and appearing externally. On occasions the blood may rupture through the membranes into the amniotic sac. If the bleeding is located more centrally the bleeding is concealed (about 10 per cent of cases have no vaginal bleeding) and some of the blood extravasates into the myometrium causing pain, uterine tenderness, and contractions. The increase in uterine tone and contractility may be due to prostaglandin release from the damaged decidual tissue. If much blood infiltrates the myometrium it may extend to, and cause port-wine discoloration of the serosal surface of the uterus. This is known as the Couvelaire uterus or utero-placental apoplexy. On very rare occasions blood may dissect through the myometrium and cause intraperitoneal bleeding. In the concealed variety decidual thromboplastins are more likely to be forced into the maternal circulation and initiate disseminated intravascular coagulation.

The combination of Couvelaire uterus and disseminated intravascular coagulation make post partum haemorrhage a significant threat. In this respect it is the coagulation defect that is most important: a Couvelaire uterus alone rarely interferes with uterine contractility. There is an intense vasoconstriction that accompanies the hypovolaemic shock with abruptio placentae. The kidneys are particularly vulnerable and any prolongation of the renal arteriolar spasm can lead to tubular and cortical necrosis with ultimate renal failure.

CLINICAL FEATURES

The majority of cases are of the mild, revealed type-sometimes referred to as a marginal separation. These patients may present like placenta praevia with painless bleeding and a soft, non-tender uterus. Usually, however, there is some pain, the uterus is irritable and there may be an area of localised uterine tenderness. In severe cases of concealed haemorrhage there is no external bleeding, but the patient presents with an acute abdomen and profound shock. There is severe and continuous abdominal pain. The uterus is woody hard and tender all over. The fetus dies. Disseminated intravascular coagulation may ensue. Oliguria and proteinuria develop. Cases of mixed haemorrhage may present anywhere along the clinical spectrum between the above two extremes.

MANAGEMENT

Treat Hypovolaemia

It must be stressed that under-transfusion is almost always a factor in these cases. Even with a loss of up to one-third of their blood volume, patients may maintain a normal pulse and blood pressure. Therefore, all patients require intravenous fluids to avoid hypovolaemia. In shocked patients, immediate and rapid infusion of crystalloid and colloid, followed by blood transfusion is essential to maintain tissue, especially renal, perfusion. The adequacy of circulation should be followed by continuous monitoring of urinary output (keep output >30 ml/hour). If available, in severe cases, central venous pressure measurement is ideal (see Chapter 24).

Disseminated intravascular coagulation should be sought and treated (see Chapter 8).

Obstetric Management

If the bleeding is slight and if there is no uterine tenderness expectant treatment, along the lines described for placenta praevia, may be followed in cases under 37 weeks' gestation. Ultrasound may help confirm the diagnosis but can be misleading ,with both false positive and false negative results.

If a definite diagnosis of abruptio placentae is made steps are taken to effect delivery. Many patients are already in labour at the time of diagnosis. Amniotomy is performed either to induce or accelerate labour. It also has the desirable effect of reducing intrauterine tension and possibly lessens the chance of extravasation of blood and thromboplastins into the myometrium and maternal circulation.

The fetal heart should be monitored continuously. Caesarean section should be selectively but liberally used and is considered for the following cases:

1. All moderate or severe cases when the fetus is mature enough and alive.
2. Any case with fetal distress.
3. The patient is unfavourable for induction.
4. Failed induction or inadequate progress of labour after 6-8 hours.

UNCLASSIFIED ANTEPARTUM HAEMORRHAGE

For a definite diagnosis of placenta praevia to be made the placenta must be felt to encroach on the lower uterine segment. Similarly there must be evidence of retroplacental clot at delivery to confirm abruptio placentae. In about half of all cases of antepartum bleeding there is no such evidence and the cases are designated as unclassified or of

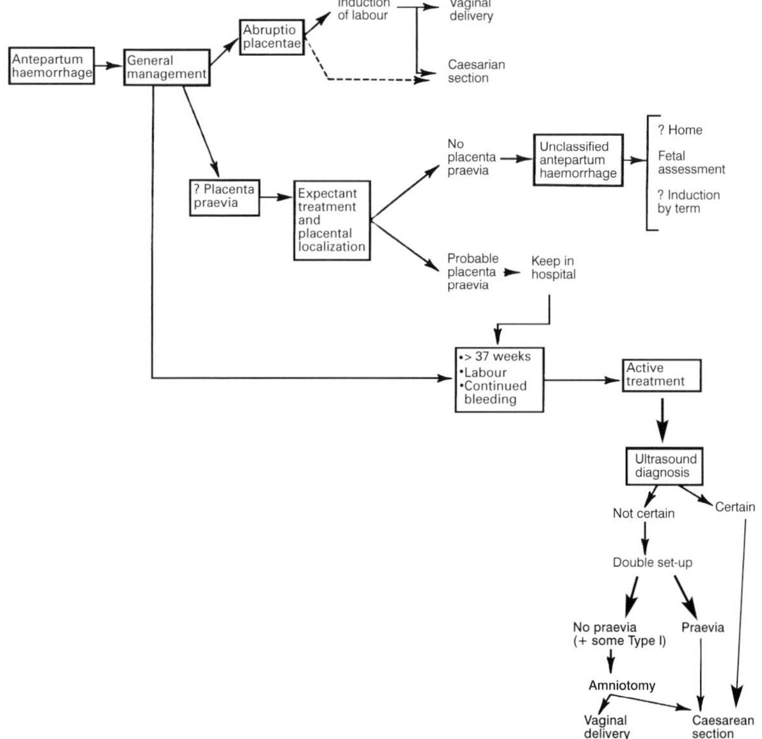

Figure 6.3 Management scheme for antepartam haemorrhage.

unknown origin. It is likely that many of these cases are due to the rupture of small blood vessels in the cervix and isthmus during formation of the lower uterine segment. Some are probably caused by minor but unconfirmed degrees of placenta praevia and abruptio placentae.

In cases managed expectantly, if the bleeding settles and ultrasound examination rules out placenta praevia, the patient is mobilised and may be discharged from hospital after a few days. These patients also have an increased perinatal loss and must be watched carefully. Fetal growth and assessment of well-being should be carefully followed and induction of labour close to term considered.

A management schema for patients with antepartum haemorrhage is outlined in Figure 6.3

REFERENCES

1. Lamb CS, Wong SF, Chow KM, Ho LC. Women with placenta praevia and antepartum haemorrage have a worse outcome than those who do not bleed before delivery. J Obstet Gynaecol 2000;20:27-31.
2. Lurie S, Appelman Z, Katz Z. Intractable postpartum bleeding due to placenta accreta: local vasopressin may save the uterus. Br J Obstet Gynaecol 1996;103:1164.
3. Estella NM, Berry DL, Baker BW, Wali A, Belfort MA. Normovolaemic hemodilution before cesarean hysterectomy for placenta percreta. Obstet Gynecol 1997;90:669-70.
4. Lisander B. Preoperative haemodilution. Acta Anaesthesiol Scand 1988;32(suppl)89:63-70.
5. Loendersloot EW. Vasa previa. Am J Obstet Gynecol 1979;135:702-3.
6. Lee W, Lee VL, Kirk JS, Sloan CT, Smith RS, Comstock CH. Vasa previa: prenatal diagnosis, natural evolution and clinical outcome. Obstet Gynecol 2000;95:572-6.

BIBLIOGRAPHY

American College of Obstetricians and Gynecologists. Committee Opinion No 266. Placenta accreta. Washington DC: ACOG, 2002.(Obstet Gynecol 2002;44:169-70.)

Ananth CV, Smulian JC, Vintzileos AM. The association of placenta previa with history of cesarean delivery and abortion: a meta-analysis. Am J Obstet Gynecol 1997;177:1071-8.

Ananth CV, Smulian JC, Vintzileos AM. Incidence of placental abruption in relation to cigarette smoking and hypertensive disorders during pregnancy: a meta-analysis of observational studies. Obstet Gynecol 1999;93:622-8.

Clark SL, Koonings PP, Phelan JP. Placenta previa/accreta and prior cesarean section. Obstet Gynecol 1985;66: 89-92.

Craigo S. Placenta previa with suspected accreta. Curr Opinion Obstet Gynecol 1997;9:71-5.

Crane JMG, Van den Hof M, Dodds L, Armson BA, Liston RM. Maternal complications with placenta previa. Am J Perinatol 2000;17:102-4.

D'Angelo L, Irwin L. Conservative management of placenta previa: a cost benefit analysis. Am J Obstet Gynecol 1983;149:320-6.

Dougall A, Baird CH. Vasa praevia-report of three cases and review of literature. Br J Obstet Gynaecol 1987;94:712-5.

Druzin ML. Packing of lower uterine segment for control of postcesarean bleeding in instances of placenta praevia. Surg Gynecol Obstet 1989;169:543-5.

Fung TY, Lau TK. Poor perinatal outcome associated with vasa previa: Is it preventable? A report of three cases and review of the literature. Ultrasound Obstet Gynecol 1998;12:430-3.

Herd WW, Miodovnik M, Hertzberg V. Selective management of abruptio placentae: a prospective study. Obstet Gynecol 1983;61: 467-73.

Hladky K, Yankowitz J, Hansen WF. Placental abruption. Obstet Gynecol Surv 2002;57:299-305.

Hudan L, Belfort MA, Broome DR. Diagnosis and management of placenta percreta: a review. Obstet Gynecol Surv 1998;53:509-17.

Kayani SI, Walkinshaw SA, Preston C. Pregnancy outcome in severe placental abruption. Br J Obstet Gynaecol 2003;110:679-83.

Matsuda Y, Maeda T, Kouno S. Comparison of neonatal outcome including cerebral palsy between abruptio placentae and placenta previa. Eur J Obstet Gynecol Reprod Biol 2003;106:125-9.

Nielson E, Varner M, Scott J. The outcome of pregnancies complicated by bleeding during the second trimester. Surg Gynecol Obstet 1991;173:371-4.

Neilsen TF, Hagberg H, Ljungblad U. Placenta previa and antepartum hemorrhage after previous cesarean section. Gynecol Obstet Invest 1989;27: 88-90.

Royal College of Obstetricians and Gynaecologists. Guideline No. 27. Placenta praevia: diagnosis and management. London: RCOG, 2001.

Timor– Trisch IE, Yunis RA. Confirming the safety of transvaginal sonography in patients suspected of placenta previa. Obstet Gynecol 1993;81:742-4.

CHAPTER 7

Severe pre-eclampsia and eclampsia

Hypertensive disease in pregnancy is one of the main causes of maternal and perinatal mortality in both developed and developing countries. It is not the purpose of this chapter to discuss the problem of hypertension in pregnancy as a whole – a topic full of variables and unresolved controversy. We are here concerned with the acute problem of the eclamptic and severely pre-eclamptic patient.

PREDISPOSING FACTORS

Certain patients have a greater risk of developing pre-eclampsia (pregnancy-induced hypertension):

- Family history
- Primigravidae
- Reproductive age extremes: < 20 years and > 35 years
- Multiple pregnancy
- Diabetes mellitus
- Chronic hypertension
- Gestational trophoblastic disease
- Hydrops fetalis

PATHOPHYSIOLOGY

The aetiology of pre-eclampsia is unknown but the main pathological effect is vascular spasm which may lead to a number of manifestations associated with alteration in regional blood flow.

The **blood volume** is reduced and haemoconcentrated but fills the available intravascular space which is smaller due to the generalised vasoconstriction. Pre-eclamptic patients therefore tolerate badly either haemorrhage or the loss of fluid from diuretic administration. On the other hand, attempts to expand the blood volume with intravenous fluid can easily overload the reduced vasoconstricted intravascular space and lead to pulmonary oedema. If the vasoconstriction is relaxed by antihypertensive drugs or regional anaesthesia, extra intravenous fluids will be needed to fill the expanded intravascular space.

Coagulation changes occur in some, but by no means all patients with severe pre-eclampsia/eclampsia. It may be that the vasospasm interferes with the circulation in the vasa vasorum leading to hypoxia and damage of the endothelial wall. This promotes adherence of platelets and fibrin deposition in the small vessels. Thrombocytopenia, usually mild, is not uncommon, but it is unusual for the full picture of microangiopathic haemolytic anaemia or disseminated intravascular coagulation to develop.

The characteristic **renal** lesion is glomerular endotheliosis. The capillary endothelial cells are swollen, narrowing the lumen of the capillaries and this, allied to the vasospasm, leads to glomerular ischaemia. The end result is reduced glomerular filtration and tubular ischaemia which cause oliguria and proteinuria.

Blood flow to the **hepatic** sinusoids may be reduced due to intravascular fibrin deposition leading to periportal haemorrhagic necrosis and elevation of serum liver enzymes. Haemorrhage can occur under the liver (Glisson's) capsule and on rare occasions may rupture with catastrophic intraperitoneal haemorrhage (see Chapter 5).

The ultimate **cerebral** manifestation is the eclamptic fit. It is not known whether the convulsions are due to cerebral oedema, ischaemia secondary to vasospasm or microhaemorrhages. Cerebral haemorrhage is one of the main causes of maternal death in eclampsia.

The **heart** may reveal subendothelial haemorrhages and focal necrosis. The **lungs** usually have diffuse haemorrhagic areas. In fatal cases of eclampsia cardio-pulmonary failure is a common cause of death.

Utero-placental blood flow, and therefore perfusion of the intervillous space, is reduced. This may lead to fetal intrauterine growth restriction and hypoxia. The risk of abruptio placentae is increased.

Pyrexia may occur in cases of eclampsia with repeated convulsions or coma and is presumably due to dysfunction of the central temperature regulating system.

CLINICAL FEATURES

The classical triad of signs of pre-eclampsia is hypertension, proteinuria, and oedema.

1. **Hypertension** is usually sustained at ≥ 160/110 mmHg for the diagnosis of severe pre-eclampsia to be established.
2. **Proteinuria** will usually exceed 1g/24 hours (2 +) and often ≥ 5g/24 hours (4 +).

3. **Oedema** may be absent. When present it is usually most marked in the face and hands. Occult fluid retention is often manifest by a marked weight gain before the development of hypertension or proteinuria.

It is essential to realize that no exact measurement of blood pressure or proteinuria can define the severity of pre-eclampsia or the risk of eclampsia. The young primigravid woman whose normal blood pressure is 90/60 mmHg may have a convulsion with a blood pressure of 140/90 mmHg. Therefore additional features must be assessed before deciding on the severity of the pre-eclampsia and the appropriate treatment. These include:

- Headache
- Visual disturbances-scotomata, blurred or double vision
- Epigastric and right hypochondrial pain
- Nausea and vomiting
- Fundoscopy-retinal oedema and retinal artery spasm
- Brisk deep tendon reflexes and sustained ankle clonus
- Oliguria
- Thrombocytopenia
- Pulmonary oedema
- Raised liver enzymes

Always remember that pre-eclampsia is a disease of signs and that symptoms are the hallmark of imminent eclampsia.

Eclampsia is defined as the presence of convulsions in addition to preeclampsia. About 40 per cent of cases occur antepartum, 20 per cent intrapartum, and 40 per cent post partum. In the vast majority of cases, eclampsia is preceded by several days, and often weeks, of clinically evident pre-eclampsia. In a very few cases an unheralded, fulminant onset occurs.

Just before the convulsion, the patient may exhibit premonitory signs such as restlessness, tremulousness, and facial twitching. The convulsion starts with a fixed stare and loss of consciousness followed by the typical grand mal seizure with tonic/clonic contractions. During the clonic phase of alternate muscle contraction and relaxation the jaws may badly damage the tongue. The loss of consciousness persists for a variable time after the convulsions have ceased.

HELLP Syndrome

In a small number of pre-eclamptic patients, the dominant features are haemolysis (H), elevated liver enzymes (EL), and low platelet count (LP): the so-called HELLP Syndrome. The classical presentation is with the signs of severe pre-eclampsia associated with nausea, vomiting, epigastric and right hypochondrial pain. In a small number, clinical jaundice may be evident. In addition to elevated liver enzymes, asparate and alanine transaminases (AST, ALT), and thrombocytopenia, there is evidence of disseminated intravascular coagulation (DIC) and haemolysis due to microangiopathic haemolytic anaemia (see Chapter 8).

This disease process has a very broad clinical-pathological spectrum with variable clinical manifestations. There may be subtle changes without clinical signs of pre-eclampsia and some cases initially manifest themselves as a gastro-intestinal disturbance and are investigated as gall bladder dysfunction. At the other extreme, the patient is acutely ill with a fulminant severe pre-eclampsia/eclampsia, jaundice, DIC and the potential for rupture of a subcapsular hepatic haematoma. Some may manifest a severe DIC with minimal signs of pre-eclampsia.

The management depends on the severity, but almost always involves the same treatment as for severe pre-eclampsia/eclampsia in addition to controlling the DIC (see Chapter 8).

MANAGEMENT

Eclampsia carries a serious risk of maternal and perinatal mortality. Severe pre-eclampsia is but one step from eclampsia and, while the severity of complications and the degree of urgency are not quite so marked, the potential for eclampsia is ever present and therefore the principles of management must be the same. With good antenatal care cases of eclampsia are rarely seen and even severe pre-eclampsia is not common. It is thus unusual for any individual doctor or nurse to be frequently involved in the management of such cases. It is therefore advisable for each hospital to develop guidelines and apply a uniform approach and therapeutic regime.

The principles of management are as follows:

1. CONTROL OR PREVENTION OF CONVULSIONS

Over the years many different drugs have been used to control eclamptic convulsions. Various drug routines have gained acceptance in different countries. Recent studies have settled the argument over the safest and best drug for the control and prevention of convulsions.[1,2] Magnesium sulphate has been shown in randomised trials to be effective, safer and superior to the other commonly used anticonvulsants: chlormethiazole, diazepam and phenytoin. In addition, magnesium sulphate prophylaxis has been shown to provide maternal and perinatal benefit with severe pre-eclampsia.[3,4]

Magnesium Sulphate

The exact mode of action is unknown but it is thought to impede acetylcholine release and decrease the sensitivity of the motor end plate to acetylcholine. It may also have a central anticonvulsant effect. It has the additional desirable side effect of dilating the cerebral and uterine arteries. The advantages include the absence of cerebral depression and the retention of intact cough and gag reflexes.

Intravenous Routine

The **initial dose** is 4grams IV given as 20ml of a 20 per cent solution over 10-15 minutes. The 20 per cent solution is made by adding 8ml (4g) of 50% Mg SO4 solution to 12ml normal saline.

The **maintainence dose** is 1-3 grams of magnesium sulphate hourly: the exact dose depending on biological and biochemical monitoring (see below). This can be made up as 50ml (25 g) of 50% Mg SO4 solution added to 250 ml normal saline. Using an infusion pump set the rate at 12 to 36 ml/hour (each 12ml contains 1gram Mg SO4). This volume of fluid must be included in the overall calculation of fluid balance (see later).

Intramuscular Routine

In many hospitals an intramuscular routine is followed. This is particularly suitable for stabilisation and transportation from rural areas. The initial dose is 10 grams of magnesium sulphate (20 ml of a 50 percent solution) by deep intramuscular injection with a 3 inch (7 cm) 20 gauge needle. This is given as two injections of 10 ml each. The maintenance dose is 5 grams (10 ml of a 50 per cent solution) every four hours. This is a very painful injection and the addition of 1 ml of 1 per cent lidocaine (lignocaine) to each injection dose is advisable.

Monitoring Magnesium Sulphate Therapy

If the level of magnesium sulphate exceeds the therapeutic range fatal respiratory and cardiovascular depression may occur. It is therefore essential that careful biological, and in some cases biochemical, monitoring is undertaken as follows:

1. Respiratory rate hourly: if < 14 per minute the magnesium sulphate must be reduced or withheld.
2. Patellar reflexes hourly: absent or reduced reflexes mean the magnesium sulphate must be withheld or reduced. On the other hand

hyper-reflexia is not an indication to increase the dose, as the reflexes may remain brisk even with therapeutic magnesium levels. If epidural analgesia is used the deep tendon reflexes can be followed using the biceps tendon.
3. Oliguria < 25 ml per hour indicates a need to reduce the dose. Magnesium sulphate is excreted solely by the kidneys.
4. Ideally serum magnesium levels should be done 1 hour after the initial dose and thereafter every 4-6 hours. Adjust the dose to keep the magnesium level between 4 and 8 mEq/1. If the facilities to estimate serum magnesium levels are not available careful biological monitoring will suffice.

Antidote to Magnesium Sulphate

This should always be available at the bedside. Calcium gluconate 1 gram (10 ml of 10 per cent solution), given intravenously over 3-5 minutes, effectively reverses the effects of magnesium toxicity.
Magnesium sulphate can cause neonatal depression but this is rare if the maternal levels are appropriately controlled as outlined above.

Recurrent Seizures

If there are recurrent seizures give a furthur bolus of magnesium sulphate, 2-4 grams IV over 5-10 minutes. The dose depends on the weight of the patient and the previous loading and maintenance doses of magnesium sulphate.

A reasonable alternative is to give **diazepam** 10mg intravenously over one minute. Diazepam can also be used initially if the patient is first seen during a seizure.

On very rare occasions, a patient may have repeated convulsions uncontrolled by the above anticonvulsant therapy**-status eclampticus**. It is possible to manage such patients by using muscle relaxants to achieve paralysis and control respiration by intermittent positive pressure ventilation.

2. TREATMENT OF HYPERTENSION

Anticonvulsant drugs do not have a marked or sustained hypotensive effect. Reduction of blood pressure is an urgent priority undertaken to protect the mother from cerebral haemorrhage. Against this goal, one has to balance the interests of the fetus and not lower the blood pressure so much as to critically reduce the utero-placental blood flow. The principles are to use antihypertensive drugs if the systolic blood pressure is > 170 mm Hg or the diastolic is sustained at ≥ 105-110 mmHg and to reduce the pressure by only 15-20 per cent into the 90-100 mmHg diastolic range.

Hydralazine is the drug of choice for acute hypertension. It reduces peripheral resistance, and increases cardiac output and renal and cerebral blood flow. The initial dose is 5-10 mg intravenously, given over 3-5 minutes to avoid acute hypotension. A continuous infusion at 5 mg per hour is then set up and adjusted up or down to maintain the diastolic blood pressure at about 95 mmHg. Others give intermittent 5mg boluses as needed.

Labetalol, a combined alpha- and beta-adrenergic blocker, reduces blood pressure, apparently without diminishing utero-placental blood flow. It may be used as an alternative to hydralazine or in combination to combat hydralazine-induced tachycardia. The initial dose is 20-40 mg given intravenously over two minutes and repeated in 20 minutes if needed. It can also be given by continuous infusion of 200mg labetalol in 200ml saline, starting at 40mg/hour and adjusting to achieve appropriate blood pressure control.

3. FLUID BALANCE

Beware of fluid overload: pulmonary oedema is one of the main causes of maternal morbidity and mortality in severe pre-eclampsia/eclampsia. The aim is to provide intravenous fluids to cover the insensible loss plus urinary output. A practical working figure for insensible loss is 50 ml per hour – an amount which should be increased if the patient is in labour or hyperthermic. It is therefore reasonable to start the intravenous crystalloid at 100 ml per hour. The urinary output should be monitored through an indwelling Foley catheter and the rate of intravenous infusion adjusted accordingly(urinary output in previous hour plus 50ml). This is adequate in most patients but in more severe cases, particularly those complicated by pulmonary oedema or severe oliguria, central venous pressure and even pulmonary wedge pressure monitoring through a Swan-Ganz catheter is required for ideal management. If peripheral vasodilatation is produced by hypotensive drugs or epidural analgesia, the intravenous fluids must be increased to fill the expanded intravascular space.

Diuretics should not be used unless there is evidence of pulmonary oedema.

4. NURSING CARE

A nurse must be in constant attendance. The patient should be nursed in a quiet dimly lit room. It is often stated that the room should be darkened, but this should not be taken to extremes because clinical appraisal of, for example cyanosis or a convulsion, can be compromised. This is certainly not a condition where the attendants should be stumbling around in the dark either figuratively or literally.

A mouth gag should be available at the bedside to place between the jaws to protect the tongue should a convulsion occur.

The patient's reflexes, respiratory rate, and urinary output should be checked hourly.

During the initial stages of antihypertensive therapy the blood pressure and pulse should be taken every 5-10 minutes and later every 30 minutes as conditions stabilise.

5. OBSTETRIC CARE

It is a truism that the only cure for severe pre-eclampsia/eclampsia is delivery of the fetus and placenta. All of the treatment outlined above is merely a holding action in an effort to protect the mother until this can be accomplished. The dilemma arises when the fetus is very premature (< 32 weeks). There is a temptation to try and gain time for the fetus with conservative management. In some cases a delay of 48 hours may be feasible and allow corticosteroids time to act and reduce the risk of neonatal RDS. However, if the patient is severely pre-eclamptic the fetus usually gains nothing by delay, and indeed often deteriorates along with the mother. As a guiding rule, if the pre-eclampsia is severe enough to warrant parenteral anticonvulsant and antihypertensive therapy, the patient should be delivered.

It is worth stressing that with modern neonatal care these infants do well if they are delivered unasphyxiated and are not poisoned by the drugs used to control maternal convulsions. When possible these patients should be transferred, after initiation of anticonvulsant treatment, and delivered in a hospital with neonatal intensive care facilities.

If conditions are favourable **induction of labour** should be undertaken by amniotomy and intravenous oxytocin. The fetus should be monitored during labour.

Caesarean section is appropriate if the patient is unfavourable for induction or if the progress of labour is unsatisfactory 8-12 hours after induction.

The most appropriate **analgesia** for labour is epidural. Before institution of the block the antihypertensive drugs are reduced and the patient is given a pre-load of about 500-1000 ml of intravenous crystalloid. It is also wise to check the coagulation profile before giving the epidural block. The advantages of epidural analgesia in these patients are enormous and obvious.

If general anaesthesia is required it must be remembered that magnesium sulphate potentiates the effects of muscle relaxants and the dose should be adjusted accordingly.

Ergometrine should not be given to these patients because of its propensity to worsen the hypertension (see Chapter 20).

The complications of abruptio placentae and disseminated intravascular coagulation are more common in these patients and are dealt with in Chapters 6 and 8.

6. POST PARTUM CARE

The anticonvulsant therapy should be continued for 24 hours and occasionally 48 hours post partum. It is very rare for eclampsia to occur more than 24 hours after delivery and almost never after 48 hours. The blood pressure will often return close to normal in a few days. On occasion an oral antihypertensive may be needed to maintain the diastolic pressure below 100 mmHg for the first 2-4 weeks post partum.

It is essential for each unit to agree on a standard approach and apply it carefully and consistently so that the staff become familiar with it. This will achieve the best results and is a most important principle when dealing with an uncommon condition that carries such risk to mother and fetus.

REFERENCES

1. The eclampsia trial collaborative group. Which anticonvulsant for women with eclampsia? Evidence from the Collaborative Eclampsia Trial. Lancet 1995;345:1455-63.
2. Chien PFW, Khan KS, Arnott N. Magnesium sulphate in the treatment of eclampsia and pre-eclampsia: an overview of the evidence from randomised trials. Br J Obstet Gynaecol 1996;103:1085-91.
3. Coetzee EJ, Dommisse J, Anthony J. A randomised controlled trial of intravenous magnesium sulphate versus placebo in the management of women with severe pre-eclampsia. Br J Obstet Gynaecol 1998;105:300-3.
4. The Magpie Trial:The Magpie Trial Collaborative Group. Do women with pre-eclampsia, and their babies, benefit from magnesium sulphate? a randomised placebo-controlled trial. Lancet 2002;359:1877-90.

BIBLIOGRAPHY

American College of Obstetricians and Gynaecologists. Practice Bulliten No33. Diagnosis and management of preeclampsia and eclampsia. Washington DC: ACOG, 2002.(Obstet Gynecol 2002;99:159-67).

Douglas KA, Redman CWG. Eclampsia in the United Kingdom. BMJ 1994;309:1395-1400.

Idama TO, Lindow SW. Magnesium sulphate: a review of clinical pharmacology applied to obstetrics. Br J Obstet Gynaecol 1998;105:260-8.

Isler CM, Barrilleaux PS, Rinehart BK, Magann EF, Martin JN. Postpartum seizure prophylaxis: using maternal clinical parameters to guide therapy. Obset Gynecol 2003;101:66-9.

Lee W, O'Connell CM, Baskett TF. Maternal and perinatal outcomes of eclampsia: Nova Scotia, 1981-2000. J. Obstet Gynaecol Can 2004; 26:140-3.

Moodley J, Daya P. Eclampsia: a continuing problem in developing countries. Int J Gynecol Obstet 1993;44:9-14.

Paterson-Brown S, Robson SC, Redfern N, Walkinshaw SA, deSwiet M. Hydralazine boluses for the treatment of severe hypertension in pre-eclampsia. Br J Obstet Gynaecol 1994;101:409-13.

Perry KG, Martin JN. Abnormal hemostasis and coagulopathy in preeclampsia and eclampsia. Clin Obstet Gynecol 1992;35:338-50.

Roberts JM, Villar J, Arulkumaran S. Preventing and treating eclamptic seizures. BMJ 2002;325:609-10.

Royal College of Obstetricians and Gynaecologists. Guideline No 10. Management of eclampsia. London: RCOG,1999.

Sheth SS, Chalmers I. Commentary: Magnesium for preventing and treating eclampsia: time for international action. Lancet 2002;359:1872-3.

Sibai BM. Diagnosis and management of gestational hypertension and preeclampsia. Obstet Gynecol 2003;102:181-92.

Sidhu H. Pre-eclampsia and eclampsia. In: Johanson R, Cox C, Grady K, Howell C(eds). Managing Obstetric Emergencies and Trauma. London: RCOG Press, 2003 pp 135-47.

Van Pampus MG, Wolf H, Westenberg SM et al. Maternal and perinatal outcome after expectant management of the HELLP syndrome compared with pre-eclampsia without HELLP syndrome. Eur J Obstet Gynecol Reprod Biol 1998;76:31-6.

Walker JJ. Severe pre-eclampsia and eclampsia. Best Prac Res Clin Obstet Gynaecol 2000;14:57-71.

Weinstein L. Syndrome of hemolysis, elevated liver enzymes and low platelet count: a severe consequence of hypertension in pregnancy. Am J Obstet Gynecol 1982;142: 159-64.

Young P, Johanson R. Haemodynamic, invasive and echocardiographic monitoring in the hypertensive parturient. Best Prac Res Clin Obstet Gynaecol 2001;15:605-22.

CHAPTER 8

Disseminated intravascular coagulation in pregnancy

Disseminated intravascular coagulation (DIC), also known as consumption coagulopathy, is a syndrome of abnormal coagulation and fibrinolysis produced in response to certain obstetric complications.

CAUSES

- Abruptio placentae
- Intrauterine death
- Missed abortion
- Amniotic fluid embolism
- Ruptured uterus
- Eclampsia/pre-eclampsia
- Hypovolaemic shock/massive blood transfusion
- Trophoblastic disease
- Saline abortion
- Sepsis

In obstetric patients DIC is always secondary to another condition. The method of activation of the clotting system may be:

1. **Release of thromboplastins** into the maternal circulation from placental and decidual tissue. This may happen suddenly in cases of abruptio placentae, amniotic fluid embolism, ruptured uterus, etc., and more insidiously in the case of intrauterine death and missed abortion. In pregnancies complicated by abruptio placentae with enough severity to cause fetal death, DIC will supervene in about 25 per cent of patients. In patients with intrauterine death or missed abortion about 25 per cent will develop DIC 5-6 weeks after fetal demise, with subtle laboratory changes evident earlier in some cases. With earlier diagnosis by ultrasound and the use of prostaglandins to facilitate evacuation of the uterus, missed abortion and fetal death as a cause of DIC are decreasing.

2. **Injury to endothelial cells** exposing the underlying collagen to the plasma and coagulation factors. This may be the initiating factor in some cases of eclampsia/pre-eclampsia and sepsis.
3. **Red blood cell or platelet injury** leading to release of phospholipids. This may occur in blood transfusion reactions.

PATHOPHYSIOLOGY

This is outlined in Figure 8.1. Normal haemostasis is a dynamic balance between coagulation, leading to fibrin formation, and the fibrinolytic system which acts to dispose of fibrin when its haemostatic function has been fulfilled. In DIC there is excessive and widespread coagulation due to the release of thromboplastins into the maternal circulation. This leads to consumption and depletion of the coagulation factors resulting in a haemorrhagic diathesis. In response to the widespread coagulation and fibrin deposition in the microvasculature the fibrinolytic system is secondarily activated. This involves conversion of plasminogen to plasmin which breaks down fibrin to form fibrin degradation products (FDP). In addition plasmin depletes factors 5 and 8 and disrupts platlelet surface receptors. Fibrin degradation products have anticoagulant properties, inhibiting both platelet function and the action of thrombin, thus further aggravating the coagulation defect.

The haemorrhagic diathesis is the main problem in most cases, but in some the widespread microvascular thrombosis can cause organ ischaemia and infarction. This may be an accessory factor in the genesis of renal cortical necrosis, lung damage and Sheehan's syndrome in cases with severe abruptio placentae.

CLINICAL FEATURES

1. Often the main symptoms and signs are those of the obstetric complications causing the DIC.
2. The haemorrhagic manifestations may be relatively subtle with bruising, purpuric rash, epistaxis and venipuncture oozing, or more dramatic, with profuse bleeding from operative sites and post partum haemorrhage.
3. Thrombotic sequelae rarely present in acute DIC as they are overshadowed by the haemorrhagic diathesis. The most common thrombotic manifestations are renal, hepatic, and pulmonary dysfunction.

DIAGNOSIS

Awareness of the obstetric conditions that may trigger DIC and the presenting clinical features is essential. Often the urgency of the situation and lack of sophisticated laboratory facilities preclude definitive

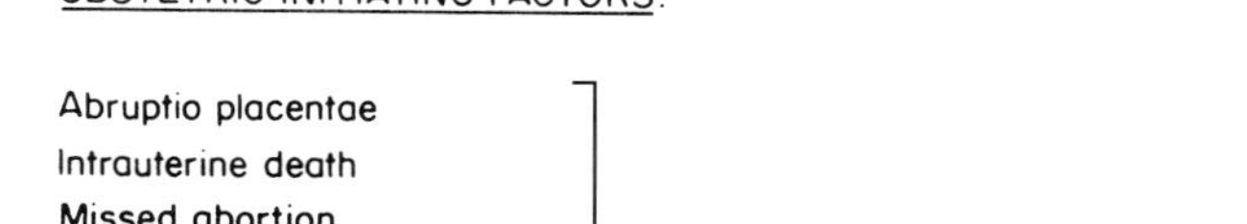

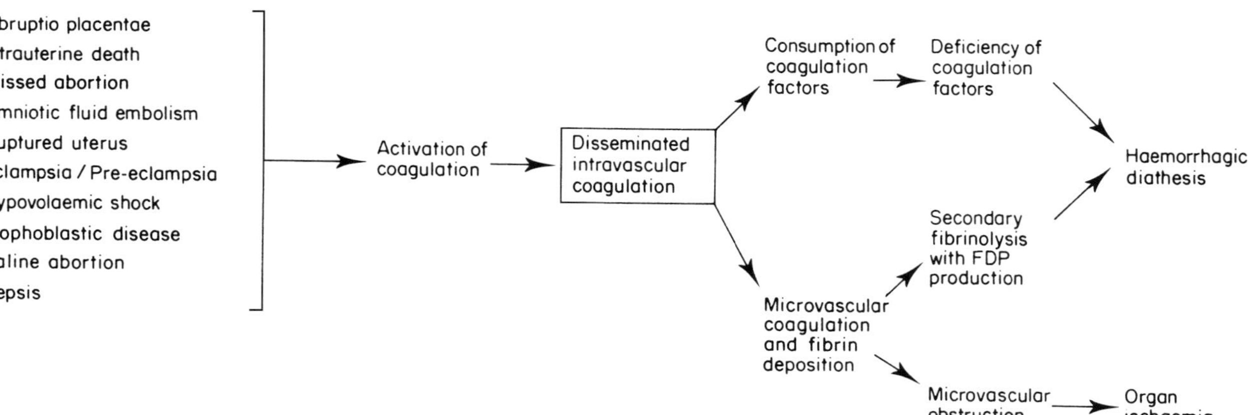

Figure 8.1 Causes and pathophysiology of disseminated intravascular coagulation.

haematological tests. Interpretation of tests may also be difficult as the process of DIC is so dynamic that results, when available, will often not reflect the current status of the patient. In severe cases of DIC virtually all of the tests of coagulation and fibrinolysis will be abnormal, but in milder cases the results are variable.

Partial thromboplastin time is variable and may only be prolonged later in the process when the clotting factors are severely depleted.
Prothrombin time usually becomes prolonged.
Thrombin time is usually prolonged and is one of the more valuable tests.
Platelet levels may be low or fall progressively .
Fibrinogen levels are normally increased in pregnancy to 400-650mg/dl. In DIC the level falls but may be in the normal non-pregnant range. With severe DIC the fibrinogen levels usually fall below 150mg/dl.
Fibrinogen-fibrin degradation products (FDP): Levels of > 80 ug/ml confirm the diagnosis of DIC. However, these elevated levels will remain for 24-48 hours after the DIC has been controlled.
A blood smear may show abnormally shaped ('helmet' or 'tear'-shaped) and fragmented red blood cells-*schistocytes*. These are formed by the alteration of normal red blood cells as they are forced through the fibrin mesh in the obstructed capillary bed.
Haemolysis and haemoglobinuria can occur if there is widespread red blood cell destruction-a condition known as **microangiopathic haemolytic anaemia**.

MANAGEMENT

In most obstetric situations DIC develops rapidly. Treatment must be prompt. Often both time and facilities do not permit the luxury of thoroughly delineating the deficient clotting mechanisms. The process and progress of DIC is so dynamic that laboratory results may not reflect the current situation. This does not mean that one should not try and follow the laboratory aspects of the coagulopathy and enlist the aid of a haematologist if available. It does mean, however, that even without detailed haematological evaluation, one must have a rational plan of management that will cover most of the problems encountered in this potentially disastrous complication.

TREAT THE INITIATING CAUSE

It should be remembered that until the obstetric complication leading to DIC supervenes, most of these patients are healthy young women. As such they have a great ability to recover rapidly and completely once the initiating cause is removed. In most cases this entails emptying the uterus. The method of doing this, and the other aspects of treating the obstetric cause of the DIC will vary (as outlined in specific chapters), but this basic principle should not.

MAINTAIN ORGAN PERFUSION

In patients in whom the cause, or result, of DIC is haemorrhage, this is the most urgent and important principle to follow. This is best accomplished by:

- Oxygen by face mask or by endotracheal intubation and intermittent positive pressure ventilation if necessary, to achieve satisfactory arterial oxygenation.
- Rapid infusion of crystalloid and colloid.
- Rapid replacement with blood. Fresh whole blood is best, but almost never available because it cannot be screened for infection. Stored whole blood loses some procoagulants, such as factors five and eight, very rapidly. Thus, in practice, packed red cells are provided and specific procoagulants added as required (see later).
- Monitor the above by a central venous pressure line if possible and/or aim to keep the urinary output at least 30-60 ml/hour and the haematocrit > 30 per cent.
- If an effective circulation is maintained the fibrin degradation products will be efficiently cleared, largely by the liver, aiding haematological homeostasis and recovery.

REPLACEMENT OF PROCOAGULANTS

The use of these is best guided by a haematologist. Provided the initiating cause of DIC has been dealt with, it is quite logical to replace critically low levels of procoagulants to facilitate haemostasis and the adage of merely 'adding fuel to the fire' does not apply:

- Fresh frozen plasma has all the clotting factors without the red cells and platelets. However, these are not in concentrated form and it is therefore hard to raise the circulating levels. As a working rule, give one unit after the initial 5-6 units of blood and thereafter, one unit for every two units of blood required.
- Cryoprecipitate is prepared by thawing a unit of fresh frozen plasma. The resultant precipitate is rich in fibrinogen, Von Willebrand factor, and factors 8 and 13. It may be given for severe hypofibrinogenaemia (< 100mg/dl)

- Platelet transfusion may be required for severe thrombocytopenia (< 50,000). One unit of platelets will raise the platelet count by approximately 5000-10,000.
- Antithrombin 111 concentrate may be given if the levels are low.
- Recombinant activated Factor 7a combines with tissue factor to enhance thrombin generation and stabilise fibrin formation. It was originally used in haemophilia, but has shown promise in non haemophiliac coagulopathies. It is given as an intravenous injection of 60-80 μg/kg. Limiting factors are its expense and short half life. Trials of its potential use in obstetric haemorrhage are underway.

INHIBITION OF DIC AND FIBRINOLYSIS

The use of heparin has been advocated as a method of blocking DIC by inhibiting the coagulation sequence.

Epsilon aminocaproic acid (EACA) and tranexamic acid inhibit the conversion of plasminogen to plasmin, and their use has been suggested as a means to counteract the secondary fibrinolysis.

It is doubtful whether these agents are ever justified in obstetric patients with acute DIC. Their use is to a large extent theoretical and wide practical experience with them is lacking. Their potential for worsening the haemorrhagic diathesis is very real. An exception may possibly be justified in the patient with intrauterine death, who is not bleeding, but has strong laboratory evidence of DIC and coagulation factor deficiency. In these rare cases, under the guidance of an expert haematologist, one may consider an intravenous infusion of 1000 units of heparin per hour, until the clotting factors are restored to normal levels. Steps can then be taken to empty the uterus.

It should be reiterated that in most patients swift treatment of the initiating cause and maintenance of organ perfusion are all that is required. Once the cause has been removed the liver will replenish adequate levels of most coagulation factors within 24 hours. The platelet count may take 5-6 days to become normal, but will probably reach adequate levels for haemostasis within 24 hours.

BIBLIOGRAPHY

Bouwmeester FW, Jonkhoff AR, Verheijen RHM, van Geijn HP. Successful treatment of life-threatening hemorrhage with recombinant activated Factor V11. Obstet Gynecol 2003;101:1174-6.

Branch DW, Rodgers GM. Recombinant activated factor V11: a new weapon in the fight against hemorrhage. Obstet Gynecol 2003;101:1155-6.

Bucur SZ, Levy JH, Despotis GJ et al. Use of antithrombin 111 concentrate in congenital and acquired deficiency states. Transfusion 1998;38:481-98.

Clark SL, Cotton DB, Hankins GDV, Phelan JP, (eds).Disseminated intravascular coagulation. In: Critical Care Obstetrics. 3rd ed. Oxford: Blackwell Science, 1997.pp 551-63.

Hedner V, Erhardsten E. Potential role for r F V11a in transfusion medicine. Transfusion 2002;42:114-24.

Letsky EA. Disseminated intravascular coagulation. Best Prac Res Clin Obstet Gynaecol 2001;15:623-44.

Lurie S, Feinstein M, Mamet Y. Disseminated intravascular coagulation in pregnancy: thorough comprehension of etiology and management reduces obstetricians' stress. Arch Gynecol Obstet 2001;263:126-30.

Naumann R0, Weinstein L. Disseminated intravascular coagulation -the clinician's dilemma. Obstet Gynecol Surv 1985;40:487-92.

O'Riordan MN, Higgins JR. Haemostasis in normal and abnormal pregnancy. Best Prac Res Clin Obstet Gynaecol 2003;17:385-96.

Weiner C P. The obstetric patient and disseminated intravascular coagulation. Clin Perinatol 1986;13: 705-17.

Zupanic SS, Sololic V, Vishovic T, Sanjug J, Simic M, Kastelan M. Successful use of recombinant factor V11a for massive bleeding after caesarean section due to HELLP syndrome. Acta Haematol 2002;108:162-3.

CHAPTER 9

Preterm labour and prelabour rupture of the membranes

PRETERM LABOUR

Preterm (premature) labour is defined as labour before 37 completed weeks of gestation. About 6-10 per cent of all deliveries are preterm and of these some two-thirds occur between 34 and 37 weeks' gestation. All infants born weighing < 2500 g were formerly classified as premature but are now designated as low birth weight.

The very low birth weight (< 1500g) represent about 1-1.5 per cent of all deliveries. It is now recognised that about one-third of low birth weight infants are not preterm but growth restricted, although the two may coexist.

The importance of preterm delivery is underlined by the fact that 60-70 per cent of all perinatal deaths and, when lethal anomalies are excluded, 80 per cent of all neonatal deaths are in preterm infants. Of the survivors, 10-15 have significant handicap. The economic consequences of prematurity to the health service and society, particularly for neonatal intensive care and handicapped survivors, are enormous.

Of all preterm deliveries about 70 per cent occur following induced or spontaneous labour associated with obstetric complications such as: severe pre-eclampsia, antepartum haemorrhage, intrauterine growth restriction, fetal anomalies, and premature rupture of the membranes. Thus, the incidence of spontaneous, otherwise uncomplicated, preterm labour is only about 2-3 per cent.

PREDICTION

If prevention of preterm delivery is feasible, it would only be applicable to the above-mentioned group with spontaneous, otherwise uncomplicated preterm labour. The main factors associated with spontaneous preterm labour are:

1. **Socio-economic:** The main correlation is with the following factors: young maternal age, unmarried, low maternal weight, smoking, cocaine use, limited antenatal care, and low socio-economic class.

Although there is a relationship between these factors and pre-term labour it is not sensitive or specific enough to be of practical help in clinical practice.

2. **Reproductive history:** A previous spontaneous preterm delivery is strongly correlated with the risk of a repeat performance. The risk can be up to 70 per cent if there have been two or more previous spontaneous preterm births.[1] Spontaneous second trimester abortion is also a significant risk factor. Induced abortion has an inconsistent relationship with subsequent preterm labour, but in general the later in gestation the abortion, the higher the risk. First trimester abortion is not a significant factor.
3. **Uterine structural factors:**
   - **Congenital uterine anomalies** slightly increase the risk of preterm labour.
   - **Uterine fibroids** are not usually associated with preterm labour unless they are submucosal.
   - **Cervical incompetence** may be idiopathic or secondary to obstetrical or surgical trauma or *in utero* exposure to diethylstilboestrol. Overall, cervical incompetence is a very rare contributor to preterm delivery.
7. **Multiple pregnancy:** About 50 per cent of multiple pregnancies end in perterm delivery. They account for one percent of all pregnancies but contribute about 10 per cent of the preterm births. Assisted reproductive technology has increased the incidence of multiple pregnancy, and is one of the main reasons the number of preterm births is rising.
8. **Infection:** There is increasing evidence that maternal cervical and vaginal infection is associated with an increased risk of spontaneous preterm labour and premature rupture of the membranes. The association has been described in women with cervical colonisation of *N gonorrhoeae, Chlamydia, trachomatis, ureaplasma, Trichomonas vaginalis, bacterial vaginosis, and group B streptococcus*. Many of these infections are linked to socio-economic factors and the exact correlation between individual organisms and preterm labour has not been established.

There is a small but definite association between recurrent urinary tract infection, pyleonephritis and preterm labour.

Antenatal identification of patients at risk of preterm labour has been tried by screening with risk scoring systems. In general, these tend to identify too large a potential risk group to be of practical help. Overall, the sensitivity of these scoring systems is less than 50 per cent and the positive predictive value less than 20 per cent.[2,3] At a practical level by far the strongest predictors for preterm labour are multiple pregnancy, a previous spontaneous preterm delivery and a previous second trimester abortion, either spontaneous or induced. Because of the importance of the past obstetric history, risk scoring of primigravid women is of limited value.

PREVENTION

General Measures

Appropriate general advice about diet, smoking, adequate rest and sleep should be given. For women at risk for preterm labour some advocate reduced work, increased rest, and patient education regarding the early symptoms and signs of labour. Women are instructed to palpate the uterus regularly for contractions and early assessment and admission is facilitated for any suspicious symptoms. These measures have not been proven effective in prospective randomised trials.

An extension of these principles has been to apply home monitoring to high-risk outpatients using a portable tocodynamometer on the grounds that true preterm labour is preceded by several weeks of increased uterine activity. However, home uterine monitoring programmes are expensive and in randomised control trials have not been shown to confer benefit.[3,4]

Seeking and treating asymptomatic bacteriuria will cut down the incidence of pyelonephritis in later pregnancy with its concomitant risk of premature labour.

Tocolytic Treatment

Trials with prophylactic administration of oral beta-adrenergic drugs have not shown any significantly improved perinatal outcome or prolongation of pregnancy.[5]

Cervical Cerclage

Randomised trials have shown cervical cerclage to be of no benefit in preventing preterm labour.[6,7] Its only application is in those rare patients in whom the past history and clinical findings indicate cervical incompetence.

Multiple Pregnancy

This represents the classic and easily identified risk factor for preterm labour. Unfortunately no prospective randomised trials have shown any benefit from prophylactic tocolytic drugs, cervical cerclage or increased bed rest in this group of patients.

Work leave

Data suggests that antenatal work leave reduces the incidence of preterm birth. However, this has not been shown in randomised controlled trials and not at the most important very preterm (< 30 weeks) gestation. From a practical point of view it seems clear that long, fatiguing, work hours should be avoided.

Psycho-social support

Maternal psychological stress is a risk factor for premature labour. This is a fairly nebulous entity and there are no good studies to show that specific interventions are of help. Again, common sense measures should prevail.

Fetal fibronectin test

Fetal fibronectin is a glycoprotein in the matrix of the decidua basalis adjacent to the intervillus space and cytotrophoblast. The presence of fetal fibronectin on a cervico-vaginal sample after 20 weeks and up to term is a marker of decidual disruption and associated with an increased risk of premature labour. An enzyme linked immunosorbent assay is commercially available.[8] The main value of this test is its very high negative predictive ability.[9]

As mentioned, the problem with identification scores and markers for premature labour is that they are too insensitive and nonspecific. Furthermore, for a screening programme for premature labour to be relevant and effective, interventions to alter the development of premature labour when it's increased risk has been identified are lacking. Until the definitive trials are performed the most sensible approach to the prediction and prevention of preterm labour is to avoid unproven and potentially dangerous treatment. One is therefore left applying methods that have some rationale and are not disrupting or unsafe for the patient. The following seems a reasonable plan:

The most productive risk groups upon which to focus attention are those with a previous preterm birth or second trimester abortion, women with multiple pregnancy, and others who have been identified in high risk screening programmes. In this group of women the following endeavours may be undertaken:

- These women should be advised to **increase the amount of rest** and sleep normally advocated in pregnancy.
- Screen for and **treat lower genital tract infections** such as: chlamydia, gonorrhoea, trichomonas, group B streptoccous and bacterial vaginosis.

- Instruction should be given regarding abdominal palpation and **early symptoms** of premature labour.
- From 26 weeks gestation an **assessment of the cervix** should be performed each week. In centres where this is available assessment of premature funnelling, effacement and dilatation of the cervix using transvaginal ultrasound. If ultrasound is not available gentle digital examination is a second choice.
- A change in the state of the cervix or warning symptoms of early labour necessitate admission for **bed rest and observation**. In certain premium pregnancies a case, albeit empirical, can be made for bed rest in hospital between the critical 24 and 32 weeks gestation.
- **Cervical cerclage** should be reserved for those few patients with incompetent cervix.
- **Supplemental progesterone:** Recent randomised trials suggest that women with risk factors for preterm delivery may benefit from supplemental progesterone in the form of weekly vaginal progesterone (100mg) suppositories or 17α–hydroxyprogesterone injections. These showed a significant reduction in preterm birth but not in perinatal mortality.[10-12] Further studies are underway to help delineate the potential role of this preventive treatment.

The prevention of premature labour remains a frustrating clinical area with no significant improvement over the past twenty years.

MANAGEMENT

TRANSFER OF PATIENT

The decision whether or not to transfer a patient with real or suspected preterm labour depends on the following factors:

- The presence or absence of facilities for neonatal care
- Available transportation
- Travel time
- Risk of journey
- Parity
- State of cervix
- Contractions
- Response to tocolysis

} Assessment of these factors will give a guide to the expected time of delivery

The least desirable outcome is that the patient delivers en route, so that the above factors have to be weighed carefully before risking transfer. Before transfer an intravenous drip should be established and tocolytic therapy started if appropriate (see later). The patient should be accompanied by an attendant capable of managing a tocolytic infusion and conducting the delivery and immediate newborn care. There is no doubt that the preterm infant, especially those below 34 weeks' gestation, are best delivered in a large hospital with immediate neonatal intensive care available. The avoidance of hypoxia and hypothermia in the first few minutes of life is crucial in reducing subsequent morbidity and mortality. No neonatal transport system, no matter how sophisticated, comes close to achieving the results of those preterm infants born in the larger hospital with the immediate availability of high level neonatal care.

TOCOLYTIC THERAPY

Over the past decade enormous quantities of tocolytic agents have been given in attempts, mostly futile, to arrest preterm labour. The following tocolytic drugs are in use or under evaluation:

Beta – adrenergic agonists

These include isoxuprine, salbutamol, terbutaline and ritodrine. Beta-adrenergic agents act mainly on the beta adrenoreceptors of which there are two types: β^1 and β^2. The main effects of β^2 are relaxation of the arteriolar and uterine smooth muscle and stimulation of glycogenolysis, while the β^1 receptors increase the rate and strength of heart contraction. None of these drugs is free from some β^1 effect but ritodrine seems mainly to stimulate the β^2 receptors.

The **side effects** of these drugs are potentially very serious and have been reviewed:[13]

- Cardiac – palpatations, tachycardia, arrhythmias, and ischaemia (myocardial infarction has been reported).
- Hypotension – mostly maternal but also occasionally in the neonate.
- Pulmonary oedema – the exact pathophysiology is unknown. Twin pregnancies with a higher maternal blood volume may be at increased risk. There is a suggestion that the concomitant adminstration of corticosteroids, with their mineralocorticoid activity causing salt and fluid retention, may compound the effect of the beta-adrenergic drug - although this has largely been discounted. Pulmonary oedema can progress quite rapidly, and any dyspnoea, dry cough or chest pain should prompt immediate discontinuation of the infusion.
- Glycogenolysis leading to hyperglycaemia and the potential for neonatal hypoglycaemia.
- Hypokalaemia due to a shift of circulating potassium into the cells.

- Lipolysis leading to increased serum lactate.
- Fetal effects include tachycardia and increased plasma glucose, insulin and lactate.

The most commonly used beta-adrenergic agonists are ritodrine and terbutaline.

Ritodrine is given as an intravenous infusion of 150 mg in 500 ml starting at 100μg every 15 minutes until contractions abate. The maximum rate is 350μg/min, or less if the maternal pulse reaches 120 b.p.m.

Terbutaline is administered by subcutaneous injection in doses of 0.15-0.5 mg every four hours.

Calcium channel blockers

Nifedipine acts by inhibiting the influx of calcium ions through the cell membrane's calcium channels thereby reducing the build up of calcium ions in the myometrial cells necessary for contraction. The dose is 10 mg orally every 15 minutes up to four doses or until contractions cease. The maintenance dose is 10-20 mg every eight hours. Side effects include hypotension, tachycardia, flushing and headaches. Nifedipine appears to be as, or more effective than beta – adrenergic agonists.[14]

Oxytocin antagonists

Atosiban inhibits uterine contractions via competitive binding with oxytocin receptors. It has similar efficacy to the beta – adrenergic agonists with less cardiovascular side effects.[15] The initial dose is 6.75 mg intravenously followed by 300μg/min for three hours and a maintanance dose of 100μg/min for 48 hours. The side effects are nausea, dizziness, headaches and flushing.

Prostaglandin synthetase inhibitors

These drugs inhibit the cyclo-oxygenase (COX 1 and 2) enzymes that help synthesise prostaglandins. The most often used, indomethacin, is an effective tocolytic. Unfortunately, it has been shown to have adverse fetal effects, including: premature closure of the patent ductus arteriosus, intraventricular haemorrhage, necrotising enterocolitis and reduced renal function leading to oligohydramnios.[16] These fetal effects are mostly with long term use. Some advocate short term use with a 100mg rectal suppository to allow transfer from a smaller hospital. The use of selective COX 2 inhibitors such as rofecoxib, which may have less fetal side effects, is being studied.

Magnesium sulphate

This is as, or slightly less, effective than the other tocolytics. However, it has the advantages of availability and familiarity and, when used appropriately, a low side effect profile. It is therefore used in many hospitals and is given in the same manner as for the prevention of convulsions in severe pre-eclampsia (see Chapter 7).

Nitric oxide donors

Nitric oxide donors facilitate smooth, including uterine, muscle relaxation. Glyceryl trinitrate is under study using a 10mg slow release transdermal patch. Hypotension is a potentially troublesome side effect.

One of the major problems in selecting patients for tocolysis is the difficulty in making the diagnosis of progressive premature labour. The clinical signs are regular uterine contractions associated with progressive cervical effacement and dilatation. One has to chart a course between over reaction and over treatment, and excessive delay leading to failed treatment.

In the prediction of those likely to go on to labour the combination of a negative fibronectin assay and normal cervical length (>30 mm) can be helpful. If both are normal, their negative predictive value is so high (99%), that active treatment can be withheld.

It is important to stress that in the majority of cases of preterm labour tocolytic therapy is contraindicated. Often the fetus is better to escape from the inhospitable uterine environment and seek refuge in the nursery. Indeed, if tocolytic drugs were more effective it is possible we would get many fetuses into trouble by attempting to keep them *in utero* whereas they are more safely delivered. Therefore, before giving tocolytic drugs a careful assessment of the following factors should be undertaken:

- Gestational age
- Estimation of fetal weight
- Fetal presentation } Ultrasound may help
- Fetal anomaly } delineate these factors
- Multiple pregnancy
- Fetal well-being can be evaluated by the non-stress test or contraction stress test as part of the initial assessment of uterine activity by cardiotocography.
- Are corticosteroids indicated? (see later)
- Is the fetus safer delivered than remaining *in utero*? For example: antepartum haemorrhage, hypertensive disorders, premature rupture of the membranes, intrauterine growth restricition, and abnormal tests of fetal well-being.

- When the cervix has reached 4 cm dilatation it is usually futile to attempt tocolysis.

Indications for Tocolysis

Randomised controlled trials have shown that the main achievement of tocolytics is to pospone delivery for up to 48 hours compared to placebo or no treatment. This is fortuitous as this time delay allows for maternal transfer and the administration of corticosteroids (see below). The most valid indication for tocolysis is to allow transfer of the mother, with the fetus *in utero*, from a small hospital to one with neo natal intensive care facilities. This may be required in pre-term labour up to 36 weeks gestation depending on the level of neonatal care available.

- Between 24 and 34 weeks gestation the main reason for using tocolytic drugs is to forestall delivery for 24-48 hours after the administration of corticosteroids.
- After 34 weeks gestation, in a hospital with good neonatal care, there is no benefit from attempting to stop preterm labour. This group of patients, between 34 and 37 weeks' gestation, constitutes the majority of patients (about two-thirds) with preterm labour. Between 32 and 34 weeks gestation the decision to use tocolytic drugs will depend upon local experience with neonatal outcome.

ANTENATAL CORTICOSTEROIDS

These agents have been widely used in an attempt to reduce the incidence of neonatal respiratory distress syndrome (RDS) in preterm infants. Corticosteroids act by accelerating the maturation of enzyme systems in the fetus, including those involved in pulmonary surfactant production. There are many other variables involved in the development of RDS such as: fetal sex, route of delivery, perinatal hypoxia, duration of ruptured membranes, intrauterine growth restriction, and the standard of immediate neonatal care. However, recent reviews of the evidence from controlled trials confirms that corticosteroids, irrespective of the above factors, significantly reduce the incidence of RDS, intraventricular haemorrhage and neonatal death.[17]

Long-term follow-up of infants exposed to one dose of antenatal corticosteroids has been reassuring, showing no effect on neurological, pulmonary or somatic development.[18,19] The decision will depend on local experience, in particular the morbidity and mortality figures from RDS at different periods of gestation. The following principles should guide their use:

1. The maximum benefit is between 24 and 34 weeks gestation.

2. The effect of corticosteroids is optimum between 24 hr and 7 days after treatment, although even shorter treatment is better than nothing. All the trials showing benefit are based on a single treatment, and one should not repeat corticosteroids at intervals for recurrent or continued risk of preterm delivery.[20]
3. Contraindications to corticosteroids include: peptic ulceration, viral keratitis, and patients already on steroids for other medical diseases.
4. Different corticosteroid regimes have been used. The most commonly prescribed is betamethasone 12 mg by intramuscular injection on two occasions 12 hours apart.

The antenatal use of corticosteroids has produced a considerable lowering of neonatal mortality and morbidity.

LABOUR AND DELIVERY

The lower limit of gestation at which one regards the fetus as viable depends greatly on local experience. In most hospitals with neonatal intensive care this is 25-26 weeks' gestation, although the mortality and morbidity in the survivors at this gestation is high even with good neonatal care. The medical and ethical aspects of interventions and intensive care on behalf of the very preterm fetus and neonate are considerable. Modern technical advances, especially in neonatal intensive care, have led to an impressive reduction in neonatal mortality and produced more intact survivors. Unfortunately, it may also lead to more handicapped survivors. The decisions regarding intervention on behalf of the extremely preterm (24-27 weeks) fetus and neonate must be considered in the context of the available facilities, the couple's circumstances and, above all, their understanding and wishes. The sometimes unavoidable and inexorable downside of neonatal intensive care should not be underestimated. The following principles are relevant:

- Avoid depressant analgesia in labour. Inhalation (Entonox) or regional (epidural) analgesia are the most suitable.
- Monitor the fetal heart rate in labour. Asphyxia and prematurity are a bad combination.
- Consider caesarean section if the fetus is in breech presentation. Circumstantial, but not conclusive evidence suggests that in many obstetricians' hands these infants suffer less trauma when delivered by caesarean section.
- For the fetus in cephalic presentation the guiding principle is the gentle delivery of the fragile head. It is often advised that forceps be used routinely to cradle and deliver the head of the preterm fetus. This advice is based on the fact that the preterm fetal head is very susceptible to the compression and decompression forces

offered by the perineum. Unless well controlled, the compression of the fetal head by the pelvic floor and perineum, followed by the sudden decompression at the point of delivery, can lead to tentorial tears and intracranial haemorrhage. The correct application of low forceps may help protect the fetal head from these forces in selected cases. However, most obstetric forceps are designed for the term fetus and fit badly around the very small fetal head. Often the premature head will descend to the perineum in the transverse position. In many instances, therefore, a carefully controlled spontaneous delivery of the head, combined with an appropriate episiotomy to relieve soft tissue resistance, is the method of choice.

PRELABOUR RUPTURE OF THE MEMBRANES

In about 10 per cent of pregnancies, the membranes rupture spontaneously before the onset of labour (PROM) Most of these, 7-8 per cent, occur at 37 weeks or beyond (term PROM) .However, pre-term (<37 weeks' gestation) rupture of the membranes (preterm PROM) only occurs in 2-3 per cent of pregnancies, complicating about one-third of all preterm deliveries.

The cause is usually unknown, but can be associated with polyhydramnios or cervical incompetence. The role of bacterial colonisation of the vagina and cervix in premature rupture of the membranes and preterm labour as a whole is emerging as an important association. Implicated are cervical-vaginal infections (e.g. chlamydia, group B streptococcus, bacterial vaginosis, mycoplasma). Whether this is related to an alteration in vaginal pH or the production of proteases that weakens the membranes is not proven. Nor have studies consistently shown that screening for infection and treatment with antibiotics will reduce subsequent preterm birth or PROM, although this remains a promising area of investigation.[21]

DIAGNOSIS

HISTORY

Most patients will give a clear history of sudden uncontrolled loss of fluid from the vagina. In others the presentation is more of an insidious 'dampness'. Urinary incontinence can be interpreted as vaginal fluid by some patients, and vice versa.

STERILE SPECULUM EXAMINATION

This is usually required to confirm the diagnosis with certainty.

- When the speculum is passed fluid may be obviously draining through the cervical os, or this may be provoked by gentle movement of the presenting part.
- The **nitrazine test** involves placing a piece of nitrazine paper in the pool of fluid. If the paper turns blue, the fluid is alkaline and suggests that it is amniotic fluid. Urine and normal vaginal secretions are acidic and will not turn the paper blue. However, this test is not specific for amniotic fluid and can be positive in the presence of antiseptics, blood, serum, semen, and vaginal infection.
- **Ferning** is the definitive test. A drop of the fluid is placed on a clean slide, allowed to dry, and examined under a microscope. If ferning is observed (Figure 9.1), due to crystals of sodium and potassium chloride, the presence of amniotic fluid is confirmed. Make sure that the slide used is clean, as sodium chloride from the sweat of a fingerprint can produce atypical ferning.[22] The absence of ferning does not prove that there is no amniotic fluid, as ferning can be inhibited by blood and serum.
- For inconclusive cases it has been suggested that amniocentesis be performed and indigo carmine dye instilled in the amniotic fluid to confirm leakage. This is cumbersome, invasive and rarely, if ever, indicated.

It must be stressed that the first person to see the patient has the best chance of confirming the diagnosis of ruptured membranes. After some hours there may be no fluid in the vagina and one is left with a suggestive history but no means of clinching the diagnosis. As the management decisions have far-reaching implications, it is crucial that every attempt be made to confirm the diagnosis. Ferning is the best test, and even if a microscope is not available some fluid can be put on a slide, dried and sent along with the patient.

MANAGEMENT

The essence of the management decision in PROM is the balance between the risks of developing chorioamnionitis if the fetus remains *in utero* and the hazards of prematurity if the baby is delivered. Other factors influencing this decision are the standard of neonatal facilities, the risk of infection based on local experience, hazards of induction, and fetal presentation.

TERM PROM

There are two approaches to term PROM: **active** – induction of labour, or **expectant** – awaiting spontaneous onset of labour for up to 72 hours. In fact, nature will take control in most cases with 75–85 per cent of women going into spontaneous labour and delivering within 24 hours of spontaneous rupture of the membranes.The maternal and perinatal outcome of these two approaches is similar and so it is appropriate to be guided by the women's wishes. The following guidelines are reasonable:

- Confirm the diagnosis with speculum examination, take cultures for group B streptococcus and, if expectant management is chosen, try and avoid digital examination.
- Confirm the otherwise normal condition of the mother and fetus.
- If active management is chosen, start intravenous oxytocin induction at the next opportune time. This will depend on the labour ward census and is often most practical the next morning. Even in the active arm of management there is much to be said for waiting 12 hours, by which time half of the women will already be in spontaneous labour.

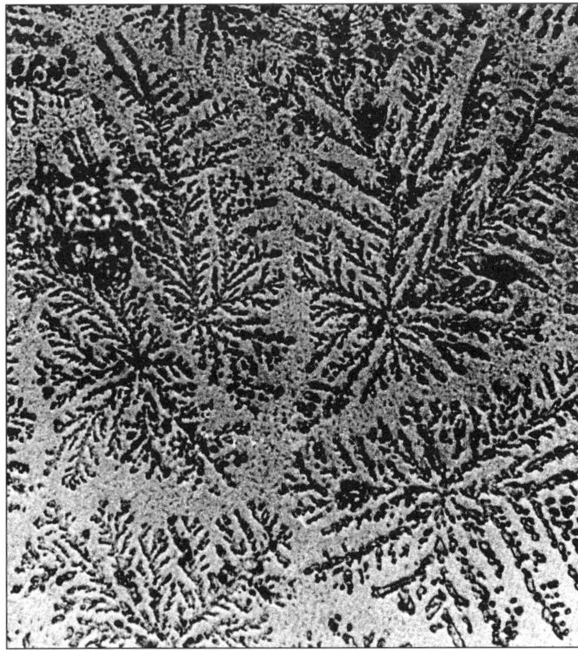

Figure 9.1 The ferning test to confirm the presence of amniotic fluid.

- If expectant management is chosen the decision for home or hospital stay will depend on local conditions and the women's preference. For the few who remain undelivered by 48-72 hours, induction with intravenous oxytocin is undertaken. In fact, most women choose not to wait much beyond 24 hours.
- If membranes are ruptured ≥24 hours at the time of spontaneous labour or induction, or if group B streptococcus positive, cover labour with appropriate antibiotic prophylaxis.

PRETERM PROM

In a hospital with neonatal intensive care facilities the balance is in favour of induction and delivery of babies >34 weeks gestation, although if local experience shows low infection rates, conservative management may be justified. An untraumatised, uninfected, unasphyxiated infant of this gestation will almost always have a good outcome in a neonatal intensive care unit. In a hospital with incomplete neonatal facilities these patients should be transferred before delivery.

Generally speaking those cases below 34 weeks gestation are best managed expectantly with the following guiding principles:

- The **speculum examination** is performed for diagnosis purposes as noted above. In addition, appropriate cultures are taken for chlamydia, gonorrhoea, and group B streptococcus. A digital examination is not performed as it may facilitate ascending infection.
- The patient is **admitted to hospital** and observed for any signs of developing chorioamnionitis. The clinical signs are pyrexia, uterine tenderness and irritability, and a purulent vaginal discharge. Unfortunately, early warning tests such as white cell counts are not helpful. If chorioamnionitis develops, the patient is started on intravenous antibiotics and steps taken to deliver the fetus, either by induction or caesarean section. In fact, in many instances one of the earliest signs of infection is the onset of labour.
- The use of amniocentesis has been advocated to gain information about fetal pulmonary maturity and the risk of infection by Gram stain and culture of the amniotic fluid. The value of this invasive intervention has not been proven and would seem to have a very limited, if any, role.
- **Corticosteroids** should be given to patients between 24 and 34 weeks gestation. The evidence shows that this reduces neonatal mortality and the associated morbidity of RDS, intraventricular haemorrhage and necrotising enterocolitis.

- There is now clear evidence that **antibiotics** in patients with preterm PROM prolong pregnancy, reduce perinatal morbidity in the form of sepsis, intraventricular haemorrhage and necrotising enterocolitis, as well as lowering the maternal morbidity of chorioamnionitis and postpartum endometritis.[23] Among the more common antibiotic routines is initial intravenous ampicillin followed by the oral route for a total of seven days.
- **Tocolytic** drugs to try and prolong pregnancy for a significant duration in the presence of ruptured membranes do not work. Early chorioamnionitis is one of the commonest reasons for patients with PROM to come into labour and for this reason tocolytic drugs are usually contraindicated. The only valid indications for tocolysis are to try and gain enough time to transfer the mother to a hospital with neonatal intensive care facilities and to allow corticosteroid administration.
- **Fetal assessment:** a detailed ultrasound examination of the fetus should be performed to rule out structural fetal anomaly. Remember that abnormal fetuses do abnormal things, including rupture their membranes prematurely. Ultrasound **amniotic fluid volume assessment** should be carried out twice a week. The institution of other tests ; such as the NST and biophysical profile, to assess fetal well being should only occur when one is willing to act upon the results. Thus, with few exceptions, these would not be necessary before 28 weeks gestation. In addition, the interpretation of these tests in the very premature fetus with ruptured membranes is contraversial. There is a small but increased risk of abruptio placentae in these patients.
- If conservative management is followed and no infection develops in the first 48-72 hours, the outlook for safe prolongation of pregnancy is quite good. In some cases the leakage of fluid stops, the amount of fluid around the fetus in normal, and the patient remains dry for several days. Such a patient is presumed to have had a hind-water leak that has sealed and can be allowed home. She should avoid intercourse and watch closely for any signs of leakage.
- In many cases fluid continues to leak but the amount of amniotic fluid around the fetus remains normal. These patients should be kept in hospital and, if there are no signs of sepsis, induced and delivered by 35-37 weeks.
- In a small number of patients with PROM, the fluid leak continues and oligohydramnios develops. This can best be evaluated by ultrasound. These fetuses are at risk of developing pulmonary hypoplasia and positional limb deformities – the so-called 'fetal crush syndrome'. The development of pulmonary hypoplasia is more likely if fetal breathing movements are persistently absent

and if the fetal chest circumference is reduced. The potential role of amniocentesis and amnioinfusion in these cases is unclear. The ideal management of these patients has yet to be determined.

The area of premature labour and PROM and its management is evolving. A number of large randomised trials are underway to help delineate the ideal management. Thus, readers are encouraged to use the Cochrane Database for the latest relevant information.

REFERENCES

1. Kierse MJN, Rush RW, Anderson ABM et al. Risk of pre-term delivery in patients with a previous pre-term delivery and/or abortion. Br J Obstet Gynaecol 1978;55: 81-5.
2. Iams JD,Goldenberg RL, Mercer BM et al. The preterm prediction study: recurrence risk of spontaneous preterm birth. Am J Obstet Gynecol 1998;178:1035-40.
3. Iams JD. Prediction and early detection of preterm labour. Obstet Gynecol 2003;101:402-12.
4. Blondel B, Breart G, Berthoux Y et al. Home uterine monitoring in France: a randomized controlled trial. Am J Obstet Gynecol 1992;167:424-9.
5. Macares GA, Berlin M, Berlin JA. Efficacy of oral beta-agonist maintainence therapy in preterm labour: a meta-analysis. Obstet Gynecol 1995;85:313-7.
6. Rush RW, Asaacs S, McPherson K et al. A randomised controlled trial of cervical cerclage in women at high risk of spontaneous preterm delivery. Br J Obstet Gynaecol 1984;91: 724-30.
7. Lazar P, Gueguen S, Dreyfus J et al. Multicentred controlled trial of cervical cerclage in women at moderate risk of preterm delivery. Br J Obstet Gynaecol 1984;91: 731-5.
8. Faran G, Boulvain M, Irion O et al. Prediction of preterm delivery by fetal fibronectin: a meta-analysis. Obstet Gynecol 1998;92:153-8.
9. Shellhaas CS, Iams JD. The diagnosis and management of preterm labor. J Obstet Gynaecol Res 2001;27:305-11.
10. da Fonseca EB, Bittar RE, Carvalho MHB, Zugaib M. Prophylactic administration of progesterone by vaginal suppository to reduce the incidence of spontaneous preterm birth in women at increased risk: a randomised placebo-controlled double-blind study. Am J Obstet Gynecol 2003;188:419-24.
11. Iams JD. Supplemental progesterone to prevent preterm birth. Am J Obstet Gynecol 2003;188:303.
12. Spong CY. Recent developments in preventing recurrent preterm birth. Obstet Gynecol 2003;101:1153-4.
13. Hill WC. Risks and complications of tocolysis. Clin Obstet Gynecol 1995;38:725-45.
14. Tsatsaris V, Popatsonics D, Goffinet F, Carbonne B. Tocolysis with nifedipine or beta-adrenergic agonists: a meta-analysis. Obstet Gynecol 2001;97:840-7.
15. Moutquin JM, Cabrol D, Fisk NM et al. Effectiveness and safety of the oxytocin antagonist atosiban versus beta-adrenergic agonists in the treatment of preterm labour. Br J Obstet Gynaecol 2001;108:133-42.
16. Norton ME, Mevrill J, Cooper BAB et al. Neonatal complications after the adminstration of indomethacin for preterm labor. N Engl J Med 1993;329:1602-7.
17. NIH Consensus Development Panel. Effect of corticosteroids for fetal maturation on perinatal outcomes. JAMA 1995;273:413-8.
18. Collaborative Group on Antenatal Steroid Therapy. Effects of antenatal dexamethasone adminstration in the infant: Long-term follow-up. J Pediatr 1984;104:259-67.

19. Smolders-de Haas H, Neuvel J, Schmand B et al. Physical development and medical history of children who are treated antenatally with corticosteriods to prevent respiratory distress syndrome: a 10 to12 year follow-up. Pediatrics 1990;86:65-70.
20. Guinn DA, Atkinson MW, Sullivan L, et al. Single vs weekly courses of antenatal corticosteroids for women at risk of preterm delivery: a randomised controlled trial. JAMA 2001;286:1581-7.
21. Schoonmaker JN, Lawellin DW, Lunt B et al. Bacteria and inflammatory cells reduce chorioamniotic membrane integrity and tensile strength. Obstet Gynecol 1989;74:590-6.
22. Lodeiro JG, Hsieh KA, Byers JH et al. The fingerprint, a false-positive fern test. Obstet Gynecol 1989;73:873-4.
23. Kenyon SL, Taylor DJ, Tarnow-Mordi W. Broad-spectrum antibiotics for preterm, prelabour rupture of fetal membranes: the ORACLE I randomised trial. Lancet 2001;357:979-88.

BIBLIOGRAPHY

American College of Obstetricians and Gynecologists. Practice Bulliten No.38.Perinatal care at the threshold of viability. Washington DC: ACOG, 2002. (Obstet Gynecol 2002;100:617-24.)

American College of Obstetricians and Gynaecologists. Practice Bulliten No.43. Management of preterm labour. Washington DC: ACOG, 2003. (Obstet Gynecol 2003;101:1039-46.)

Goldenberg RL. The management of preterm labor. Obstet Gynecol 2002;100:1020-37.

Goldenberg RL, Rouse DJ. Prevention of premature birth. N Engl J Med 1998;339:313-20.

Hannah ME, Ohlsson A, Farine D et al. Induction of labor compared with expectant management for prelabor rupture of the membranes at term. N Engl J Med 1996;334:1005-10.

Husslein P, Lamont R.(eds). Strategies to prevent the morbidity and mortality associated with prematurity. Br J Obstet Gynecol 2002;110(Suppl 20)pp1-135.

Lamont RF. New approaches in the management of preterm labour of infective aetiology. Br J Obstet Gynaecol 1998;105:134-7.

Lamont RF. The pathophysiology of pulmonary oedema with the use of beta-agonists. Br J Obstet Gynecol 2000;107:439-44.

Lee SK, McMillan DD, Ikkssin A et al. The benefit of preterm birth at tertiary centres is related to gestational age. Am J Obstet Gynecol 2003;188:617-22.

Maconer GA, Marder SJ, Clothier B, Stannilio DM. The controversy surrounding indomethacin for tocolysis. Am J Obstet Gynecol 2001;184:264-72.

McClure BG, Bell AH. The edge of viability. In: Sturdee D, Olah K, Keane D,(eds). Yearbook of Obstetrics and Gynaecology. London:RCOG Press.2001;9:289-94.

McCormick MC. Has the prevalence of handicapped infants increased with improved survival of the very low birth weight infant? Clin Perinatol 1993;20:263-77.

Mercer BM. Preterm premature rupture of the membranes. Obstet Gynecol 2003;101:178-93.

Morrison JJ, Rennie JM. Clinical, scientific and ethical aspects of fetal and neonatal care at extremely preterm periods of gestation. Br J Obstet Gynaecol 1997;104:1341-50.

Rand L, Norwitz ER. Current controversies in cervical cerclage. Semin Perinatol 2003;27:73-85.

Royal College of Obstetricians and Gynaecologists. Clinical Guideline No.1(B). Tocolytic drugs for women in preterm labour. London: RCOG,2002.

Society of Obstetricians and Gynaecologists of Canada. Committee Opinion No.122. Antenatal corticosteroid therapy for fetal maturation. J Obstet Gynaecol Can 2003;25:45-8.

Wood NS, Marlow N, Costeloe K et al. Neurologic and developmental disability after extremely preterm birth. N Engl J Med 2000;343:378-84.

CHAPTER 10

Emergency uterine relaxation

There are a number of clinical situations in obstetrics in which rapid, short lived, but profound uterine relaxation is necessary. In the past one had to resort to the induction of general anaesthesia and administration of halogenated agents to achieve uterine relaxation. This was attended by an element of delay, the requirement for facilities and personnel, and the potential dangers of general anaesthesia. For several years amyl nitrate was used to achieve short term uterine relaxation. It is a highly volatile, flammable liquid which was administered by inhalation. However, it was cumbersome to administer, unpleasant to inhale, and produced inconsistent results. The development of beta-adrenergic drugs, and most recently nitroglycerin, has improved our ability to provide rapid uterine relaxation.

INDICATIONS

Emergency uterine relaxation may be required in the following situations:

Acute fetal distress associated with uterine hypertonus

This may occur *de novo* in spontaneous labour but is more likely to be in response to oxytocic drugs: oxytocin and prostaglandins. It is less likely to be required in response to oxytocin stimulation due to the short half life of this drug. Most cases are associated with the use of prostaglandins for cervical ripening and induction of labour.

Fetal entrapment during delivery of malpresentations

This may occur with delivery of the after coming arms and head of a **breech presentation** during both vaginal and caesarean delivery. It is most commonly encountered at the time of caesarean section for a premature breech when, following delivery of the fetal trunk through the uterine incision, the uterine muscle clamps down around the fetal head which is larger than the trunk in the premature infant. Unless rapid uterine relaxation is forthcoming, the fetus may sustain asphyxia and trauma, even though caesarean section was chosen as the method of delivery to reduce these very same risks.

In both vaginal and caesarean **delivery of the second twin** uterine relaxation may be required to assist external version or internal version and breech extraction if there is a persistent transverse lie. (See Chapter 15)

Despite effective epidural anaesthesia in the above situations the uterus may not relax adequately. In contrast to general anaesthesia with halogenated agents, epidural anaesthesia has no inherent uterine relaxation properties. Those with experience of intrauterine fetal manipulation under both general and epidural anaesthesia can attest to the much greater degree of uterine relaxation achieved with the former.

Cephalic replacement

In the very rare case of **severe shoulder dystocia**, in which cephalic replacement (Zavanelli manoeuvre) may be possible if aided by rapid tocolysis. (See Chapter 12)

Third stage of labour

In cases of a **retained but separated placenta** due to a uterine contraction or retraction ring, uterine relaxation may allow assisted or manual removal of the placenta without having to resort to general anaesthesia. On other occasions it may be necessary to relax the uterus even though epidural anaesthesia is in place.

Manual replacement of **acute uterine inversion** may be facilitated by uterine relaxation. (See Chapter 20)

TOCOLYTICS

Nitroglycerin

Nitroglycerin is an ester of nitric acid. When administered systemically it produces smooth muscle relaxation. The drug is rapidly metabolised by the liver with a half life of 2-2.5 minutes. It has a molecular weight of 227 and crosses the placenta easily but no adverse fetal or neonatal effects have been observed. Maternal blood pressure may fall significantly due to peripheral vasodilatation and reduced venous tone. However, in therapeutic doses, without preexisting hypovolaemia or hypotension, this has not been clinically relevant. The peripheral vasodilation and uterine relaxation respond to ephedrine and oxytocin respectively.

Beta-adrenergic drugs

The characteristics of these agents are covered in Chapter 9. Those most commonly used for the management of uterine hypertonus are ritodrine and terbutaline. Magnesium sulphate has also been used for this purpose but has been found to be inferior to the beta-adrenergic agents.

ADMINISTRATION

Nitroglycerin can be administered by the sublingual or intravenous routes. The aerosol spray is given by the sublingual route in doses of 400 µg. While this has been used occasionally in obstetrics the mucosal absorption may not be as predictable and precise as the intravenous route, although the simplicity of administration is attractive. There is more experience in obstetrics with intravenous administration.

Nitroglycerin for intravenous administration comes in an ampoule containing a solution of 5 mg in 1 ml. Individual hospitals will have their own routine, but one practical way of making up this solution for administration is to add 1 ml (5 mg) to a 100 ml bag of normal saline. This produces a solution of 50 µg/ml. Drawing this solution into a 20ml syringe, allows one to give accurate aliquots of 50 µg per ml.

The intravenous route rapidly achieves a high concentration and, along with the rapid degradation of the drug (1-3 min), the desired response can be safely titrated. The effect is usually evident within 90 seconds of intravenous administration and lasts for about one to two minutes.

The dose should be titrated depending on the situation and the initial response. For fetal entrapment and cephalic replacement one needs rapid action and it is therefore reasonable to start with an initial dose of 200 µg and repeat this at one to two minute intervals until adequate uterine relaxation occurs. For cases of retained placenta, the degree of urgency is less and one can start with a lower dose, say 100 µg, and work up until the desired relaxation is achieved. Higher doses of nitroglycerin may be needed if oxytocin has already been given.

Nitroglycerin has been used in small doses, 50-100 µg, for the initial management of uterine hypertonus. However, the beta-adrenergic drugs are more often used for this purpose.

Nitroglycerin may produce transient maternal hypotension which is usually not clinically important. However, hypovolaemia should be avoided or corrected with appropriate intravenous fluids. Obviously in patients with hypovolaemic shock associated with third stage accidents, the hypovolaemia must be corrected before administering nitroglycerin.

Beta-adrenergic drugs are the most frequently used tocolytics for uterine hypertonus. The most common clinical situation is possible fetal distress manifest by fetal heart rate abnormality associated with uterine hyperstimulation caused by oxytocic agents. This is usually initiated by vaginal prostaglandins for cervical ripening or induction of labour. Less commonly it is in response to oxytocin augmentation of labour. The initial management involves the obvious discontinuation of the oxytocic involved: either stop the intravenous administration of oxytocin or remove and wipe out any residual prostaglandin vaginal gel.

Depending on one's familiarity with and availability of the drug, either ritodrine or terbutaline can be used. With **ritodrine**, 6 mg is drawn up in 10 ml normal saline and administered over two to three minutes. **Terbutaline** is given in a dose of 250 μg either subcutaneously or intravenously in 5ml saline over five minutes. In many reports this has caused cessation of the uterine hyperstimulation, restoration of a normal fetal heart rate, and allowed labour to continue. On other occasions it may just allow temporary improvement before caesarean section.

BIBLIOGRAPHY

Altabef KM, Spencer JT, Zinberg S. Intravenous nitroglycerin for uterine relaxation of an inverted uterus. Am J Obstet Gynecol 1992;166:1237-8.

Campbell DC, Epp A, Turnell R. Emergent uterine relaxation with intravenous nitroglycerin for a vaginal breech delivery: clinical report and review. J Soc Obstet Gynaecol Can 1997;19:415-20.

DeSimone CA, Norris MC, Leighton BL. Intravenous nitroglycerin aids manual extraction of a retained placenta. Anesthesiology 1990:773-87.

Dufour P, Vinatier S, Puech F. The use of intravenous nitroglycerin for cervico-uterine relaxation: a review of the literature. Arch Gynecol Obstet 1997;261:1-7.

Dufour PH, Vinatier S, Vanderstichele S, Ducloy AS, Depret, Monnier JC. Intravenous nitroglycerin for intrapartum podalic version of the second twin in transverse lie. Obstet Gynecol 1998;92:416-9.

Greenspoon JS, Kovacic A. Breech extraction facilitated by glyceryl trinitrate sublingual spray. Lancet 1991;338:124-5.

Lau LC, Adaikau PC, Arulkumaran S, Ng SC. Oxytocics reverse the tocolytic effect of glyceryl trinatrate on the human uterus. Br J Obstet Gynaecol 2001;108:164-8.

Magann EF, Cleveland RS, Dockery JR. Acute tocolysis for fetal distress: terbutaline versus magnesium sulfate. Aust NZ J Obstet Gynaecol 1993;33:362-5.

Mayer DC, Weeks SK. Antepartum uterine relaxation with nitroglycerin at caesarean delivery. Can J Anaesth 1992;39:166-9.

Mercier FJ, Dounas M, Bouoziz H. Intravenous nitroglycerin to relieve intrapartum fetal distress related to uterine hyperactivity: a prospective observational study. Anesth Analg 1997;84:1117-20.

Morgan PJ, Kung R, Tarshis J. Nitrogylcerin as a uterine relaxant: a systematic review. J Obstet Gynaecol Can 2002;24:403-9.

O'Grady JP, Parker RK, Patel SS. Nitroglycerin for rapid tocolysis: development of a protocol and a literature review. J Perinatol 2000;1:27-33.

Riley ET, Flanagan B, Cohen SE. Intravenous nitroglycerin: A potent uterine relaxant for emergency obstetric procedures. Review of literature and report of three cases. Int J Obstet Anesth 1996;5:264-8.

Shekarloo A, Mendez-Bauer C, Cook V, Freese V. Terbutaline (intravenous bolus) for the treatment of acute intrapartum fetal distress. Am J Obstet Gynecol 1989;160:615-8.

Straszak-Suri M, Nimrod C. Medical management of uterine hyperstimulation. J Soc Obstet Gynaecol Can 1992;9:59-65.

Wessen A, Elowesson P, Axemo P. The use of nitroglycerin for emergency cervico-uterine relaxation. Acta Anesthesiol Scand 1995;39:847-9.

CHAPTER 11

Non-progressive labour: dystocia

INTRODUCTION

Prolonged labour used to be defined as lasting more than 24 hours. A passive 'hands off' attitude prevailed. The original work of Friedman,[1,2] in the 1950s showed that normal labour was much shorter, and that plotting labour in a graphic manner promoted a more logical view of its progressive nature. Thus, we no longer think of abnormal labour, or dystocia, as a defined passage of time, but as non-progressive labour.

The scope of this problem is considerable and carries an increased risk to both mother and infant. Over the last 30 years delivery by caesarean section has increased world wide, with rates increasing four to five-fold in some countries.[3,4] The main rise was due to repeat caesarean section. However, dystocia is the indication for about half of all primary caesarean sections and, as the vast majority of these are in nulliparous women, it is also the largest contributor to those destined to have repeat caesarean section in subsequent pregnancies. Thus, directly or indirectly, dystocia accounts for almost two-thirds of all caesarean sections. Neglected dystocia leading to obstructed labour and uterine rupture is a major cause of maternal death in developing countries. In addition, perinatal morbidity and mortality are increased with abnormal labour.[5]

Friedman developed labour curves for nulliparous and multiparous women by plotting cervical dilatation against time in labour, taking time zero as the onset of regular contractions (Figure 11.1).

He divided the first stage of labour into the **latent phase**, during which the cervix effaced and dilated slowly, and the **active phase**, when dilatation was rapid. He found that the average duration of the latent phase was 6.4 hours in nulliparae and 4.8 hours in multiparae and defined the latent phase as prolonged if it exceeded 20 hours and 14 hours respectively. He subdivided the active phase of labour into the **acceleration phase** (as the rate of dilatation increased), the **phase of maximum slope** (the maximum rate of dilatation), and the **deceleration phase** (at 8-9 cm the dilatation rate slowed slightly and the rate of fetal descent increased). During the phase of maximum slope the

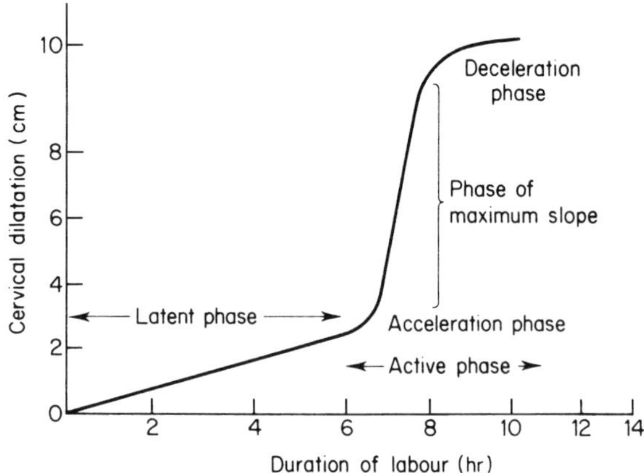

Figure 11.1 Friedman's curve

average dilatation rate was 3 cm/hour in nulliparae and 5.7 cm/hour in multiparae: with abnormally slow rates defined as less than 1 and 1.5 cm/hour respectively. During the deceleration phase the rate of fetal descent averaged 3.3 cm/hour in nulliparae and 6.6 cm/hour in multiparae: with the slower limits of normal defined as 1 cm/hour and 2 cm/hour respectively.

Friedman divided the abnormal, non-progressive labours into three groups, which he felt allowed the most accurate diagnosis and rational management.[2]

1. **The prolonged latent phase** was often associated with an unfavourable cervix at the onset of labour and/or heavy sedation. Some patients in this category eventually turn out to be in false labour.
2. **The protraction disorders** (protracted dilatation and protracted descent). These included patients with malpresentation, malposition, heavy sedation, conduction anaesthesia, and disproportion.
3. **The arrest disorders:** secondary arrest of dilatation in the active phase of labour and failure, or arrest, of descent were commonly associated with disproportion and ineffective uterine action.

Much of Friedman's work has been questioned by others who have tended to disregard the latent phase of labour, at least as far as the practical management of labour is concerned. Indeed, it has been shown that even in different parts of the world, the majority of patients arrive at hospital in labour with the cervix at least 2-3 cm dilated. In the clinical management of labour it is usually not possible to divide the active phase of labour into the three subdivisions suggested by Friedman. What is practical and reasonable, is to expect normal progress of 0.5-1 cm/hour in labour.

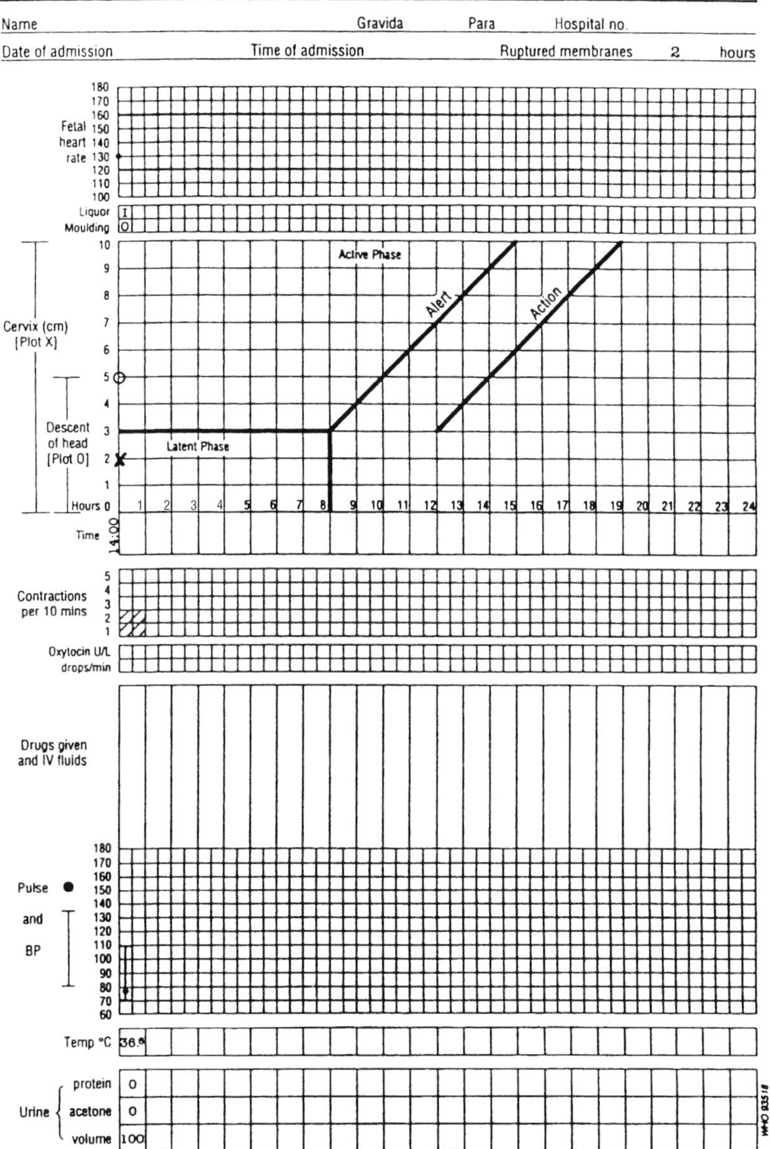

Figure 11.2 World Health Organisation – partogram

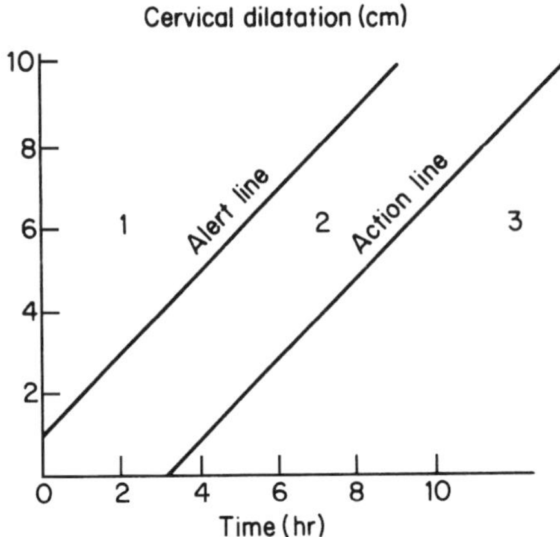

Figure. 11.3 Philpott's cervicograph with alert and action lines. Reproduced from Philpott and Castle (1972), by permission of the *British Journal of Obstetrics and Gynaecology.*

The graphic representation of labour has been expanded by others to include additional events in labour, but the central theme remains cervical **dilatation** and fetal **descent**. Philpott[6] incorporated alert and action lines into his partogram to assist midwives working in outlying areas in the selection of women in non-progressive labour for referral to the larger hospital (Figure11.3). This principle has been incorporated into the WHO partogram (Figure 11.2)[7] O'Driscoll has also developed a partogram with a line plotted to separate normal from abnormal progress in labour[8] (Figure 11.4). The principle behind these partograms is that the normally progressive labour should plot to the left of the diagonal line: if it does not, abnormal progress is spotted early allowing transfer of the woman and/or initiation of active treatment. This approach has shortened the duration of labour and reduced the need for instrumental and caesarean delivery in many units. In all of these partograms time zero is taken as the point of admission to hospital.

This partographic charting of labour is very helpful, ensuring a systematic and logical appraisal of labour. Depending on the type of hospital in which one works it can be an invaluable guide in the appropriate selection of women for transfer to a larger hospital or for active treatment in the form of amniotomy and/or oxytocin augmentation.

CAUSES OF NON-PROGRESSIVE LABOUR

It is important to try and determine the cause of non-progressive labour. One should avoid the all too common and slovenly term – 'Failure to

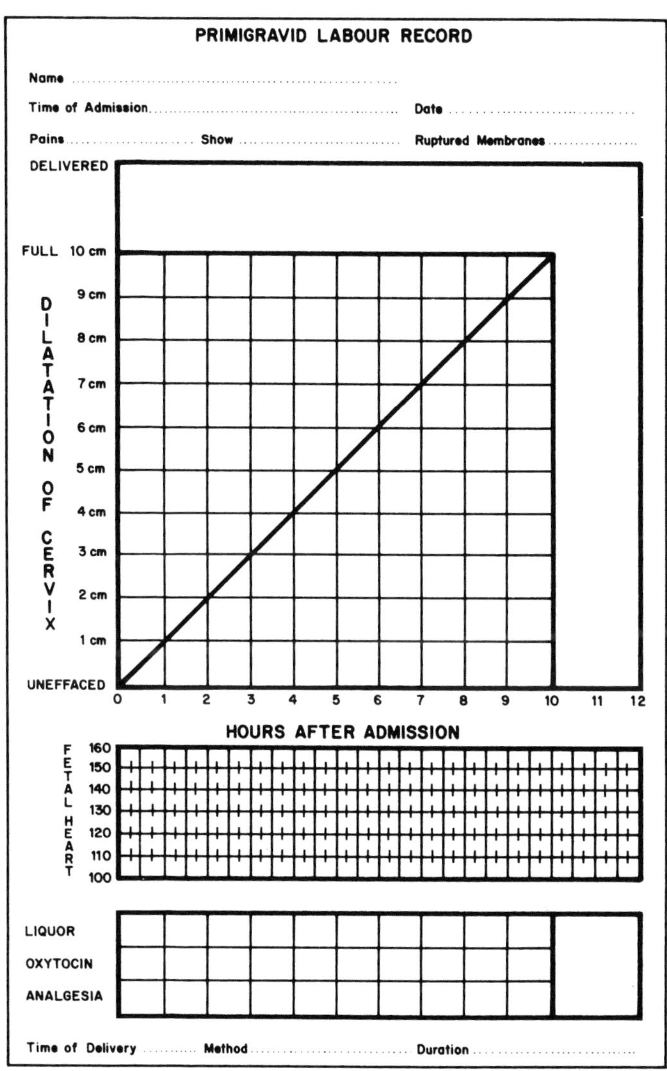

PRIMIGRAVID LABOUR RECORD

Name ....

Time of Admission.......... Date ....

Pains.......... Show .... Ruptured Membranes..........

DELIVERED	
FULL 10 cm	
DILATATION OF CERVIX	9 cm, 8 cm, 7 cm, 6 cm, 5 cm, 4 cm, 3 cm, 2 cm, 1 cm
UNEFFACED	

0 1 2 3 4 5 6 7 8 9 10 11 12

HOURS AFTER ADMISSION

FETAL HEART: 160, 150, 140, 130, 120, 110, 100

LIQUOR

OXYTOCIN

ANALGESIA

Time of Delivery .... Method.......... Duration..........

Figure 11.4 Partogram used in the National Maternity Hospital, Dublin. Reproduced from O'Driscoll and Meagher (1980), by permission of W. B. Saunders Co. Ltd.

progress' – as though this of itself was an adequate diagnosis upon which to base treatment. Only by trying to pinpoint the reason for the failure to progress can one hope to institute rational and successful management.

There is still much to be said for the traditional approach of the three Ps – the powers, the passages, and the passenger – remembering that it is often a combination of these factors at fault:

1. **The powers**
   In the past attempts were made to try and classify various types of abnormal and incoordinate uterine action and included: hypertonic lower uterine segment, colicky uterus, asymmetrical uterine action. It is more practical to judge uterine action on the basis of its ability to produce cervical effacement and dilatation, which is after all the *raison d'etre* of uterine contractions. Failure to do so amounts to **ineffective uterine action**.
2. **The passages**
   - Bony obstruction (e.g. contracted pelvis, previous fracture of pelvis)
   - Soft tissue obstruction (e.g. cervical fibroid)
3. **The passenger**
   - Big baby
   - Malpresentation
   - Malposition
   - Fetal anomaly

CLINICAL ASSESSMENT OF THE PATIENT IN LABOUR

There are three main considerations in the assessment of the labouring woman: (1) progress of labour, (2) maternal condition, and (3) fetal condition. Each time one evaluates a woman in labour these factors should be systematically assessed and recorded.

1. **PROGRESS OF LABOUR**
   Uterine contractions
   - Frequency.
   - Duration.
   - Strength.

   State of the cervix
   - Effacement.
   - Dilatation.
   - Position: anterior or mid-position in early labour is most favourable.
   - Consistency: a soft distensible cervix is a favourable sign. Thickening and oedema of the cervix as labour advances is a poor sign.

   Presenting part
   - Station: relationship to the ischial spines.
   - Presentation: vertex, face, brow, etc.

- Position: occipito-anterior, -transverse or -posterior.
- Synclitism: posterior asynclitism is unfavourable.
- Caput: rather subjective, expressed as: none, +, + + or + + +
- Moulding:

none =	bones normally separated.
+ =	bones touching.
++ =	bones overlapping but easily separated on digital pressure.
+++ =	bones overlapping and not separable on digital pressure.

Bony pelvis

Clinical pelvimetry, despite its limitations, is worthwhile. Measurement of your own fingers and fist will allow you to assess the following points:

Pelvic assessment	**Normal findings**
Diagonal conjugate	At least 12 cm
Curve of sacrum	Curved and lower end not inclined anteriorly
Pelvic side walls	Should be parallel and not converge
Ischial spines	Blunt and not prominent
Sacro-spinous ligaments	Two fingerbreadths + (4 cm)
Subpubic arch	Not narrowed
Inter-tuberous diameter	At least 10 cm

2. MATERNAL CONDITION

- Morale
- Pain relief
- Hydration/ketosis
- Temperature
- Bladder } If these are full they may interfere with effective uterine action
- Rectum }

3. FETAL CONDITION

- Fetal heart rate
- Amniotic fluid: volume, meconium.

(This is covered in Chapter 16, 'Intrapartum fetal monitoring')

Most of the above information is best incorporated into a partogram. However, periodic brief notes summarising the situation should also be made. This ensures a concise reappraisal of the woman and her labour leading to a logical management plan.

MANAGEMENT

Diagnosis of labour:

One of the most important practical problems is the diagnosis of the onset of true labour. Most women presenting at hospital, believing themselves to be in labour, are indeed in labour, with an effaced cervix at least 2-3 cm dilated. The problem is in trying to distinguish between early labour and false labour in those women who arrive with a partially effaced, undilated cervix. Generally those women with regular, painful contractions, associated with a 'show', or ruptured membranes, are in labour. The importance of establishing a correct diagnosis of labour cannot be overemphasised. If a woman is falsely diagnosed as being in labour, a prolonged, demoralising and unproductive sequence of events can be initiated which may culminate in unnecessary operative delivery. Most women are either clearly in labour, or not, when initially assessed. However, in about 10-15 per cent one cannot be sure and it is quite legitimate and honorable to admit this and tell her that a period of observation is required in order that she may 'declare herself'. If there is doubt it is reasonable to encourage the woman to walk about, or rest, whichever is most acceptable to her. An interval of 4-6 hours will usually distinguish between those in false labour and those with a prolonged latent phase. This period of observation is best done away from the active labour suite, and may involve the women returning home for a few hours.

The main elements in managing non-progressive labour are as follows:

1. **Establish the cause** of the failure to progress. Malpresentations, for example, will require definitive treatment.
2. **Transfer of the patient:** Decide whether you have adequate facilities and personnel to manage this case. As previously outlined, the partographic documentation of labour can greatly assist those working in smaller hospitals in deciding the appropriate time of transfer. If the woman has a prolonged latent phase with intact membranes, a period of rest aided by an analgesic may be acceptable. Many such women will awaken refreshed and in active progressive labour. Those who do not can be transferred to a hospital where more active treatment is possible.
3. **Correct ineffective uterine action:** This is one component of the active management of labour. As successfully practiced in Dublin, active management of labour is a comprehensive approach to the nulliparous woman, involving: antenatal education, emphasis on the correct diagnosis of labour, continuous nursing support, early detection of non-progressive labour by partograph, and correction of ineffective uterine action by amniotomy and/or oxytocin augmentation. In many but not all units this approach has shortened labour and

reduced operative delivery.[9-12] It is very important not to embark upon active intervention in the nulliparous woman until she is established in labour with an effaced cervix $\geq$3cm dilated. Before this she should be encouraged to walk or sit in a lounge with her companion away from the active labour ward.

It must be emphasized that nulliparous and multiparous women are quite different in their behaviour in labour. The cause of non-progressive labour in the nullipara is usually a combination of uterine, fetal, and pelvic factors. Often this is due to a deflexed occipito-posterior position, presenting a bigger diameter than the well flexed occipito-anterior vertex, combined with a borderline pelvis for this sized infant, and poor uterine action. If uterine action can be improved the result will often be rotation and flexion of the fetal head, with safe descent and vaginal delivery. Provided reasonable safeguards are applied, the nulliparous uterus can be stimulated with oxytocin without fear of rupture.

This is not the case with the multiparous patient in whom uterine action is usually efficient and nonprogressive labour rare: when it occurs one must exclude malpresentations and disproportion as probable causes. Oxytocin augmentation in the multiparous patient, in the face of disproportion, carries a serious risk of uterine rupture. *Thus, oxytocin augmentation of labour in the multiparous patient should only be undertaken by the experienced after careful consideration.*

The simplest way to improve uterine action, and the first step, is **amniotomy**. If this fails to produce adequate uterine action in one to two hours intravenous **oxytocin augmentation** should be started. This is given by a constant infusion technique starting at 0.5-1.0 milliunits/min with incremental increases every 30 minutes until effective uterine contractions are achieved. The efficacy of uterine contractions is judged by progressive dilatation of the cervix at a rate > 0.5-1 cm/hour in the first stage, and progressive descent of the presenting part in the second stage of labour. The limiting factors are that contractions should be no more frequent than every two minutes and should not cause fetal heart rate abnormality. It is rare to require more than 30 milliunits/min infusion rates. Uterine activity can be monitored by the midwife and only in selected cases is an intrauterine pressure catheter necessary.

4. **Fetal condition**: Continuous electronic fetal heart rate monitoring is advisable in cases of non-progressive labour, particularly when oxytocin augmentation is utilised. Excessive uterine activity, in response to oxytocin stimulation, is one of the commonest causes of iatrogenic fetal distress.
5. **Maternal condition**
   - Nursing care: An important factor is the continuous presence of a competent nurse/midwife.
   - Morale: Explanation of events and the plan of management

should be outlined to the woman along with sustaining and encouraging words.

- Analgesia: Adequate pain relief is essential, particularly when one is going to increase the frequency and strength of the uterine contractions with oxytocin. In many of these women epidural analgesia is appropriate.
- Companion: Randomised trials have shown that continous support and explanation, not necessarily from a professional or family member, shortens labour, lessons analgesia requirements and reduces operative delivery.[13]
- Intravenous fluids: Avoid dehydration and ketosis.
- Bladder: This should be kept empty.
- Position: When possible, the woman should be up and walking during the first stage of labour. It is important to avoid the supine position in labour and the woman should be nursed in semi-erect lateral, or other reasonable position of her choice. This improves the efficiency of uterine action and avoids the possibility of aorto-caval compression that can lead to reduced utero-placental perfusion.

6. **Relative's condition**: Whether the accompanying relative is the husband or other family member, it can be a very harrowing experience to watch a loved one going through the tribulations of a non-progressive labour. Explanation and support for them are very necessary.
7. **Progress of labour**:
   - Once an active policy of labour augmentation has been adopted, the progress of labour should be reassessed every 1-2 hours. If the clinical pelvimetry does not reveal any gross abnormality of the bony pelvis then X-ray pelvimetry will not be of value.[14] The imponderables of fetal size, flexion and moulding of the fetal head, and efficiency of uterine action are more important than bony measurements. Ian Donald's comment is apt: '... good contractions are worth half an inch of true conjugate'.[15]
   - If, despite good uterine contractions there is slow dilatation and slow, or no, descent of the presenting part, along with the progressive development of other unfavourable signs, which include thickening of the cervix, increasing caput and moulding, then the diagnosis of cephalo-pelvic disproportion is confirmed and delivery should be by caesarean section.
   - In neglected cases there may be accentuation of the physiological retraction ring that forms at the junction of the contracting upper uterine segment and the passive stretched lower uterine segment. This pathological ring (Bandl's ring) may be palpable per abdomen as an indentation between the upper segment and the thinned, ballooned lower segment.

8. **Delivery**:
   - The elements of the **second stage of labour** are descent, flexion and anterior rotation of the fetal head. These are accomplished by effective uterine action, aided by maternal expulsive efforts. There are two phases to the second stage: the first, **passive phase**, in which uterine action alone brings the head down to the pelvic floor and the second, **active phase**, during which maternal effort is added. In the multiparous woman the passive phase can be very brief as the head often descends rapidly to the pelvic floor after full cervical dilatation. In the nulliparous woman, however, the head is often close to the level of the ischial spines at full dilatation, so that time and uterine work alone are needed to bring it down to the pelvic floor.
   - It is important to recognise that **in normal spontaneous labour there is an increase in the endogenous production of oxytocin in the second stage**, serving to augment uterine action and aid descent of the presenting part. Nature, as it were, actively manages the second stage of labour. This increase of oxytocin production during the second stage of labour is blocked by epidural anaesthesia, presumably due to the interruption of Ferguson's reflex.[16] As a result, the duration of the second stage is likely to be prolonged and the need for instrumental delivery increased when epidural analgesia is used. Thus, it is often necessary to initiate oxytocin, or increase the amount of the already existing oxytocin augmentation, during the second stage of labour. This can apply to patients with or without epidural analgesia-though it is more likely to be required in the former. In addition to denying the patient her own physiological endogenous oxytocin infusion in the second stage, epidural reduces the bearing down reflex and may blunt the effectiveness of maternal expulsive efforts. However, with skilled, selective, epidural anaesthesia, maternal effort need not be blocked.
   - **Maternal effort**: Based on the above rationale the correct timing of maternal effort becomes obvious. Just because full dilatation has been reached does not mean that the woman should be encouraged to make expulsive efforts. Indeed, particularly in nullipara, the opposite is true. In the early second stage it is best to allow uterine work to cause fetal descent and save maternal effort until later when it will be more productive. One of the most demoralising things for the woman is to be directed to expend her efforts in the early second stage when the fetal head is in the mid pelvis. The result is often unproductive and the resource of maternal effort has been squandered unnecessarily.
   - **The maternal position** during bearing-down efforts can be of her choosing but is best guided to the more upright stance. The

supine, 'stranded beetle', pushing-uphill, position should be avoided as mechanically illogical, and is associated with potential aorto-caval compression, fetal heart rate abnormalities, and lower Apgar scores.

- **The type of maternal effort** should be of several 4-6 second efforts during a contraction, rather than the excessively coached and sustained Valsalva manoeuvres of 10-12 seconds – often accompanied by enthusiastic loud encouragement more suited to a sports arena. The excessively extended Valsalva manoeuvre increases intrathoracic pressure, decreases venous return and cardiac output, which may reduce utero-placental circulation. Furthermore, the sustained increase of intrauterine pressure augmented by maternal effort may further reduce intervillous blood flow. The net result is more fetal heart rate abnormalities and lower cord pH.
- **Duration of second stage**: The progressive nature of the second stage is important, rather than a fixed time limit. A working definition of **arrest of progress** in the second stage is: no descent after 30 minutes in multipara and 60 minutes in nullipara. **Protracted progress** is <2cm descent per hour in multipara and <1cm in nullipara.

A reasonable guide in nullipara (in whom the vast majority of cases of dystocia occur) is to allow one hour after full dilatation without maternal effort. If the head remains in the midpelvis, start oxytocin augmentation. After an hour of effective uterine contractions, or before if the head has come down low in the pelvis, start maternal bearing down efforts. This means that by about three hours in the second stage the clinical decision should be clear. This time frame is not rigid and will be influenced by the effect of epidural analgesia, the rate and continuity of progress, fetal condition, and the wishes and morale of the woman. There are those who advocate a protracted second stage of several hours if the fetal and maternal condition warrant. I think that with some exceptions, given effective timing and use of oxytocin augmentation and maternal effort, there is rarely a lot to be gained by going much beyond three hours. In the broader picture of the woman's health the potential detrimental effect of a protracted second stage, particularly with active maternal effort, on subsequent pelvic floor function should be considered.[17]

- Most cases will declare themselves as cephalo-pelvic disproportion requiring caesarean section or descend to a spontaneous or low forceps/vacuum assisted delivery. The real problem cases are those that arrest in the mid or low-mid pelvis (spines→spines +2cm). It is here that the finest judgement is required and the potential for fetal damage is highest. If one works in a hospital where skill in mid pelvis assisted vaginal deliveries is not available then caesarean section is the safest choice.[18]

- If vaginal delivery of a mid pelvis arrest is contemplated it should be carried out as a formal **Trial of Forceps or Trial of Vacuum**. This entails taking the patient to the operating theatre where all is set up and ready for an immediate caesarean section. In this setting, along with careful explanation to the patient beforehand, the obstetrician declares in advance that the delivery may not be safely feasible by the vaginal route, thereby removing any subtle pressure that may cause him/her to try too hard to achieve vaginal delivery. In this environment the obstetrician can back off at any stage if vaginal delivery seems inappropriate and move straight to caesarean section without loss of face. Often vaginal delivery can be easily and safely achieved, saving the mother the risks of caesarean section and greatly enhancing and safeguarding her future obstetric career. It is very rare for harm to befall the baby if this formal 'trial' approach is undertaken correctly. Its importance at the end of an abnormal labour, which can leave both patient and attendants exhausted, cannot be overemphasised.

It is again stressed that by ensuring adequate uterine action with oxytocin augmentation in the nullipara and by withholding maternal effort until later in the second stage when it is productive, the need for assisted mid pelvis delivery will be greatly reduced.

One of the most cogent guiding principles put forward by the Dublin group is that propulsion is more effective and less traumatic than traction and extraction.[19]

Active management of labour has been consistently shown to reduce the duration of labour, and in some trials it has also reduced operative, including caesarean, delivery. However, in other studies it has not affected operative delivery rates or improved neonatal outcome. The resources needed to properly conduct active management of labour (especially skilled, motivated, one-to-one nursing) are not always available. In addition, such active intervention in spontaneous labour is not acceptable to some – both patients and those who care for them in labour. A flexible approach to the couple's wishes, allied to the principles of management of non-progressive labour here outlined is recommended.

REFERENCES

1. Friedman EA. Primigravid labor-a graphiostatistical analysis. Obstet Gynecol 1955;6: 567-89.
2. Friedman EA. Labor management updated. J Reprod Med 1978;20:59-60.
3. Curtin SC, Kozak LJ, Gregory KD. U.S. cesarean and VBAC rates stalled in the mid-1990s. Birth 2000;27:54-7.
4. Notzon FC, Cnattingius S, Bergsjo P et al. Cesarean section delivery in the 1980s: international comparison by indication. Am J Obstet Gynecol 1994;170:495-504.
5. Van Roosmalen J. Perinatal mortality in rural Tanzania. Br J Obstet Gynaecol 1989;96:827-34.
6. Philpott RH, Castle WM. Cervicographs in the management of labour in primigravidae (1 and II). J Obstet Gynaecol Br Commonw 1972;79:592-602.
7. World Health Organisation partograph in management of labour. Lancet 1994;343:1399-1404.
8. O'Driscoll K, Stronge JM, Minogue M. Active management of labour. BMJ 1973;3:1325-7.
9. Thornton JG. Active management of labour. BMJ 1996;313:378.
10. Sadler LC, Davison T, McCowan LME. A randomised controlled trial and meta-analysis of active management of labour. Br J Obstet Gynaecol 2000;107:909-15.
11. Tabowei TO, Oboro VO. Active management of labour in a district hospital setting. J Obstet Gynaecol 2003;23:9-12.
12. Pattinson RC, Howarth GR, Mdluli W, MacDonald AP, Makin JD, Funk M. Aggressive or expectant management of labour: a randomised clinical trial. Br J Obstet Gynaecol 2003;110:457-61.
13. Kennell J, Klaus M, McGrath S et al. Continuous emotional support during labour in a US hospital. JAMA 1991;265:2197-2201.
14. O'Brien WF, Cefalo RC. Evaluation of X-ray pelvimetry in abnormal labour. Clin Obstet Gynecol 1982;25:157-64.
15. Donald I. In:Practical Obstetric Problems. 5th ed. London: Lloyd-Luke, 1979.p 606.
16. Goodfellow CF, Howell MGR, Swaab DF et al. Oxytocin deficiency at delivery with epidural analgesia. Br J Obstet Gynaecol 1983;90: 214-9.
17. Sultan AH, Kamn MA, Hudson CN. Pudendal nerve damage during labour: prospective study before and after childbirth. Br J Obstet Gynaecol 1994;101:22-8.
18. American College of Obstetricians and Gynecologists. Practice Bulliten No 17. Operative vaginal delivery. Washington DC: ACOG,2000.(Obstet Gynecol 2000;95:No6.)
19. O'Driscoll K, Meagher D, Robson H. Active Management of Labour. 4th ed.St Louis: Mosby, 2003.

BIBLIOGRAPHY

Albers LL, Schiff M, Gorwoda JG. The length of active labor in normal pregnancies. Obstet Gynecol 1996;87:355-9.

Arulkumaran S, Symonds IM. Psychosocial support or active management of labour or both to improve the outcome of labour. Br J Obstet Gynaecol 1999;106:617-9.

Bates RG, Helm CW, Duncan A, Edwards DK. Uterine activity in the second stage of labour and the effect of epidural analgesia. Br J Obstet Gynaecol 1985; 92: 1246-50.

Hansen SL, Clark SL, Foster JC. Active pushing versus passive fetal descent in the second stage of labor: a randomised controlled trial. Obstet Gynecol 2002;99:29-34.

Impey L, Boylan P. Active management of labour revisited. Br J Obstet Gynaecol 1999;106:183-7.

Jong PR, Johanson RB, Baxen P, Adrian VD, Van der Westhuisens S, Jones PW. Randomised trial comparing the upright and supine positions for the second stage of labour. Br J Obstet Gynaecol 1997;104:567-71.

Lavender T, Alfirevic Z, Walkinshaw S. Partogram action line study: a randomised trial. Br J Obstet Gynaecol 1998;105:976-80.

Lowe B. Fear of failure: a place for the trial of instrumental delivery. Br J Obstet Gynaecol 1987; 94: 60-6.

Murphy DJ. Failure to progress in the second stage of labour. Curr Opin Obstet Gynaecol 2001;13:557-61.

Nielsen TF, Olausson PO, Ingemarsson I. The cesarean section rate in Sweden: the end of the rise. Birth 1994;21:34-48.

O'Driscoll K, Foley M, MacDonald D. Active management of labor as an alternative to caesarean section for dystocia. Obstet Gynecol 1984;63: 485-90.

Plunkett BA, Lin A, Wong CA, Grobman WA, Peaceman AM. Management of the second stage of labor in nulliparas with continuous epidural analgesia. Obstet Gynecol 2003;102:109-14.

Royal College of Obstetricians and Gynaecologists. Guideline No. 14. Pelvimetry-clinical indications. London: RCOG,1998.

Saunders NJS, Spiby H, Gilvert L et al. Oxytocin infusion during second stage of labour in primiparous women using epidural analgesia: a randomised double-blind placebo controlled trial. BMJ 1989; 299: 1423-6.

Siraj N, Johanson R. The second stage of labour. In: Studd J. (ed). Progress in Obstetrics and Gynaecology. Edinburgh: Churchill Livingstone. 2000;14:170-87.

Sizer AR, Evans J, Bailey SM, Weiner J. A second-stage partogram. Obstet Gynecol 2000;96:678-83.

Socol ML, Peaceman AM. Active management of labor. Obstet Gynecol Clin North Am. 1999;26:287-94.

Zhang J, Bernasko JW, Leybovich E et al. Continuous labor support from labour attendant for primiparous women: a meta-analysis. Obstet Gynecol 1996;88:739-44.

CHAPTER 12

Shoulder dystocia

Shoulder dystocia exists when the head of the baby is born but the shoulders cannot be delivered by the usual means. The incidence is 1 in 100 to 1 in 400 cephalic vaginal deliveries – the wide range reflecting the subjective nature of the diagnosis. It is predictable that anyone providing obstetrical care will encounter shoulder dystocia. Perinatal death is rare, but morbidity due to associated asphyxia and trauma is still common, carrying both clinical and medicolegal implications.

MECHANISM

Normally the shoulders enter the pelvic brim in the oblique diameter. If the bisacromial diameter is broad and attempts to enter the pelvis in the antero-posterior diameter the posterior shoulder will usually descend below the sacral promontory, but the anterior shoulder will become impacted behind the pubic symphysis. After the head has delivered the uterus contracts down and this leads to a reduction or cessation of blood flow to the placenta. This, allied to the fact that the fetal chest is compressed impeding adequate respiratory effort, leads to progressive asphyxia. Unless delivered expeditiously the baby will die or suffer hypoxic brain damage.

COMPLICATIONS

Fetal

- Brachial plexus injury - Erb-Duchenne palsy.
- Fractures - clavicle, humerus, cervical spine.
- Asphyxia - hypoxic brain damage, perinatal death.

Maternal

- Genital tract lacerations.
- Post partum haemorrhage.

PREDISPOSING FACTORS

Antepartum

The factors predisposing to shoulder dystocia are mainly those associated with fetal macrosomia and include:

- Post-term pregnancy
- Maternal diabetes
- Maternal obesity
- Excessive weight gain in pregnancy
- Previous shoulder dystocia

While there is a clear association with shoulder dystocia and increasing birth weight this is not specific enough to warrant pre-emptive caesarean section on this basis alone. Furthermore, the notion that ultrasound will provide accurate prediction of birth weight is not supported in practice.[1] In the upper weight range clinical estimation of fetal weight is as accurate as ultrasound. To put the problem in perspective, about 95 per cent of all infants weighing over 4000 grams will not have shoulder dystocia.

Intrapartum

There are certain patterns of labour that increase the likehood of shoulder dystocia:

- Protraction/arrest in the late first stage of labour
- Protraction/arrest of descent in the second stage of labour
- Assisted mid pelvis delivery

However, most cases of shoulder dystocia cannot be predicted and will occur unheralded following a normal labour and spontaneous or assisted low pelvis delivery of the head. Thus, anyone who delivers babies must have a clear plan of action to deal with this potentially lethal complication.

DIAGNOSIS

Once the head has been delivered it recoils tightly against the perineum ('turtle sign'). External rotation of the head does not occur spontaneously because the perineum hugs the head like a turtleneck collar. The normal amount of traction on the head fails to deliver the anterior shoulder.

MANAGEMENT

It is important to remember that the problem lies with the shoulders at the level of the pelvic brim. Hence, attempts to correct this by twisting or pulling on the head are illogical, unsuccessful and traumatic.

After delivery of the head the supply of oxygen to the fetus is compromised and the umbilical artery pH falls at a rate of approximately 0.04 units per minute.[2] Thus, provided the fetus is not hypoxic up to delivery of the head ,there are about four minutes in which delivery of the infant can be achieved without hypoxic brain damage. Obviously this time will be shorter if the fetus has some degree of prior hypoxia. This does mean, however, that there is time to institute a logical sequence of manoeuvres to assist delivery of the fetal shoulders:

1. **Assistance** in the form of personnel to provide anaesthesia and neonatal resuscitation should be summoned. In the meantime give a brief and decisive explanation to the patient, institute inhalation analgesia, perform a generous episiotomy, and proceed with delivery.
2. **Gentle head traction** downwards and backwards (the patient being in the lithotomy position), allied to maternal effort is the normal method of delivery of the anterior shoulder. This should be abandoned early when it is clear that the shoulder is unyielding. Indeed, there is much to be said for minimal, if any, downward traction on the head in all deliveries. Either the anterior shoulder is easily accessible and can be guided out directly, or the manoeuvres listed below should be followed. Excessive persistence with downward head traction is the commonest cause of brachial plexus injury.
3. **McRoberts' manoeuvre** (exaggerated flexion of the maternal hips): If the maternal hips are hyperflexed, by bringing the knees up to the chest, the consequent rotation of the symphysis superiorly and reduction in the angle of lumbo-sacral inclination help free the impacted anterior shoulder.[3] In addition, the angle of inclination of the pelvis is reduced so that the plane of the pelvic inlet is brought perpendicular to the expulsive forces necessary for delivery. Experience with this simple manoeuvre in recent years has shown a gratifying level of success and atraumatic delivery of the fetus with shoulder dystocia. Recent data suggest that this technique reduces shoulder extraction forces and brachial plexus stretching.[4] Early recourse to this manoeuvre is strongly recommended.
4. **Suprapubic pressure** by an assistant may help dislodge the shoulder from behind the symphysis. This is best done on the back of the fetal scapula pushing the shoulder down and lateral to the larger oblique and transverse diameters of the pelvic inlet. By pushing on the back of the fetal scapula this manoeuvre helps adduct the fetal

shoulders – which, as Rubin pointed out, is a narrower diameter than abducted shoulders.[5]

5. **Rotate the fetal shoulders to the oblique diameter of the pelvic brim.** Insert a hand, or two fingers, posteriorly into the vagina and push the infant's shoulder off the midline, so that the shoulders lie obliquely with the infant's back anterior. This may be assisted by concomitant suprapubic pressure. There is an advantage in moving the shoulders into the larger oblique and transverse diameters of the pelvic inlet as a prelude to all further manoeuvres. Attempting to turn the shoulders by rotating the head is usually unsuccessful, and if tried too forcefully risks trauma to the cervical spine.
6. **Deliver the posterior arm:** The episiotomy must be generous to accommodate the whole hand posteriorly deep into the vagina and follow the fetal humerus to the elbow. Grasp the forearm and hand and sweep them anteriorly across the infant's abdomen and chest, finally delivering the whole arm. If the anterior shoulder does not deliver easily,support the posterior arm and head and rotate the body 180° bringing the released posterior shoulder to the anterior position. The remainder of the delivery can then be carried out normally, or by directly bringing down the second arm now that it is posterior, or by rotating the shoulders a further 180°.
7. **All-fours manoeuvre**: The woman is guided to the all-fours position on her hands and knees. In this posture the flexibility of the sacroiliac joints may allow a 1-2 cm increase in the antero-posterior diameter of the pelvic inlet. In addition, gravity may push the posterior shoulder forward and below the sacral promontory. In this technique the posterior shoulder is delivered first by gentle head traction. Experience with this manoeuvre is limited but promising.[6]

Any obstetrician will attest that severe shoulder dystocia is one of the most unwelcome of all intrapartum complications. The accusing presence of the increasingly cyanosed and congested face of the infant, within inches of safety, can instil panic at just the moment when calm, decisive action is vital. Many brachial plexus injuries and clavicular fractures are associated with downward traction and lateral stretching of the fetal neck. It is therefore essential to abandon downward traction early on and move to McRoberts' manoeuvre which will safely deal with most cases of moderate shoulder dystocia. If this fails it is best to go directly for the posterior arm or try the All-fours manoeuvre.

All personnel involved in the management of labour should learn the above sequence. There is much to recommend mannequin drills for this purpose. From the aspects of clinical audit and potential medico-legal review it is essential that all manoeuvres and their sequence be clearly documented in the patient's chart.

Alternative methods are available and are described below. Some involve more intricate manipulations that may be forgotten in the heat of the moment and others may only be relevant in very special circumstances.

The management of shoulder dystocia is summarised in Figure 12.1

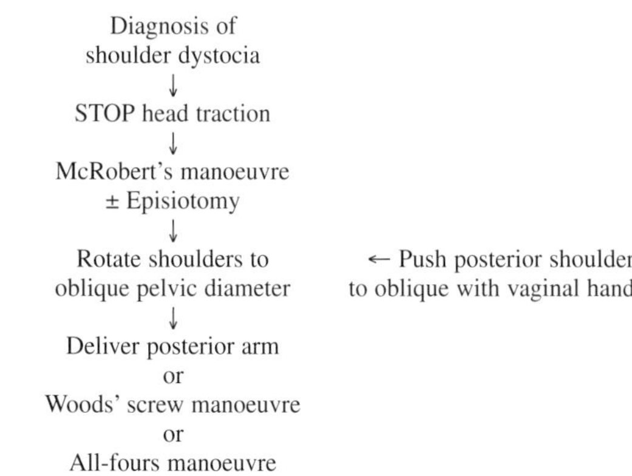

Figure 12.1 Management of shoulder dystocia

ALTERNATIVE METHODS

1. **Woods' screw manoeuvre:** Using wooden models Woods showed that the relationship between the fetal shoulders and the symphysis, sacral promontory and coccyx was like the threads of a screw. Thus, if the fetal shoulders were rotated through 180° they could be 'cork-screwed' through the pelvis without trauma.[7]

   Two fingers are placed on the anterior aspect of the posterior shoulder (use the right hand if the infant's back is on the mother's right). Pressure is exerted to rotate the baby 180° with the posterior aspect of the shoulder leading the way. Thus, the posterior shoulder, which is below the level of the pelvic brim, corkscrews under the pubic arch and can be delivered from the anterior position in the normal way. If not, the process is repeated in reverse as the infant's back will now be on the opposite side. In the hands of those with the experience and equanimity this manoeuvre works in many cases.
2. **Cephalic replacement (Zavanelli manoeuvre):** This is an unusual and rare manoeuvre that has recently been reviewed and proposed as an alternative in the very rare and desperate case in which dystocia is unresolved by the more conventional techniques.[8] As soon as the intractable nature of the dystocia is recognised, and before the infant has been traumatised, the head is grasped in the hand, flexed and returned to the vagina by reversing the mechanism of delivery. Steps

are then taken to carry out caesarean section. In some of the cases reported, this manoeuvre has been described as surprisingly easy, and followed by a normal fetal heart rate for the next 30 minutes, before intact delivery by caesarean section. Others report difficulty and tocolysis was required to assist replacement of the head (see Chapter 10). This option should be kept in mind for the exceptionally rare situation of sufficient desperation.

3. **Symphysiotomy:** In areas of the world where it is performed, symphysiotomy may have a role, albeit more in theory than in practice,in the management of severe cases of shoulder dystocia. In practiced and skilled hands subcutaneous symphysiotomy can be performed under local anaesthesia within five minutes. A two centimetre separation of the pubic bones should allow safe delivery of the impacted shoulders.[9]
4. The use of the **parallel forceps** to grasp the fetal chest and abdomen and rotate the shoulders to the optimum diameter has been described by Shute.[10] This is an option for those experienced with this instrument.
5. **Cleidotomy** in order to allow greater adduction and narrowing of the shoulders is often advocated, but is very difficult to perform in a large fetus. Access is compromised and trauma to the adjacent subclavian vessels is a real threat. Thus, this is really only practical in a dead fetus or one with a lethal anomaly (eg anencephaly).

The reccurance rate of shoulder dystocia in subsequent pregnancies has been reviewed and found to vary from 1.1 to 16.7 per cent, with an average from six series of about ten per cent.[11]

REFERENCES

1. Sherman DJ, Arieli S, Tovbin J et al. A comparison of clinical and ultrasonic estimation of fetal weight. Obstet Gynecol 1998;91:212-7.
2. Wood C, Ng K, Hounslow D, Benning H. Time: an important variable in normal delivery. J Obstet Gynaecol Br Cwlth. 1973;80:295-8.
3. Gonik B, Stringer CA, Held B. An alternative maneuver for management of shoulder dystocia. Am J Obstet Gynecol 1983;145:882-4.
4. Gonik B, Allen R, Sorab J. Objective evaluation of the shoulder dystocia phenomenon: effect of maternal pelvic orientation on force reduction. Obstet Gynecol 1989;74:44-8.
5. Rubin A. Management of shoulder dystocia. JAMA 1964;189:835-7.
6. Bruner JP, Drummond SB, Meenan AL, Gaskin IM. All-fours maneuver for reducing shoulder dystocia during labor. J Reprod Med 1998;43:439-43.
7. Woods CE. A principle of physics as applicable to shoulder delivery. Am J Obstet Gynecol 1943;45:796-805.
8. Sandberg EC. Zavanelli maneuver: twelve years of recorded experience. Obstet Gynecol 1999;312-7.
9. Hartfield VJ. Sympsiotomy for shoulder dystocia. Am J Obstet Gynecol 1986;155:228.
10. Shute WB. Management of shoulder dystocia with the Shute parallel forceps. Am J Obstet Gynecol 1962;84:936-9.
11. Baskett TF. Shoulder dystocia. Best Prac Res Clin Obstet Gynaecol 2002;16:57-68.

BIBLIOGRAPHY

Allen R, Sorab J, Gonik B. Risk factors for shoulder dystocia: an engineering study of clinician-applied forces. Obstet Gynecol 1991;77:352-5.

Allen RH, Rosenbaum TC, Ghidini A, Poggi SH, Spong CY. Correlating head-to-body delivery intervals with neonatal depression in vaginal births that result in permanent brachial plexus injury. Am J Obstet Gynecol 2002;187:839-42.

American College of Obstetricians and Gynecologists. Practice Bulletin No 40. Shoulder dystocia. Washington DC: ACOG, 2002. (Obstet Gynecol 2002;100:1045-50)

Bager B. Perinatally acquired brachial plexus palsy – a persisting challenge. Acta Pediatr 1997;86:1214-9.

Baskett TF, Allen AC.Perinatal implications of shoulder dystocia. Obstet Gynecol 1995;86:14-17.

Baskett TF. Prediction and management of shoulder dystocia. In: Bonnar J (ed). Recent Advances in Obstetrics and Gynaecology. Vol 21. Edinburgh: Church Livingstone, 2001 p 45-54.

Beall MH, Spong CY, Ross MG. A randomised controlled trial of prophylactic maneuvers to reduce head-to-body delivery time in patients at risk for shoulder dystocia. Obstet Gynecol 2003;102:31-5.

Dimitry ES. Cephalic replacement-a desperate solution for shoulder dystocia. J Obstet Gynecol 1989;10: 49-50.

Gherman RB. Shoulder dystocia: an evidence-based evaluation of the obstetric nightmare. Clin Obstet Gynecol 2002;45:345-62.

Gherman RB. A guest editorial: New insights to shoulder dystocia and brachial plexus palsy. Obstet Gynecol Surv 2002;58:1-2.

Goodwin TM, Banks E, Miller LK, Phalen JP. Catastrophic shoulder dystocia and emergency symphysiotomy. Am J Obstet Gynecol 1997;177:463-4.

Leigh TH, James CE. Medico-legal commentary: shoulder dystocia. Br J Obstet Gynaecol 1998;105:815-17.

Poggi SH, Spong CY, Allen RH. Prioritizing posterior arm delivery during severe shoulder dystocia. Obstet Gynecol 2003;101:1068-72.

Spellacy WN. The Zavanelli maneuver for fetal shoulder dystocia: three cases with poor outcome. J Reprod Med 1995;40:543-4.

Chapter 13

Cord prolapse

Cord prolapse occurs when part of the umbilical cord falls in front of the presenting part. The frequency is about 1 in 300 to 1 in 600 deliveries. When the same situation occurs with intact membranes, a much rarer diagnosis, it is called cord presentation.

PREDISPOSING FACTORS

Anything which interferes with the close application of the presenting part to the lower uterine segment will predispose to cord prolapse:

1. **Malpresentations** are the commonest cause. Of these, the most frequent offenders are transverse lie and breech presentation, especially the footling breech.
2. **The premature fetus** is a predisposing factor due to the small size of the presenting part and the increased likelihood of malpresentation.
3. **The abnormal fetus** may have an irregular presenting part and more often lies in abnormal positions.
4. **Multiple pregnancy** due to its association with prematurity, polyhydramnios, and malpresentations.
5. **Polyhydramnios** frequently causes the presenting part to remain high. In addition, the rush of large amounts of amniotic fluid following rupture of the membranes increases the risk of cord prolapse.
6. **Premature rupture of the membranes** and **amniotomy** may lead to cord prolapse if they occur when the presenting part is high and poorly applied to the cervix. However, the risk of cord prolapse is no greater with amniotomy than spontaneous rupture of the membranes.[1,2]
7. **Placenta praevia** due to a combination of the lower lying cord insertion and the presence of the placenta in the lower uterine segment keeping the presenting part high.
8. **Pelvic tumours** and **pelvic contraction** predispose to a high presenting part.
9. **Obstetric procedures** such as rotation of the fetal head, version, etc.

DIAGNOSIS

1. This may be dramatic with the sudden appearance of a loop of umbilical cord at the introitus, usually just after rupture of the membranes.
2. In most cases a vaginal examination is the only way to make the diagnosis. One should be suspicious in all cases with predisposing factors-particularly malpresentations. All patients with a breech presentation should have an immediate vaginal examination following spontaneous rupture of the membranes. All cases with fetal heart decelerations, particularly of the variable type, also need a vaginal examination to exclude cord prolapse.
3. On rare occasions, in cases with high risk factors, a diagnosis of cord presentation can be made using ultrasound, either before or during early labour.[3]

MANAGEMENT

The perinatal mortality associated with cord prolapse is at least 10-20 per cent in most reviews, and is related to the detection-delivery interval. Rapid decisive action, based on the following principles, is most likely to produce a favourable outcome:

1. **Relieve cord compression:** This initial treatment is required in all cases, even as the decision is being reached regarding the baby's viability. If the baby is viable, cord compression must be relieved until delivery.

   If it has prolapsed outside the introitus, **the cord is gently replaced in the vagina**. This is important because, apart from cord compression, the other threat to the circulation is spasm of the umbilical vessels due to the colder temperature outside the vagina. Spasm of the vessels may also be caused by rough handling of the cord. With the whole hand in the vagina and **the cord cradled in the palm of the hand** the tips of the fingers try and **elevate the presenting part** to alleviate or prevent cord compression (Figure 13.1).

   The **maternal position** should be adjusted. If possible the bed or stretcher should be put in the **Trendelenburg** position. The mother can be placed in either the **knee-chest** or **Sims lateral position.** The knee-chest position provides good initial elevation of the presenting part, but is a tiring posture to maintain. If any length of time is involved, the lateral Sims position with the buttocks elevated by pillows is more relaxed and dignified for the patient, and virtually as effective.
2. **Is the baby viable?** This is the immediate and pressing question. Obviously if the baby is already dead, too immature to survive, or

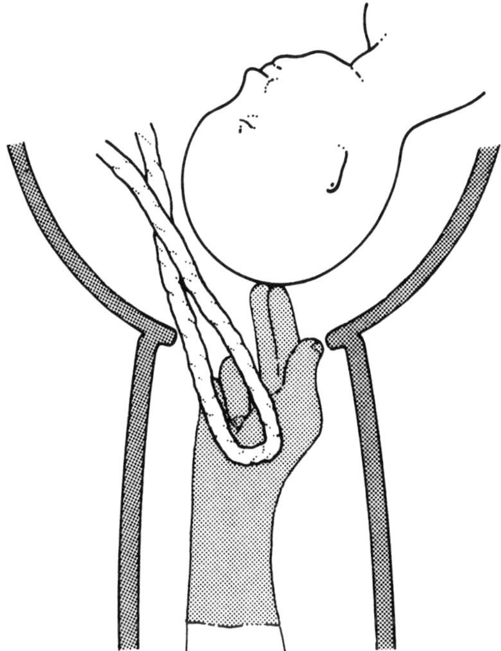

Figure 13.1 Relief of cord compression.

has a lethal anomaly, intervention for fetal reasons in not appropriate. In these cases labour is allowed to continue and the baby is delivered vaginally. The only exception would be if caesarean section is required to avoid maternal trauma, e.g. neglected transverse lie.

The quickest way to tell if the **fetus is alive** is by palpating the presence or absence of pulsations in the cord. Beware the pitfall of mistaking folds of membranes or the tips of fetal fingers and toes for the cord. Absent pulsations should be confirmed between contractions in case cord compression is released and pulsations return. Before pronouncing the baby dead the fetal heart should be sought by auscultation, doptone or electronic fetal heart monitoring via fetal electrode. If available, real-time ultrasound may show fetal heart activity when the cord is non-pulsatile.[4]

The gestation at which the baby is deemed **too immature** is a very individual decision and will depend to a large extent on the facilities available for immediate neonatal care.

In some cases one may be able to diagnose a **lethal anomaly** by pelvic examination and palpation of the presenting part, e.g. anencephaly. Usually, however, one cannot and even if an anomaly is suspected one has to give the fetus the benefit of the doubt and regard it as potentially viable.

3. **Method of delivery:** If the cervix is fully dilated and the presenting part low in the pelvis, an immediate assisted vaginal delivery is called for. The instruments and technique used will depend on the experience and preferences of the attendant and may include vacuum extraction, forceps delivery or breech extraction.

   Unless conditions are favourable for assisted vaginal delivery the baby should be delivered by immediate caesarean section.

4. **Transfer of the patient:** Although speed is of the essence in the management of cord prolapse there may be occasions when it occurs in an area where immediate caesarean delivery is impossible. In such circumstances, if initial attempts at relief or prevention of cord compression are successful, one may consider transfer of the patient to a facility where caesarean section is available. There have been cases in which relief of cord compression has been accomplished successfully for hours. This may involve transporting the patient in the Sims position after catheterising and filling the bladder to tolerance, or 500 ml, to assist elevation of the presenting part and inhibition of uterine contractions.[5,6] This is more likely to be successful in early labour or before labour is established. An extension of this method, by adding intravenous tocolytic treatment has achieved good results in one study.[7]

   An outline of the management of cord prolapse is shown in Figure 13.2.

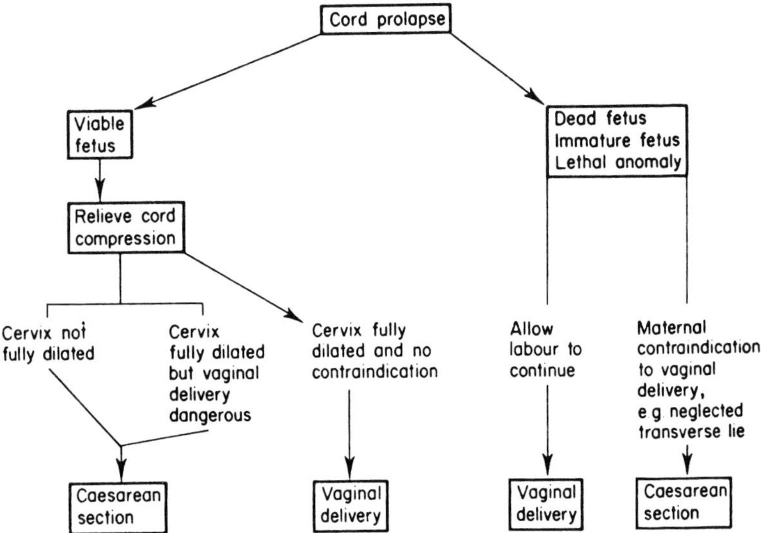

Figure 13.2 Management of the cord prolapse.

REFERENCES

1. Yla-Outinen A, Heinonen PK, Tuimala R. Predisposing and risk factors of umbilical cord prolapse. Acta Obstet Gynecol Scand 1985; 64:567-70.
2. Roberts WE, Martin RW,Roach HH, Perry KG, Martin JN, Morrison JC. Are obstetric interventions such as cervical ripening, induction of labor, amnioinfusion or amniotomy associated with umbilical cord prolapse? Am J Obstet Gynaecol 1997;176:1181-3.
3. Jones G, Grenier S, Gruslin A. Sonographic diagnosis of funic presentation: implications for delivery. Br J Obstet Gynaecol 2000;107:1055-7.
4. Driscoll JA, Sadan O, Van Gelderen CJ, Holloway GA. Cord prolapse-can we save more babies? Br J Obstet Gynaecol 1987;94:594-5.
5. Chetty RM, Moodley J. Umbilical cord prolapse. S Afr Med J 1980;57:128-9.
6. Runnebaum IB, Katz M. Intrauterine resuscitation by rapid urinary bladder installation in a case of occult prolapse of excessively long umbilical cord. Eur J Obstet Gynecol Reprod Biol 1999;84:101-2
7. Katz Z, Shoham Z, Lancet M, Blickstein J, Mogilner BM, Zalel Y. Management of labor with umbilical cord prolapse: A 5-year study. Obstet Gynecol 1988;72:278-80.

BIBLIOGRAPHY

Critchlow CW, Leet TL, Benedetti TJ, Daling JR. Risk factors and infant outcomes associated with umbilical cord prolapse: A population-based case-control study among births in Washington State. Am J Obstet Gynecol 1994;170:613-8.

Koonings PP, Paul RH, Campbell K. Umbilical cord prolapse: a contemporary look. J Reprod Med 1990;35:690-2.

Murphy DJ, Mackenzie IZ. The mortality and morbidity associated with umbilical cord prolapse. Br J Obstet Gynaecol 1995;102:826-30.

Prabulos AM, Philipson EH. Umbilical cord prolapse: Is the time from diagnosis to delivery critical? J Reprod Med 1998;43:129-32.

Usta IM, Mercer BM, Sibai BM. Current obstetrical practice and umbilical cord prolapse. Am J Perinatol 1999;16:479-84.

CHAPTER 14

Breech delivery

INTRODUCTION

Breech presentation is the commonest malpresentation, accounting for some 3-4 per cent of all deliveries. The debate over the safest method of delivery of the fetus in breech presentation has been largely answered by the international multicentre randomised trial.[1] Thus, in developed countries and where facilities exist, caesarean delivery has become the standard of care.[2,3] The trial only applied to term breech delivery, but most obstetricians were already delivering the preterm breech by caesarean – although there is no solid evidence of benefit. Indeed, despite the clear benefits to the term breech fetus demonstrated in the trial, the debate continues.[4-6]

A carefully selected and conducted vaginal breech delivery can bring good perinatal outcome with less maternal risk. Even if the decision is taken that every breech should be delivered by caesarean section, occasions will arise when one is presented with no choice but to conduct a vaginal breech delivery, such as:

- Incorrect diagnosis of the presenting part until late in the second stage of labour. Even the relatively experienced can, on examination, mistake a frank breech for a vertex.
- The patient arriving at hospital in advanced labour with the breech on the perineum.
- Labour and delivery occur in a setting where caesarean section is not available.
- The woman decides, even after being informed of the risks, that she wishes to proceed with vaginal delivery.

Thus, whether by accident or design, one may be called upon to deliver a breech vaginally and it is for this reason that the principles of breech delivery are outlined here. In particular, this section is aimed at those without sufficient practical experience in breech delivery. Indeed, with the rising rates of caesarean delivery for breech presentation, even trainees in specialist programmes may have limited exposure to vaginal breech delivery. However, it is possible to teach many of the necessary manoeuvres as the breech is delivered through the uterine incision at the time of caesarean section.[7] Adherence to the following principles, along with practice on a manikin should ensure that, on the rare occasion it is required, enough skill is retained to increase the chance of safe delivery.

The aim is to try and avoid the pitfalls and dangers to which a breech is more prone during delivery:

1. Asphyxia may be caused by cord prolapse, which is most likely in the footling breech. As the fetal head descends into the pelvic brim during delivery the cord is compressed, so that excessive delay from this point to delivery may lead to asphyxia.
2. Intra-abdominal organ damage during manipulation.
3. Limb fractures, particularly with arm entrapment.
4. Cervical spine and brachial plexus injuries from inappropriate traction and delivery of the head.
5. Compression, followed by sudden decompression ,with delivery of the head causing tentorial tears and intracranial haemorrhage.

One therefore has to try and achieve that fine balance between bringing the fetal head through the pelvis too rapidly and risking intracranial haemorrhage, and too slow a delivery leading to asphyxia from the cord compression that inevitably occurs as the head enters the pelvic brim. This requires careful timing of events and minimum interference, but with elective protection of the head at delivery.

CONDUCT OF BREECH DELIVERY

As already outlined we are concerned here with the fetus in breech presentation that reaches the second stage of labour and requires vaginal delivery. There are, however, certain aspects of the first stage of labour that should be stressed.

- A safe vaginal delivery is most likely if the first stage of labour is smooth and progressive. The frank and complete types of breech, particularly the former, are quite efficient dilators of the cervix.
- If the membranes rupture spontaneously an immediate pelvic examination should be done to exclude cord prolapse.
- Because the breech is smaller than the head it is possible to have the legs and breech visible at the introitus before full dilatation. This is especially so with the premature breech as the small body can easily slip through the incompletely dilated cervix, leaving the bigger head trapped. Some 25 per cent of breeches are < 2500 grams because of the propensity of the fetus to lie in breech presentation in earlier gestation. It is therefore a cardinal rule to be absolutely sure that the cervix is fully dilated before proceeding with delivery.

Should the occasion arise that the breech is beginning to slip through the incompletely dilated cervix, giving the patient the urge to push, all efforts must be made to prevent descent of the breech until full dilatation has been reached. The ideal in this situation is an epidural anaesthetic. When this is not available a combination of pudendal block and inhalational analgesia may reduce the patient's urge to bear down. This, allied to the attendant's hand preventing descent of the breech, may allow one to carry through until full dilatation. Fortunately in many such cases the cervical dilatation is proceeding rapidly and the above stalling action may only be required for a short time.

DELIVERY OF THE BREECH AND LEGS

- If available, epidural anaesthesia is very helpful, especially if it is of the selective type that allows retention of motor function by the mother. If not available, or if labour proceeds so rapidly that it is not feasible or necessary, a pudendal block is usually adequate. Ideally an anaesthetist should be present in case difficulty with the delivery necessitates the rapid induction of general anaesthesia.
- As the breech descends to the perineum the patient is placed in the lithotomy position and pudendal block is performed. When the anterior buttock distends and 'climbs up' the perineum so that the fetal anus is visible, the point has been reached when a generous episiotomy is needed to allow delivery of the buttocks and legs. If it is a footling breech wait until the buttocks are at the perineum before doing the episiotomy.
- The episiotomy is performed at the beginning of a contraction so that maternal effort will deliver the buttocks with this contraction.

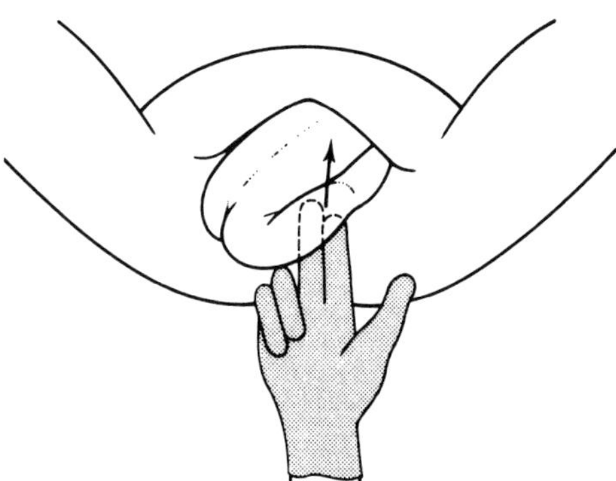

Figure 14.1 Frank breech: delivery of extended legs. Fingers splint the thigh and flex and abduct the hip.

If the legs are flexed they will fall out or be easily hooked down with a finger. If the legs are extended (frank breech) two fingers are placed behind the thigh to flex and abduct the hip (Figure 14.1). This in turn flexes the knee and allows the leg to be delivered. One has to concentrate on this manoeuvre as it is not uncommon to want instinctively to try and hook the thigh down and, by extending the hip, attempt to bend the knee in the wrong direction-an impossible and inappropriate move!

- With further maternal effort the fetal abdomen is delivered and a loop of umbilical cord is gently hooked down, so that tension on it is relieved during the rest of the delivery.
- Throughout these events the back will usually remain anterolateral. If it shows any tendency to rotate posteriorly it must be guided back to the anterior position.

DELIVERY OF THE TRUNK, SHOULDERS, AND ARMS

- At this stage the operator assumes a more active role in the delivery. As the head is entering the pelvic brim the umbilical transfer of oxygen has stopped or is greatly reduced. The rest of the delivery should therefore be accomplished within 2-3 minutes.
- The placement of the operator's hands is crucial if trauma to the abdominal contents is to be avoided. The thumbs are placed over the sacrum and the fingers around the iliac crests, so that the hands cradle the fetal pelvis and thighs (Figure 14.2). In practice, a small sterile towel wrapped around the fetal pelvis prevents this grip from slipping.
- With maternal effort the trunk should be expelled so that the lower border of one scapula is visible below the pubic arch. Up until this time traction should be avoided, otherwise it may promote exten-

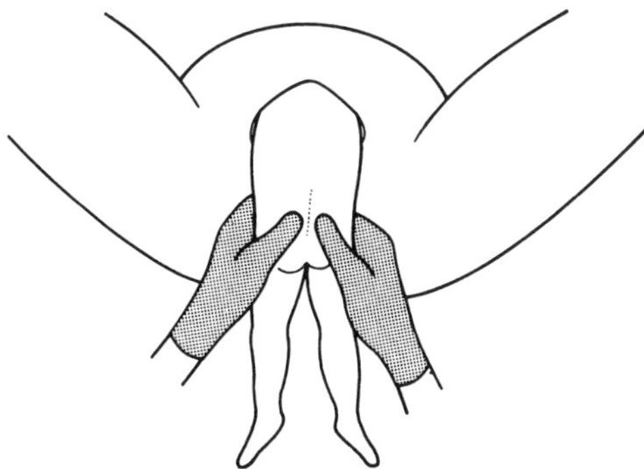

Figure 14.2 Breech delivery. The correct grip to assist delivery of the shoulders and arms.

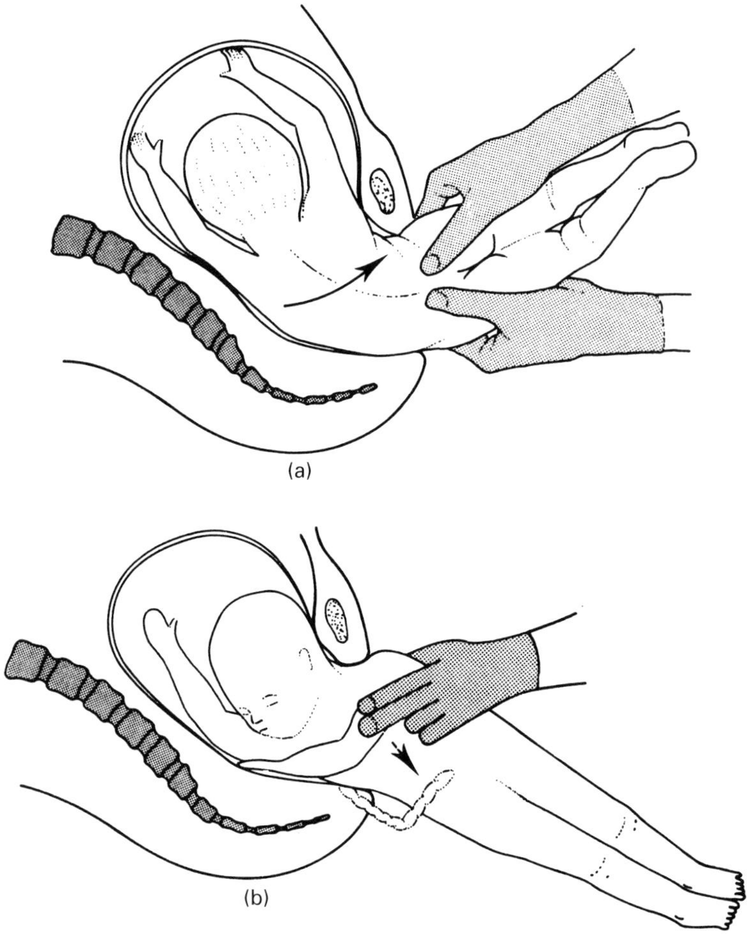

Figure 14.3 Løvset's manouvre. *(a)* Lateral flexation is exaggerated to facilitate descent of the posterior shoulder beneath the promontory. With the back uppermost the body is rotated 180°. *(b)* The posterior shoulder has now been rotated anteriorly beneath the symphysis and can be hooked down. The body is then rotated back 180° and the other arm delivered in the same way.

sion of the arms. If, however, the scapulae do not descend with matemal effort alone, gentle traction is permissible to avoid delay.

- Provided the arms have not become extended they will lie flexed in front of the baby. Pass the index and middle fingers over the shoulder, splint and sweep the humerus down across the chest. The back is rotated 90° to bring the other scapula into view and the other arm is delivered in the same fashion.

Extended arms are best dealt with by Løvset's manoeuvre. The principle is based upon the fact that with the inclination of the maternal pelvis the posterior shoulder enters the pelvic cavity before the anterior shoulder. The fetal pelvis is grasped and the body lifted to cause lateral flexion and promote descent of the posterior shoulder below the sacral promontory. Keeping the back uppermost the body is then rotated 180° so that the posterior shoulder is rotated to become the anterior shoulder (Figure 14.3). In so doing it remains below the pelvic brim and descends beneath the symphysis so the arm can be delivered in the usual fashion. The body is then rotated back through 180° bringing the other shoulder beneath the symphysis and allowing delivery of the second arm. This logical and elegant manoeuvre safely delivers the extended arms, and brings comfort and a sense of accomplishment to the accoucheur.

Nuchal arm: This is usually the result of inappropriate manoeuvres during delivery. The shoulder is extended, but the elbow is flexed so that the forearm is trapped behind the occiput. The fetal trunk is rotated in the direction of the fetal hand (Figure 14.4). The occiput should then rotate past the arm and further rotation promotes flexion of the shoulder and allows delivery of the arm. Should both arms be in the nuchal position, the trunk is rotated back the opposite way to release the other arm.

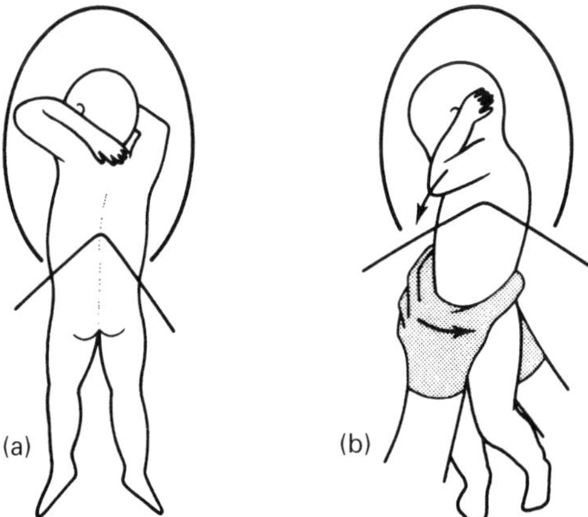

Figure 14.4 (a) Nuchal arm. (b) The body is rotated 90° freeing the forearm from behind the occiput. The friction of rotation promotes flexion of the shoulder making it accessible for delivery.

DELIVERY OF THE HEAD

Once the arms have been delivered the baby is allowed to hang by its own weight with partial support from the operator's hands. At the same time an assistant applies mild suprapubic pressure to facilitate descent and flexion of the fetal head. When the hair line on the occiput appears beneath the pubic arch the head is ready for delivery. There are many different methods described but only two will be outlined here, and they are suitable for virtually all occasions:

1. **Forceps to the aftercoming head:** This is the method of choice. The forceps cradle the fetal head and protect the brain from potential compression by the perineum and sudden decompression at the point of delivery. This 'cannonball'or 'champagne cork' delivery of the fetal head is to be avoided at all costs. In addition, the forceps encourage flexion and allow the safest form of traction on the fetal head. All other forms of traction on the fetal body are transmitted through, and risk trauma to, the fetal cervical spine.

   An assistant holds the fetal body horizontally and the operator drops to one knee (at this point all forms of assistance, including celestial, are welcome!). The forceps are therefore applied below the fetal body at the 4 and 8 o'clock positions and wandered to the sides of the fetal head (Figure 14.5). Piper's forceps were specially developed for this purpose, having a very long shank. In fact most of the normal length forceps are quite suitable. It is very important that the assistant does not raise the fetal body above the horizontal until the fetal chin is visible. If the fetal body is raised above the horizontal before this time it risks hyperextension of the fetal neck and trauma to the cervical spine. Then, as the forceps are elevated to flex and complete delivery of the fetal head, the fetal legs and body are raised in unison.

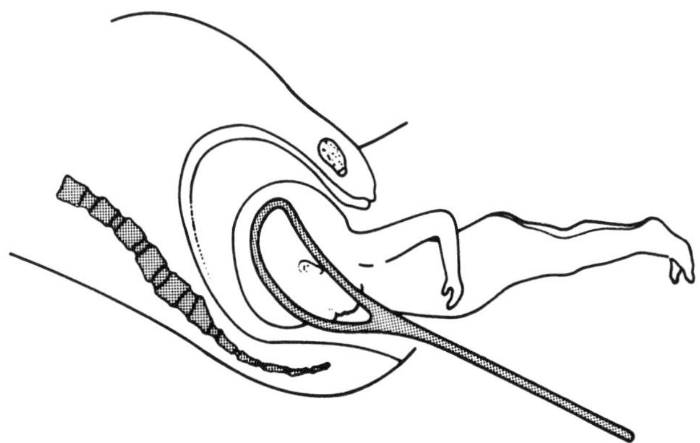

Figure. 14.5 Breech delivery. Forceps to the aftercoming head.

2. **Mauriceau-Smellie-Veit:** This method is not quite as good as the use of forceps described above. However, it can be very useful if events have progressed so rapidly that there is no time to position the patient properly and apply forceps, or if forceps are not available.

The fetal body is placed astride the operator's forearm. The forefinger and middle finger are placed on the fetal maxilla beside the nose to gently flex the head. The other hand is placed on the fetal back. The middle finger pushes upwards on the occiput, thus encouraging head flexion while the other fingers lie on the shoulders (Figure 14.6). In this way the vulnerable cervical spine is splinted and partially protected from traction. Gentle traction in a downward and backward direction may be needed until delivery of the chin. The mouth and forehead are then guided up and over the perineum. At this stage it is important to ensure a controlled release of the fetal head, rather than risk a precipitate delivery by exerting traction. Indeed, if any degree of traction is required it should be with forceps, as excessive traction with the Mauriceau-Smellie-Veit technique risks damage to the brachial plexus and cervical spine. Although this method does not have quite the same protective value as the forceps on the fetal head, it is quite acceptable and can be very useful when conditions are not ideal and the patient is uncooperative.

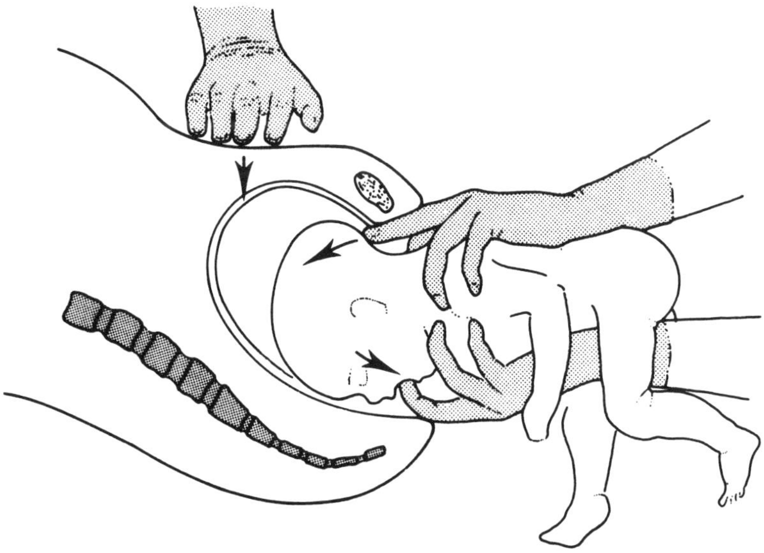

Figure 14.6 Mauriceau-Smellie-Veit manouvre.

If there is unexpected delay in delivery of the head a forceps blade may be used to retract the vagina and expose the baby's mouth and nose to permit respiration.

If, because of neglect or failure to keep the back anterior, the fetal head has been allowed to enter the pelvis in the occipito-posterior position the following methods may be tried to effect delivery.

a) The hands are placed as for the Mauriceau-Smellie-Veit manoeuvre and the fetal head is elevated and rotated to the occipito-anterior position. The head is then delivered by the Mauriceau-Smellie-Veit method or with forceps to the aftercoming head.
b) If the head is deep in the pelvis with the chin impacted behind the symphysis, and there is room in the sacral bay of the pelvis, the reverse **Prague manoeuvre** can be tried (Figure 14.7). One hand exerts traction downwards and backwards on the shoulders, while the other lifts the feet to flex the baby and aid delivery of the occiput.

While it may seem that vaginal breech delivery is obselete, obstetricians will still be faced with occasions when it is necessary and should use the opportunities outlined in the introduction to acquire and retain these skills.

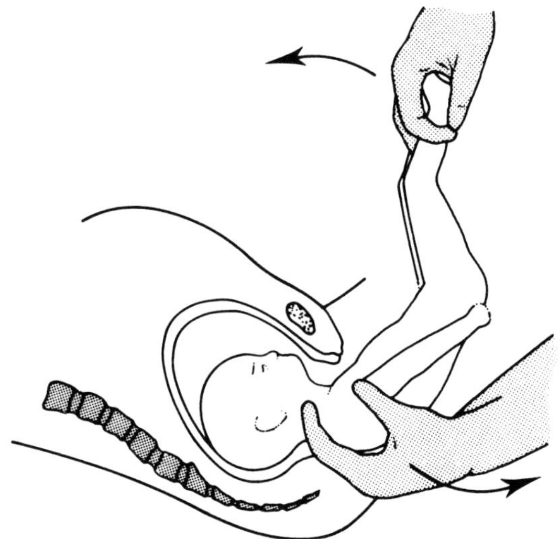

Figure 14.7 Prague manouvre.

REFERENCES

1. Hannah ME, Hannah WJ, Hewson SA, Hodnett ED, Saigal S, Willan AR. Planned caesarean section versus planned vaginal birth for breech presentation at term: a randomised multicentre trial. Lancet 2000;356:1375-83.
2. American College of Obstetrician's and Gynaecologists. Mode of term singleton breech delivery. Committee Opinion No 265. Obstet Gynecol 2001;98:1189-90.
3. Royal College of Obstetricians and Gynaecologists. The management of breech presentation. Guideline No20. London:RCOG,2001.
4. Greene MF. Vaginal breech delivery is no longer justified. Obstet Gynecol 2002;991113-5.
5. Hauth JC, Cunningham FG. Vaginal breech delivery is still justified. Obstet Gynecol 2002;99:1115-6.
6. Van Roosmalen J, Rosendaal F. There is still room for disagreement about vaginal delivery of breech infants at term. Br J Obstet Gynaecol 2002;109:967-9.
7. Baskett T F. Trends in operative obstetrical delivery: implications for specialist training. Ann R Coll Phys Surg Can 1988; 1: 119-21.

BIBLIOGRAPHY

Allardice JG, Amankwah K, Baskett TF et al. The Canadian Consensus on breech management at term. J Soc Obstet Gynaecol Can 1994;16:1839-48.

Irion O, Almagbaly PH, Morabia A. Planned vaginal delivery versus elective caesarean section: a study of 705 singleton term breech presentations. Br J Obstet Gynaecol 1998;105:710-17.

Menticoglou SM. Symphysiotomy for the trapped aftercoming parts of the breech: A review of the literature and a plea for its use. Aust NZ J Obstet Gynaecol 1990;30:1-9.

Rietberg CCT, Stinkens PME, Brand R, vanLoon AJ, Van Hemel JS, Visser GHA. Term breech presentation in The Netherlands from 1995 to 1999: mortality and morbidity in relation to the mode of delivery of 33,824 infants. Br J Obstet Gynaecol 2003;110:604-9.

Tunde-Byass MO, Hannah ME. Breech vaginal delivery at or near term. Semin Perinatol 2003;27:34-45.

Young PF, Johanson RB. The management of breech presentation at term. Curr Opin Obstet Gynecol 2001;13:589-93.

CHAPTER 15

Twin delivery

ASSESSMENT

Twins occur in about 1 per cent of all pregnancies but contribute almost 10 per cent of perinatal mortality and morbidity. In many countries the incidence of twins is increasing due to assisted reproductive technologies which account for about two-thirds of all multiple pregnancies. The main causes of mortality are intrauterine growth restriction and prematurity, but trauma and asphyxia during delivery also play their part.

Appropriate antenatal care will lead to the diagnosis of twin pregnancy and selection of those cases best delivered by elective caesarean section, which may include: monoamniotic twins, non-vertex first twin, preterm twins <32 weeks gestation, and the same indications as for singleton pregnancies. Ideally twin delivery should be conducted in a large hospital with specialist obstetric, anaesthetic, and neonatal care available.

In selecting patients suitable for labour and vaginal delivery, some authors differentiate between vertex/vertex (twin A/twin B) and vertex/non-vertex presentation at the start of labour. However, in about 10-20 per cent of cases, the presentation of the second twin will alter after delivery of the first twin. In addition, external version can be used to convert the second twin from an unfavourable presentation after delivery of the first twin. In extreme cases, the potential exists to deliver the second twin by caesarean section should unfavourable circumstances for vaginal delivery develop and persist. Thus, the presentation of twin A is the dominant factor in the decision to allow labour and vaginal delivery.

The most common presentations in twin births are, in decreasing order of frequency: vertex-vertex, vertex/breech, breech/vertex, breech/breech. These make up more than 90 per cent of the combinations, the remainder involving transverse lie of one or both fetuses. In broad terms the most common combinations are vertex/vertex 40%, vertex/non-vertex 40%, non-vertex/other 20%.

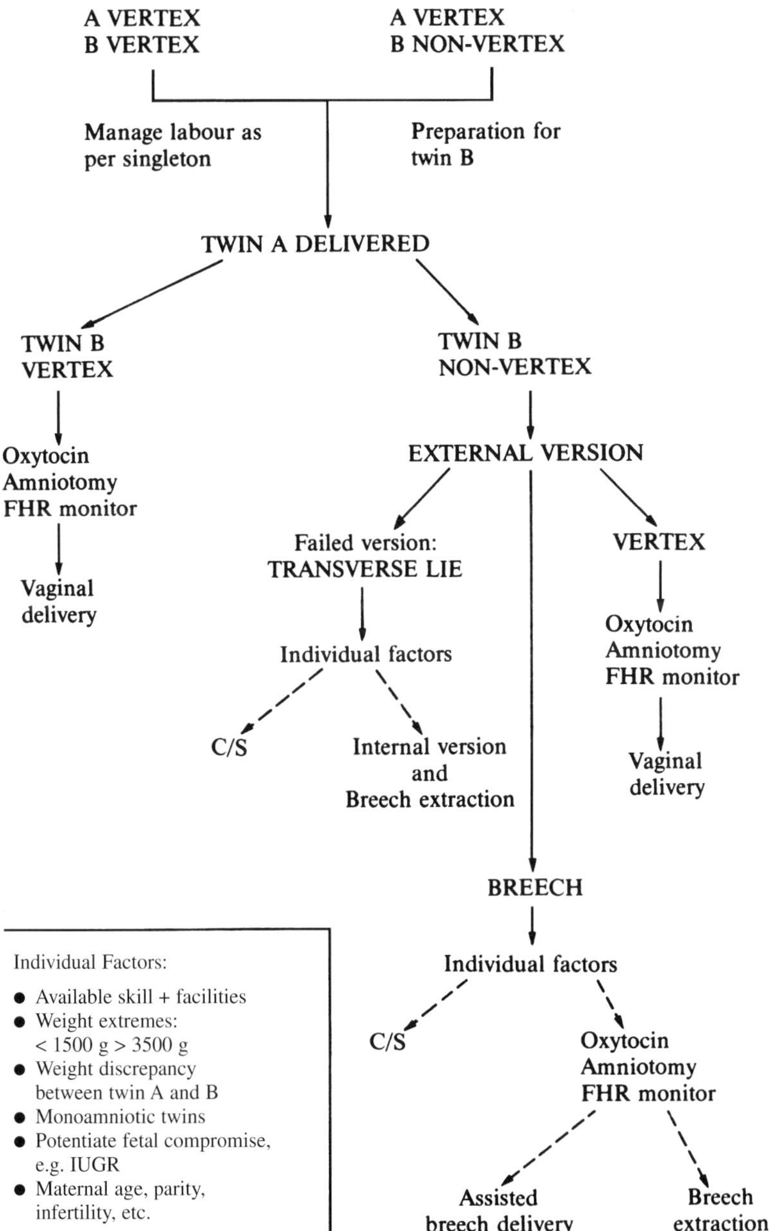

Individual Factors:

- Available skill + facilities
- Weight extremes: < 1500 g > 3500 g
- Weight discrepancy between twin A and B
- Monoamniotic twins
- Potentiate fetal compromise, e.g. IUGR
- Maternal age, parity, infertility, etc.

Figure 15.1 Twin pregnancy: intrapartum management.

The second twin faces increased risks during labour for the following reasons:

1. Once the first twin has been delivered the partial emptying of the uterus may alter the haemodynamics of the placental bed, reducing circulation and leading to fetal asphyxia.
2. Partial placental separation after delivery of the first twin may also cause asphyxia.
3. Greater risk of trauma due to more malpresentations and intrauterine manipulation.

Individual Factors

In considering the advisability of labour and vaginal delivery in twin pregnancy, individual factors involving a blend of available facilities, personnel, and clinical aspects of the patient must be carefully assessed. These include: weight extremes (< 1500 g, > 3500 g), weight discrepancy (especially twin B > twin A), monoamniotic twins, potential fetal compromise from intrauterine growth restriction or twin-to-twin transfusion, maternal age, parity and history of infertility (Figure 15.1).

An overall outline of the intrapartum management of the common combinations in twin pregnancy is given in Figure 15.1.

MANAGEMENT OF LABOUR

Overdistension of the uterus may cause ineffective uterine action, although this is usually offset by the small size of the babies.

The first twin is managed in labour as if it were a singleton. The second stage of labour may be managed under double set-up conditions in an operating theatre prepared for both vaginal and caesarean delivery. In addition to anaesthetic and neonatal personnel, it is advisable to have a knowledgeable obstetrical assistant. If available during delivery of the first twin, it may be helpful for the obstetrical assistant to follow the position of the second twin with realtime ultrasound. This should assist in the manipulation of the second twin into a favourable presentation and also reduce the rare possibility of locked twins.

Following delivery of the first twin there is usually transient uterine inertia, so that unless active measures are taken 20-30 minutes will elapse before the second twin is born. The cord of the first twin should be securely clamped in case a vascular connection exists that could allow the second twin to exsanguinate through the cord of the first. On rare occasions the placenta of the first twin will separate and deliver before the second twin.

For reasons already outlined the longer the second twin is undelivered the greater the risks, particularly if more than 15 minutes elapse. One therefore has to achieve a balance between active, and potentially traumatic extraction, and passive delay with possible asphyxia. The following course of action provides a suitable compromise:

1. During labour an intravenous infusion should be established. With the delivery of the first twin a separate infusion set with 5 units of oxytocin in 500 ml crystalloid should be mixed and made ready to 'piggy-back'on to the main intravenous line to overcome uterine inertia.
2. After the first twin has been delivered check the lie and presentation of the second twin:
   - If cephalic-hold the head over the pelvic brim, rule out cord presentation, start the oxytocin infusion, and when contractions are regular rupture the membranes.
   - If breech-hold the breech over the pelvic brim, rule out cord presentation, start the oxytocin infusion, and when contractions are regular rupture the membranes.
   - If transverse lie-perform external cephalic or podalic version, whichever is easier, and then proceed as above.

Alternatively, if the second twin is a footling breech or transverse lie, a case can be made for immediate breech extraction or internal version and breech extraction. With the recent passage of the first twin conditions are ideal for these manoeuvres, **provided the uterus is well relaxed**. (See No. 5 below for technical details). This obviates the risks associated with delay, such as cord prolapse or clamping down of the lower uterine segment and cervix. One of the reasons for the increasing trend to deliver the second twin by caesarean section is failure to grasp this opportunity.

3. The oxytocin infusion should be started at about 10 drops per minute. Provided contractions are initiated the baby usually descends rapidly during two or three contractions to allow a spontaneous vertex or assisted breech delivery. Ideally the second twin should be delivered within 15 minutes, and usually is with the above management. If not, provided the fetal heart is normal and there is no untoward bleeding, it is advisable to wait for descent of the fetus until spontaneous or an easily assisted delivery is achieved.
4. If the heart rate suggests fetal distress or there is intrapartum bleeding, cord prolapse or continued delay, the delivery should be expedited. This decision will depend on experience and facilities, with the following options:

- Forceps or vacuum extraction. The vacuum will be better at higher stations of the fetal head.
- Breech extraction
- Caesarean section

5. If the second twin is lying transversely, and external version does not succeed, internal version and breech extraction are indicated. It must be stressed that with the birth canal already distended by the passage of the first twin this is much less risky than for a singleton and is one of the only acceptable indications for internal version in modern obstetrics. Internal version should only be attempted when the uterus is relaxed.(See Analgesia below).
   - Grasp one, or preferably both feet through the membranes and pull downwards and backwards into the pelvis and out through the introitus. By keeping the membranes intact the baby turns easily to a breech before the uterus clamps down. As traction is continued the membranes rupture, but by this time the breech is on its way, cushioned by the amniotic fluid as it descends into the pelvis.
   - If the membranes are too tense to allow identification of the feet, wait and make sure this is not due to a uterine contraction. If the uterus is definitely relaxed and the membranes are still tense one has to proceed to rupture the membranes. As quickly as possible find the feet and exert traction so that the breech is 'washed' down as the amniotic fluid escapes and helps to buffer the clamping down effect of the uterus.
   - The foot is best identified by the point of the heel. If only one foot can be reached this will have to suffice. It should be the anterior foot, as traction on the posterior leg may cause the anterior buttock to be arrested astride the pubic symphysis. Thus, if the posterior leg has been brought down it should be rotated 180° in a wide arc during traction to convert it to the anterior position. The second leg is then brought down in the same way as the extended legs of a frank breech. Once the legs are delivered, traction on the thighs will deliver the abdomen. From this point the rest of the delivery is accomplished in the manner described for the assisted breech delivery in Chapter 14.

6. Although rare in modern obstetrics with almost universal antenatal ultrasound a potentially disastrous complication of undiagnosed twin pregnancy can occur when active management of the third stage of labour is practised and intramuscular oxytocin is given with the delivery of the anterior shoulder, only to find that an undiagnosed second twin remains. Obviously within 2-3 minutes the oxytocin will cause a powerful, sustained uterine contraction that may

asphyxiate the fetus. Immediate and decisive action is needed as follows:

- If cephalic-rupture the membranes and deliver with forceps as soon as the head is low in the pelvis.
- If breech-perform breech extraction.
- If transverse lie, carry out internal version and breech extraction.

Obviously prevention of this situation is desirable. This is best accomplished (when antenatal ultrasound has been omitted) by the ritual of always considering the possibility of an undiagnosed twin pregnancy before giving the oxytocin. If there is any doubt withhold oxytocin until the baby is delivered.

Locked Twins

This is extremely rare (about 1:1000 twin deliveries) and carries a high risk of asphyxia, trauma and death, particularly to the first twin. It usually occurs with the twin A breech: twin B vertex combination, and is more likely with smaller fetuses. It manifests itself when the first twin delivers normally up to the trunk and shoulders but further descent of the head is arrested. The other possible cause of an arrested after-coming hydrocephalic head should be considered. There is little time to be lost as the first infant is subjected to progressive asphyxia. Under deep general anaesthesia and supporting the body of the first twin, one can attempt to manually disimpact the head of the second twin and, if successful, proceed with breech extraction of the first infant. If gentle attempts at disimpaction fail, one should, as far as possible, elevate and return the first twin to the vagina and proceed to caesarean section-often requiring a classical uterine incision to provide adequate room. Even if the first twin is already dead, caesarean section will be necessary to avoid trauma and a similar fate to the second twin. Intricate manoeuvres have been tried in the past with variable degrees of success, including decapitation of the first dead twin to allow vaginal delivery of the second twin. These manoeuvres, with their attendant high risks of maternal and fetal trauma, are inappropriate in modern obstetrics.

Analgesia

If available, epidural anaesthesia can be very useful in twin delivery. If epidural anaesthesia is not available, a pudendal block performed just before delivery of the first twin will allow most of the vaginal manipulations required for the second twin. If internal version and breech extraction is required the uterus must be well relaxed. The one drawback to epidural is, that while it provides excellent analgesia, it does not relax the uterus. Thus, in the patient with epidural who requires internal version, one can either add a full general anaesthetic or give intravenous nitroglycerin for acute, short-term uterine relaxation. (see chapter 10)

Post partum

The risk of post partum haemorrhage is increased following twin delivery due to the tendency of the overdistended uterus to relax. Thus, with delivery of the second twin 5 units of oxytocin should be given intravenously followed by an oxytocin infusion for 8 hours.

BIBLIOGRAPHY

Adam C, Allen AC, Baskett TF. Twin delivery: influence of the presentation and method of delivery of the second twin. Am J Obstet Gynecol 1991;165:23-7.

American College of Obstetricians and Gynecologists. Education Bulletin No.253. Special problems of multiple gestation. Obstet Gynecol 1998 Vol 96, No3.

Barrett JFR, Ritchie JWK. Twin delivery. Best Prac Res Clin Obstet Gynaecol 2002;16:43-56.

Barrett J, Bocking A (eds) SOGC Consensus Statement. Management of twin pregnancies. J Soc Obstet Gynaecol Can 2000;22:519-29 and 607-10.

Benachi A, Pons JC. Is the route of delivery a meaningful issue in twins? Clin Obstet Gynecol 1998;41:31-5.

Boggess KA, Chisholm CA. Delivery of the nonvertex second twin: a review of the literature. Obstet Gynecol Surv 1997;52:728-35.

Dufour P, Vinatier D, Vanderstichele S, Ducloy AS, Monnier JC. Intravenous nitroglycerin for internal podalic version of the second twin in transverse lie. Obstet Gynecol 1998;92:416-9.

Hogle KL, Hutton EK, McBrien KA, Barrett JFR, Hannah ME. Cesarean delivery for twins: a systematic review and meta-analysis. Am J Obstet Gynecol 2003;188:220-7.

Khunda S. Locked twins. Obstet Gynecol 1972; 29: 453-9.

Leung TY, Tam WH, Leung TN, Lok IH, Lou TK. Effect of twin-to-twin delivery interval on umbilical cord blood gas in the second twins. Br J Obstet Gynaecol 2002;109:63-7.

Persad VL, Baskett TF, O'Connell CM, Scott HM. Combined vaginal-cesarean delivery of twin pregnancies. Obstet Gynecol 2001;98:1032-7.

Pschera H, Jonasson A. Is Cesarean section justified for delivery of the second twin? Acta Obstet Gynecol Scand 1988;67: 381-2.

Ramsey PS, Repke JT. Intrapartum management of multifetal pregnancies. Semin Perinatol 2003;27:54-72.

Redick L F. Anesthesia for twin delivery. Clin Perinatol 1988;15:107-22.

Saad FA, Sharara HA. Locked twins: a successful outcome after applying the Zavanelli manoeuvre. J Obstet Gynaecol 1997;17:366-7.

Stone J, Eddkeman K, Patel S. Controversies in the intrapartum management of twin gestations. Obstet Gynecol Clin North Am 1999;26:327-43.

CHAPTER 16

Intrapartum fetal monitoring

During uterine contractions of labour the intervillous blood flow is transiently halted. This reduces the supply of oxygen available for transfer to the fetus. With normal uterine contractions, placental circulation and function, the fetus withstands this repeated stress without ill effect. With certain complications this stress may progress to fetal hypoxia and acidosis.

CAUSES OF FETAL HYPOXIA

A. Decreased intervillous blood flow and placental transfer:

1. Excessive uterine action:
   - Abruptio placentae may increase uterine tone and raise the intrauterine pressure cutting down intervillous blood flow.
   - Oxytocin and prostaglandins may increase uterine tone as well as the frequency and duration of contractions.
2. Hypotension:
   - Hypovolaemia, e.g. antepartum haemorrhage.
   - Regional anaesthesia, e.g. epidural, spinal.
   - Drug reaction, e.g. narcotics, tocolytic agents.
   - Supine hypotension.
3. Vasoconstriction:

   Both chronic and pregnancy-induced hypertension may cause vasoconstriction of the placental vascular bed. Catecholamines released in response to fear or pain may also cause vasoconstriction.
4. Idiopathic:

   Some patients, with no obvious clinical cause, have placental ‘dysfunction’ leading to intrauterine growth restriction. In labour the normal uterine contractions and diminution of intervillous blood flow may cause fetal hypoxia in these patients. This is probably due to a combination of reduced placental transfer of oxygen and the fact that the growth restricted fetus, with minimal glycogen reserves, cannot metabolise anaerobically.

B. Decreased umbilical blood flow:

1. Intrauterine cord compression due to fetal cord entanglement or positional cord compression in utero, which may be aggravated by oligohydramnios.
2. Cord prolapse.

C. Decreased maternal oxygenation:

1. Cyanotic heart disease.
2. Chronic pulmonary disease.
3. Severe anaemia.
4. Eclamptic or epileptic convulsions.

D. Fetal anaemia:

1. Severe isoimmunisation.
2. Twin to twin transfusion.
3. Vasa praevia.

DIAGNOSIS OF FETAL HYPOXIA

There are three methods of fetal assessment in labour:

1. Meconium staining of the amniotic fluid.
2. Fetal heart rate monitoring.
3. Fetal blood acid-base determination.

1. MECONIUM

Approximately 10 per cent of fetuses pass meconium prior to delivery. One stimulus to the passage of meconium is fetal hypoxia which may cause hyperperistalsis of the bowel and relaxation of the anal sphincter. However, in most cases with meconium staining in labour the fetus is not hypoxic, or else the hypoxic episode was transient. On the other hand fetal hypoxia may exist without the passage of meconium, especially in the premature (<34 weeks' gestation) fetus. As the fetus in breech presentation descends in the pelvis meconium is often passed without signifying hypoxia.

In general old, thin meconium staining of the amniotic fluid does not have a strong association with hypoxia, although it is a warning to be heeded. Fresh, thick, green meconium of the 'peasoup' variety is frequently ominous and should be considered indicative of fetal hypoxia until proved otherwise.

The passage of meconium during labour should be taken as an indication for careful fetal heart rate monitoring.

2. FETAL HEART RATE (FHR) MONITORING

Auscultation

Auscultation of the fetal heart with a fetal stethoscope allows only intermittent assessment and is subject to observer error. However, skilled observers listening every 15 minutes during the first stage and with every contraction associated with maternal pushing in the second stage of labour can provide adequate fetal heart monitoring in normal patients. It is best to auscultate before, during, and after the contraction. If this is not feasible listen for one minute at the end and after the contraction. In so doing one can evaluate the baseline heart rate and any marked periodic alterations in rate (accelerations and decelerations). The baseline variability and subtle periodic alterations in heart rate cannot be assessed by auscultation.

Electronic fetal heart rate monitoring (EFM)

Electronic fetal heart monitors were developed in the 1960s.

Internal or direct monitoring of the fetal heart is achieved by attaching a bipolar electrode to the skin of the fetal scalp or buttock. The rate is derived from the R-R interval between each fetal ECG complex. This provides an instantaneous heart rate so that even the small rate difference between each heart beat is represented: the beat-to-beat, or baseline, variability. Obviously for this technique to be used the cervix has to be dilated and the membranes ruptured (Figure 16.1).

External or indirect monitoring of the fetal heart can be performed by ultrasound, fetal ECG or phonocardiography. For practical purposes, in labour, ultrasound is the method that produces the most satisfactory tracing. Ultrasound monitors use the Doppler principle but exclude the second sound of the Doppler component in order to avoid doubling the rate. For this reason heart rates over 180 may be halved and rates below 90 doubled by ultrasound fetal heart monitors. Another important deficiency of the ultrasound method is that the Doppler signal triggering the machine to record the beat is not as 'clean' as the fetal ECG signal from which the internal electrode records the rate. As a result the true beat-to-beat, baseline variability is not reproduced. Therefore the ultrasound monitor may show apparently normal baseline variability when it is in fact absent (Figure 16.2). On the other hand if the ultrasound monitor shows reduced baseline variability it is usually valid. In some of the newer FHR monitors with auto correlation the ultrasound may represent the true baseline variability.

The uterine contractions are recorded by one of two methods:

1. Internal intrauterine pressure monitoring via a fluid-filled transcervical catheter attached to a pressure transducer. Obviously the membranes need to be ruptured for this technique.

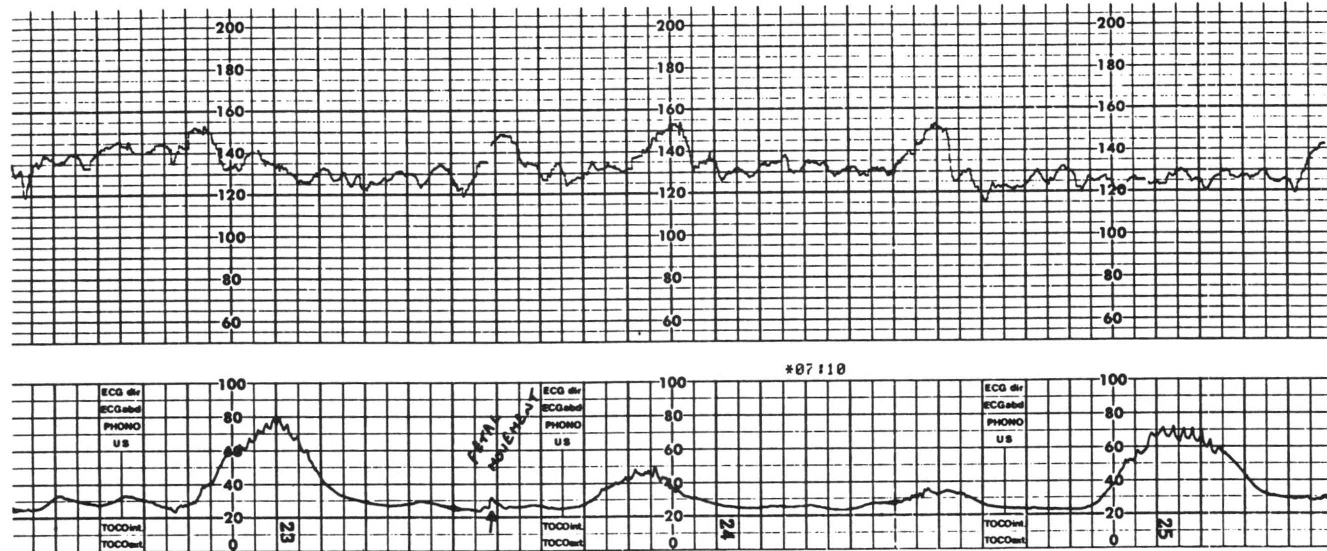

Figure 16.1 Normal fetal heart rate tracing. The rate and baseline variability are normal. Note the accelerations associated with uterine conditions and fetal movement. Such a tracing virtually precludes fetal hypoxia. (This, and all the figures in this chapter are recorded at 3cm/minute).

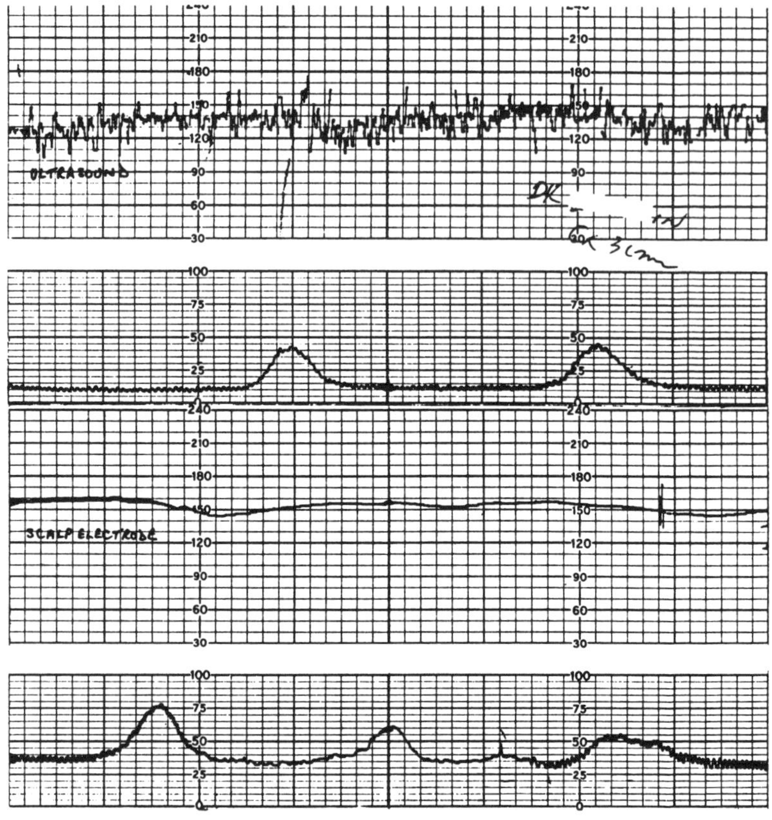

Figure 16.2 The upper panel, recorded with an ultrasound transducer, shows apparently normal baseline variability and no decelerations. The lower panel taken 15 minutes later with a scalp electrode reveals that the baseline variability is in fact absent and there are subtle decelerations. Thus, a very ominous pattern can occasionally be masked by ultrasound.

2. External tocodynamometry with a pressure transducer placed on the uterine fundus provides a measure of the frequency and duration of contractions but does not quantitate them.

Indications for electronic fetal heart rate monitoring (EFM) in labour

Whether it is ideal to provide EFM for all women in labour or only those with factors known to increase the risk of fetal hypoxia is a hotly debated issue, both in the medical and lay press.[1,2] Indeed, although the most commonly held view is that EFM is of benefit in high risk groups, this too is unproven.[3-7] In low risk groups the provision of EFM in labour does not improve perinatal outcome and in many instances is associated with an increase in instrumental, including caesarean, delivery.[8,9] The low risk woman who enters spontaneous labour, has a normal fetal heart rate on auscultation, no meconium staining of the amniotic fluid, and a normal progressive labour is extremely unlikely to deliver an asphyxiated infant. A case can be made for applying an initial 20 minute EFM screen on low risk patients in early labour (the so-called 'admission test'), to predict the likelihood of subsequent fetal hypoxia. Ingemarsson et al. found that the initial EFM screen was normal in 95 per cent of women, of whom about 1 per cent subsequently developed abnormal FHR in labour.[10] Others have not found this to be of value in reducing neonatal morbidity,[11,12] although in units with limited staff it may help direct resources. It must be emphasised that for these low risk women to achieve good results, continuous, one-to-one skilled nursing care in labour is required.

In controlled trials, EFM plus fetal scalp acid-base sampling reduced neonatal asphyctic seizures.[6] The majority of obstetricians feel that in high risk cases carefully applied EFM improves perinatal outcome. The following patients are likely to benefit from EFM in labour:

Maternal disorders:

- Hypertensive disease
- Diabetes mellitus
- Cardiac disease
- Renal disease
- Antepatum haemorrhage
- Blood group isoimmunisation

Labour complications:

- Induction of labour
- Non-progressive labour
- Oxytocin augmentation
- Premature labour
- Labour after previous caesarean section

Fetal complications:

- Suspected intrauterine growth restriction
- Previous stillbirth
- Twins
- Meconium staining
- Abnormal fetal heart on auscultation
- Prolonged pregnancy (>42 weeks)

Fetal Heart Rate Patterns

The most widely used terminology and classification of FHR patterns is that proposed by Hon,[13] and more recently in the guidelines approved by the International Federation of Gynaecology and Obstetrics (FIGO).[14]

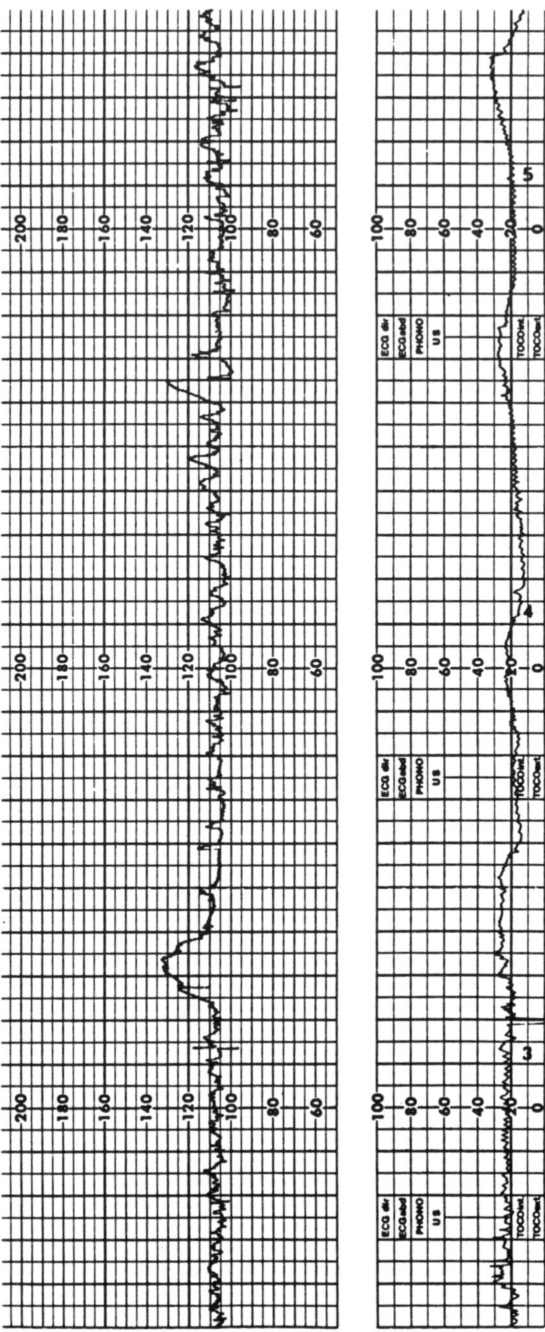

Figure 16.3 Mild bradycardia. Note the reassuring normal variability and periodic accelerations.

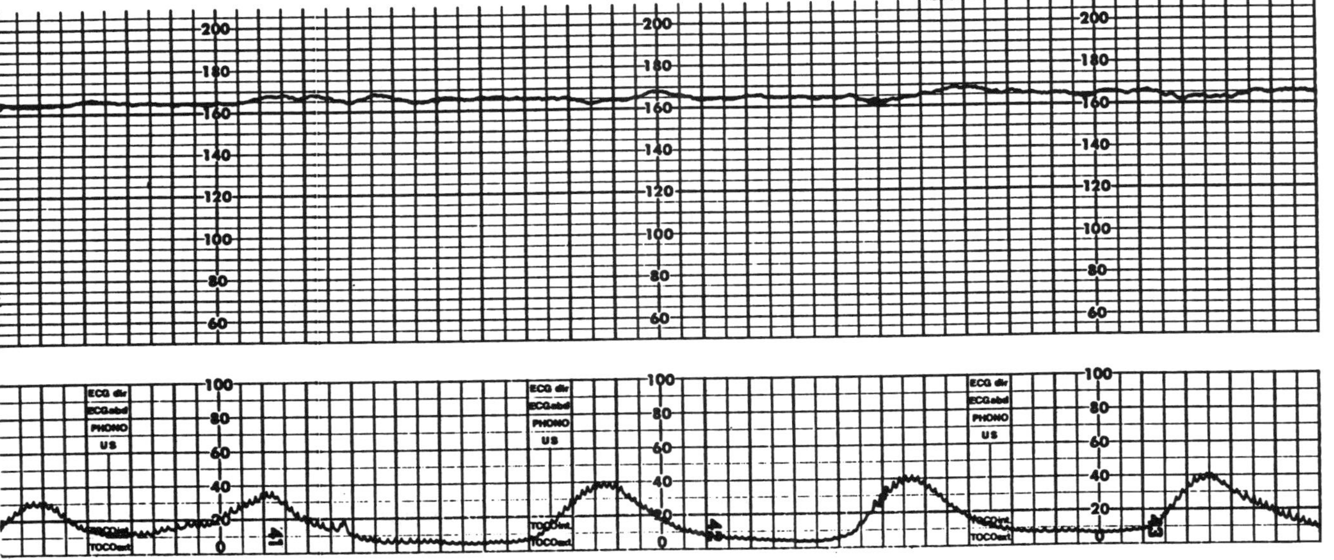

Figure 16.4 (*a*) Tachycardia with reduced baseline variability.

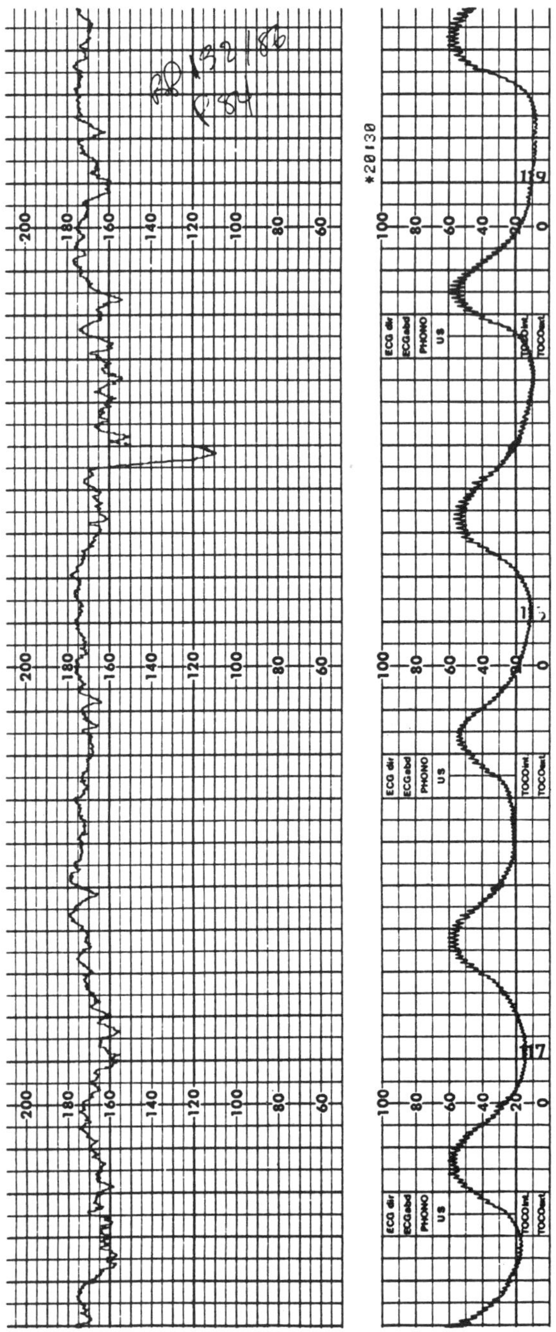

(*b*) Tachycardia with one mild variable deceleration.

FHR monitors have variable paper speeds, ranging from 1-3cm/min. With a normal tracing 1cm/min paper speed is adequate. If abnormalities occur some feel it is best to increase the speed to 2 or 3cm/minute for more precise interpretation, although in many hospitals 1cm/min is used for both screening and interpretation. Whatever paper speed is chosen, consistent training of medical and nursing staff who work on the labour ward is essential.[15,16]

Baseline FHR:

The baseline FHR is the rate recorded between contractions or other fetal stimuli. It is normally between 110 and 160 beats per minute (b.p.m.) and is usually assesed over 10-15 minute time intervals.

Bradycardia:

Persistent mild fetal bradycardia (90-110 b.p.m.) is not uncommon and is usually benign (Figure 16.3). A marked bradycardia (<90 b.p.m.) may be associated with congenital heart block. A potential pitfall exists in the presence of fetal death in that the scalp electrode can transmit the maternal heart rate, producing an apparent fetal bradycardia.

Tachycardia:

A fetal heart rate above 160 b.p.m. has many potential causes (Figure 16.4):

- Drugs – parasympatholytics, e.g. atropine and scopolamine
  – beta adrenergics, e.g. ritodrine
- Chorioamnionitis or other maternal or fetal infection
- Maternal hyperthyroidism
- Fetal anaemia and hypovalaemia
- Fetal cardiac dysrhythmia
- Fetal hypoxia
- Maternal dehydration

Variability:

Baseline, or beat-to-beat, variability is controlled by the balance of the sympathetic and parasympathetic nervous control of the heart. The normal variability is greater than 5 b.p.m. and may be reduced in the following circumstances:

- Drugs – parasympatholytics, e.g. atropine and scopolamine
  – narcotic analgesia, e.g. demerol (pethidine)
  – hypnotics and tranquillisers, e.g. barbiturates, benzodiazepines, phenothiazines

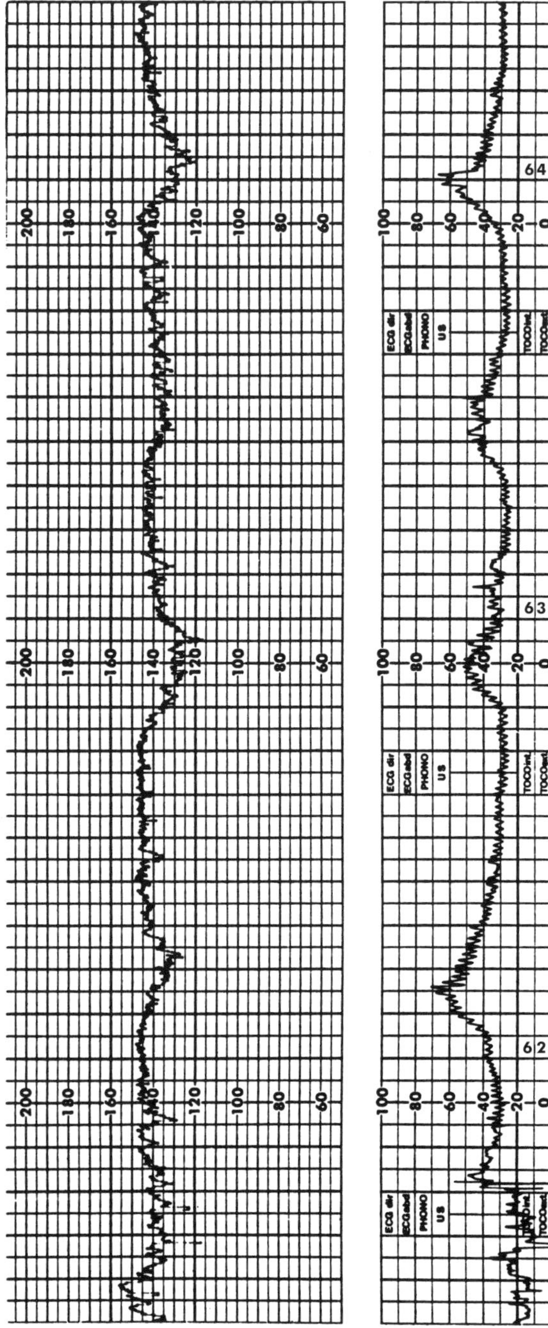

Figure 16.5 Early deceleration – an innocent pattern. The acceleration at the beginning of the panel and the normal variability are additional reassuring features.

- Physiological fetal sleep cycles may reduce, but not eliminate, baseline variability. This usually only lasts 20-40 minutes, but can rarely be as long as 90 minutes.
- Fetal hypoxia

Periodic FHR:

Periodic changes in the FHR may be either accelerations or decelerations.

Accelerations: These are often associated with fetal stimulation during movement, uterine contractions, pressure during pelvic examinations, etc. Accelerations are considered benign and indeed their presence usually indicates a well oxygenated fetus.

Decelerations: Classically three fairly well defined deceleration patterns are described: early, late, and variable. To these, in clinical practice, one can add the prolonged deceleration.

Early deceleration: These decelerations have a uniform shape, start early in the contraction, and have returned to the normal rate by the end of the contraction. The bell shape mirrors the uterine contraction (Figure 16.5). The magnitude of the deceleration is usually <40 b.p.m. These decelerations are due to head compression, are mediated by a vagal reflex, and occur during the active phase of labour. They are benign.

Late deceleration: Late decelerations have a similar shape and magnitude to early decelerations but their timing is different. They start as the contraction peaks and the rate does not return to the baseline until well after the contraction has ceased (Figure 16.6). This pattern is felt to represent reduced intervillous space blood flow and fetal hypoxia.

Variable deceleration: This is by far the most commonly seen deceleration pattern. As the name implies the shape, duration, and timing of the decelerations are variable. Both the fall and return of the fetal heart rate are abrupt (Figure 16.7). They are often preceded and followed by small accelerations, producing ‘shoulders’ for each deceleration. The magnitude of the deceleration is usually 50-80 b.p.m. which is why they are the most common pattern picked up on auscultation. Variable decelerations are due to cord compression and are vagally mediated. If the umbilical cord compression persists hypoxia supervenes, compounding the deceleration.

Mild variable decelerations last less than 30 seconds and are benign. Moderate variable decelerations last 30-60 seconds, and the severe type last > 60 seconds and fall to < 70 b.p.m.

Prolonged deceleration: Decelerations lasting two minutes or more are designated 'prolonged'. They often have characteristics similar to the variable deceleration (Figure 16.8). They can be caused by excessive uterine action, cord compression, following paracervical block, maternal hypotension, and fetal manipulation during pelvic examination. Prolonged decelerations often indicate hypoxia.

Mixed deceleration patterns: The above descriptions represent the accepted terminology of deceleration patterns. In clinical practice many decelerations defy precise classification. One of the more common mixed patterns is a variable deceleration with a late component, in which the recovery of the heart rate is slow and gradual instead of abrupt (Figure 16.9). Variable, late, and prolonged decelerations may be mixed together and often indicate fetal hypoxia.

Sinusoidal pattern: This uncommon sine wave pattern may occur in response to narcotic drugs, fetal anaemia, and fetal hypoxia. Intermittent mild episodes of a sinusoidal type pattern (psuedo-sinusoidal) are not uncommon in normal fetuses. (Figure 16.10).

3. FETAL BLOOD ACID-BASE DETERMINATION

The hypoxic fetus has to resort to anaerobic metabolism, the end result of which is lactic acid accumulation and a fall in the fetal blood pH. Access to fetal blood is obtained via an amnioscope with the patient in the left lateral position to avoid supine hypotension. The amnioscope is initially directed to the posterior fornix and then anteriorly through the cervix. The amnioscope is pressed gently but firmly against the fetal scalp and the scalp cleaned with a cotton wool swab. The scalp is then sprayed with ethyl chloride to induce hyperaemia and smeared with a thin layer of gel to promote beading of the blood after incision with a special blade. The blood is collected in a heparinised glass tube for pH analysis. The normal **fetal scalp blood pH** is >7.25. If the pH is < 7.20, and there is no maternal acidosis, the fetus should be delivered. In the intermediate zone (7.20-7.25) the fetus should either be delivered or the pH be rechecked in 10-15 minutes to establish the trend.

Recent work suggests that measuring **fetal scalp blood lactate** levels may have comparable predictive value to pH.[17] Less blood is required and the analysis of blood lactate is easier to perform. Its utility awaits furthur experience.

There are obviously limitations on the number of times and the frequency with which fetal blood sampling can be performed. Its main value is in confirmation or denial of fetal acidosis when the heart pattern suggests fetal hypoxia. Thus, the careful application of this technique can reduce the need for operative delivery with abnormal fetal heart patterns.

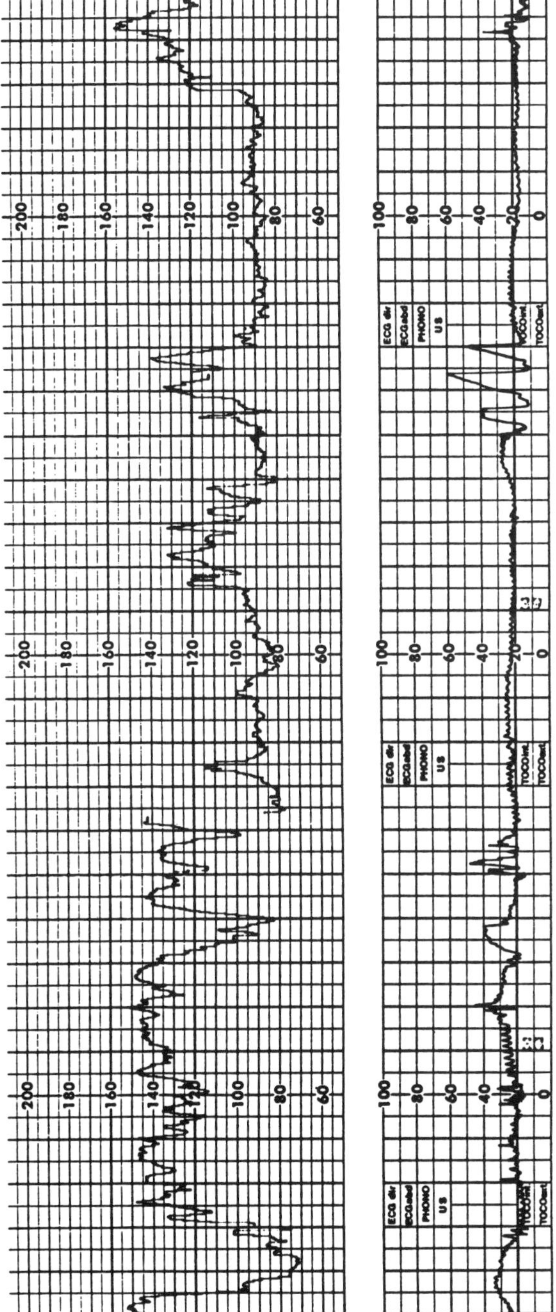

Figure 16.8 Prolonged decelerations.

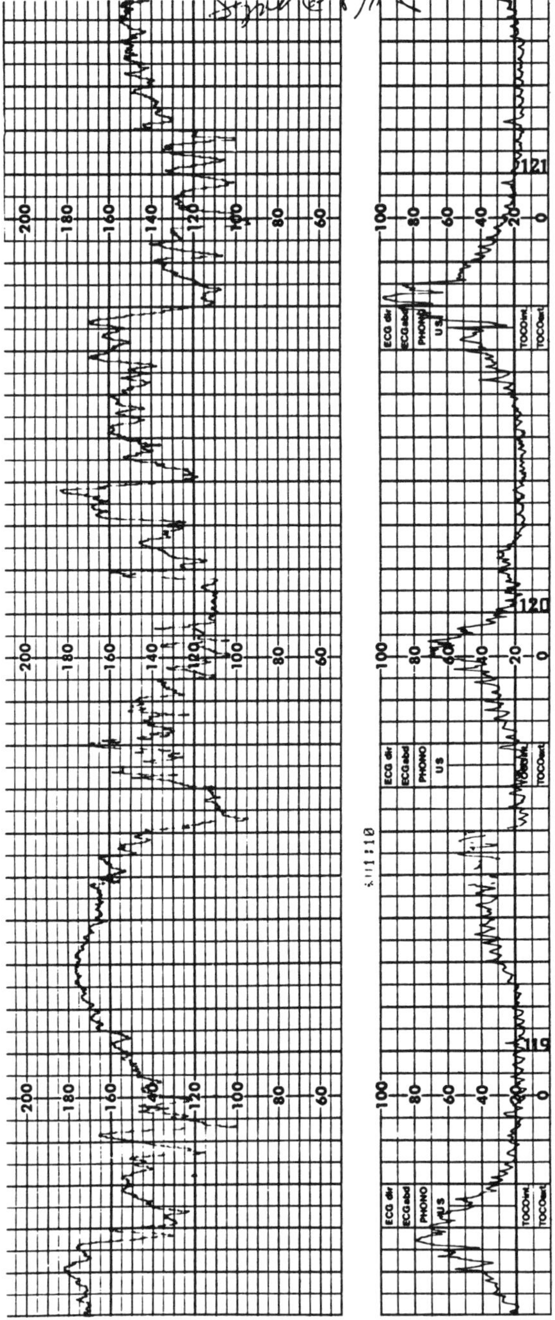

Figure 16.9 Mixed deceleration pattern: Variable decelerations with a late component.

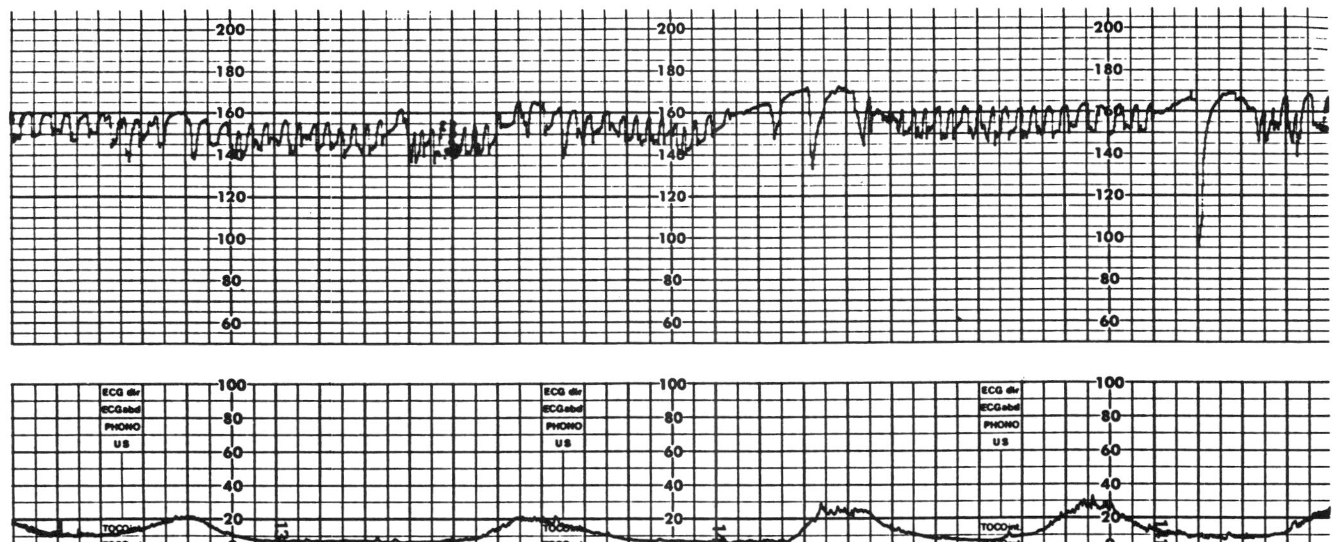

Figure 16.10 (*a*) Pseudo-Sinusoidal pattern: interspersed with accelerations. This is usually an innocent variant of baseline variability.

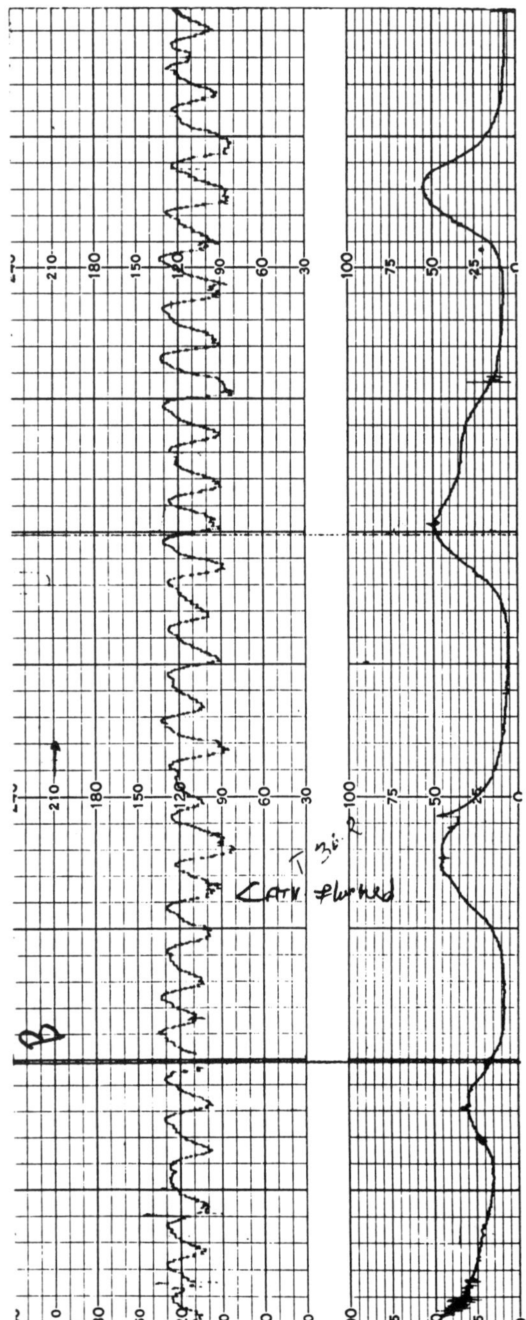

(b) True sinusoidal pattern. Rare–if not drug induced, fetal anaemia and hypoxia have to be considered.

Complications

- Bleeding-usually responds to pressure with a cotton wool swab.
- Infection-rare and usually superficial
- Falsely normal and falsely abnormal pH results occur in about 10 per cent of cases and are more likely with marked caput formation or contamination of the sample with amniotic fluid.[18]

MANAGEMENT OF ABNORMAL FHR PATTERN

The main predictive value of fetal heart monitoring is that a normal tracing virtually precludes fetal hypoxia. This is very reassuring and a valuable aid in the management of the high risk patient in labour. Unfortunately abnormal fetal heart patterns do not have the same predictive accuracy. Although there is a statistical association between certain abnormal fetal heart patterns and fetal hypoxia this is rarely specific enough to allow one to make important clinical decisions on this basis alone. Furthermore, adding to the vagaries of FHR interpretation are the different responses of the FHR depending on fetal prematurity (reduced accelerations) and intrauterine growth restriction (IUGR) (reduced variability). In addition, intra and inter-observer reliability in the interpretation of FHR patterns is often not high. To emphasise the imprecise nature of FHR pattern predictability the descriptive terms 'fetal distress' or 'abnormal' FHR pattern are being replaced by the rather cumbersome, but more medico-legally correct (as it were), 'non-reassuring' FHR pattern or 'suspected fetal compromise'. Thus, one has to seek additional information to confirm or deny the association of fetal hypoxia with the non-reassuring FHR pattern.

INTERPRETATION OF FETAL HEART RATE PATTERNS

As outlined above the significance of non-reassuring fetal heart patterns is based on probabilities, with certain patterns requiring clarification by fetal blood pH determination. In some of the potentially ominous patterns certain characteristics of the baseline fetal heart rate may help narrow down the risk of fetal hypoxia. Keep in mind that abnormal FHR patterns, of no specific type, are more common in the anomalous fetus. The following represents a guide to the clinical interpretation of non-reassuring fetal heart patterns:

Tachycardia and Decreased Baseline Variability

- These patterns are potentially important indicators of fetal health and can modify the interpretation of other deceleration patterns. Assuming that drug-induced and other causes of these patterns have been excluded one has to consider fetal hypoxia as a possible cause.

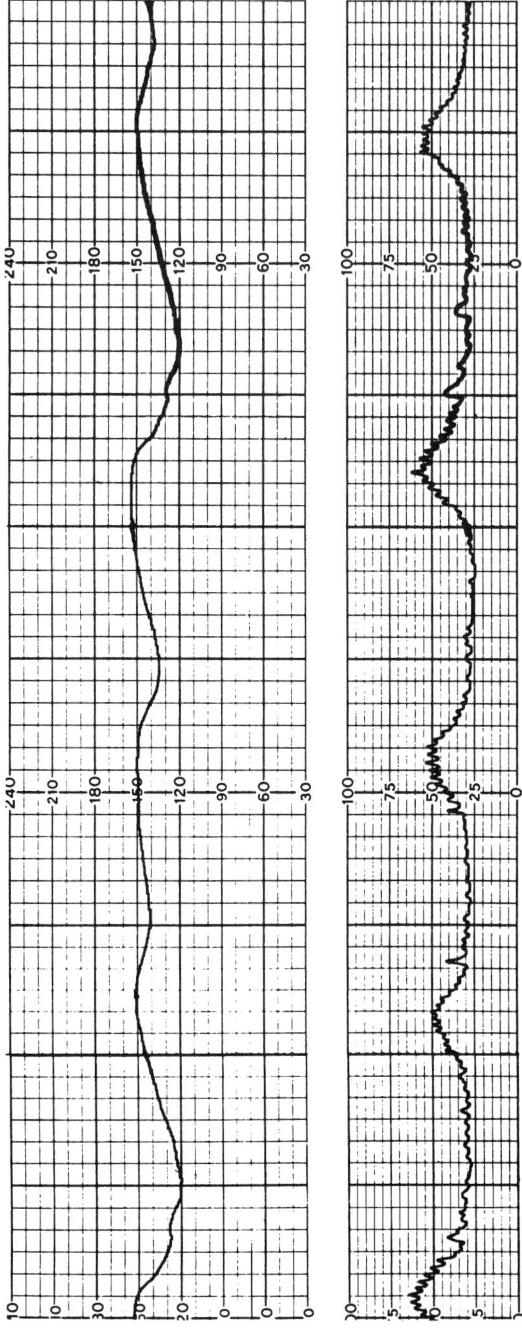

Figure 16.11 Late decelerations and absent variability. This is one of most ominous fetal heart patterns.

- Individually neither of these patterns is diagnostic of fetal hypoxia, but they are an indication for close surveillance.
- The combination of tachycardia and absent baseline variability as a persistent pattern, even in the absence of deceleration, is ominous. It should be an indication for fetal acid-base determination.
- The likihood of late or variable decelerations being associated with fetal hypoxia is increased if the baseline heart rate shows tachycardia and loss of variability.
- It is rare for fetal hypoxia to exist in the presence of normal variability. Thus, this feature of the fetal heart has a very important influence on the interpretation of abnormal patterns.

Accelerations

- Accelerations of at least 15 b.p.m. and >15 seconds duration are also a useful guide to the likelihood of fetal hypoxia with abnormal patterns. When such accelerations are present the likelihood of fetal hypoxia is low. Fetal heart acceleration is a normal response to fetal stimulation and this response is diminished or lost with hypoxia.
- The observation that FHR accelerations occurring with the stimulation of fetal scalp blood pH collection correlate with the absence of fetal acidosis has led to the development of the **fetal scalp stimulation test**.[19,20] The most practical way to perform this test is to use Allis or similar forceps to pinch the fetal scalp. Accelerations of >15 b.p.m. and >15 seconds duration correlate well, with a normal scalp pH. This may be useful as a screening test for the need to do fetal blood scalp sampling or if facilities for scalp pH are unavailable. This is a simple and underused method of clarifying non-reassuring FHR patterns. On the other hand, the absence of FHR accelerations with scalp stimulation has low specificity in predicting fetal acidosis. A similar absence of fetal acidosis has been found if FHR accelerations occur in response to vibratory acoustic stimulation.[21]

Early Decelerations, Mild-Moderate Variable Decelerations, and Bradycardia

These are almost invariably innocent and not associated with fetal hypoxia. If the baseline variability is normal and there are intermittent accelerations of the heart rate, this further confirms that no intervention is necessary

Late, Severe Variable and Prolonged Decelerations

These patterns, or a mixture thereof, are potentially ominous and a correctable cause, which is often present, must be sought. If the pattern persists the baby should be delivered, or fetal blood pH analysis carried out to confirm or deny hypoxia. The likelihood of these patterns being associated with fetal hypoxia is increased if the baseline fetal heart rate shows tachycardia and particularly if the baseline variability is reduced or absent. The combination of persistent tachycardia, absent variability, and late decelerations (however subtle) is the most predictably bad of all fetal heart patterns and dictates immediate delivery of the fetus (Figure 16.11).

ADDITIONAL TESTS OF INTRAPARTUM FETAL HYPOXIA

Fetal Electrocardiograph

Hypoxia and acidosis affect the fetal myocardium and cause depression of the ST segment of the fetal ECG. This test shows promise for improved detection and discrimination of fetal hypoxia, compared to FHR monitoring alone.

Fetal Pulse Oximetry

Sensors placed against the fetal cheek may allow continuous fetal oxygen saturation monitoring via pulse oximetry. Furthur technical advances, and experience are required to establish the role of this technique.

MANAGEMENT OF POTENTIALLY OMNIOUS FETAL HEART RATE PATTERNS

A. Look for correctable cause:

- Stop oxytocin and consider emergency tocolysis (see chapter 10).
- Correct hypotension and hypovalaemia.
- Pelvic examination:
- If cervix fully dilated, and safely feasible, carry out assisted vaginal delivery.
- Exclude cord prolapse.
- Assess cervical dilatation and likely duration of labour.
- Maternal repositioning will often relieve cord compression *in utero* and correct variable and prolonged decelerations.
- Relieve pain and fear.
- Give oxygen to the mother.

- Amnioinfusion: This simple technique has been proven to reduce the persistence of certain abnormal FHR patterns (variable and prolonged decelerations) and decrease the caesarean section rate for 'fetal distress'.[22] It has also been shown to decrease the morbidity and sequelae of meconium aspiration in the neonate, when used during labour for meconium staining of the amniotic fluid.[23] Others have used it prophylactically for patients entering labour with oligohydramnios.[24]

The fluid, normal saline at room temperature, is infused via a transcervical intrauterine pressure catheter or another simple plastic catheter, such as a number eight nasogastric tube. For abnormal FHR patterns the saline is infused at 15ml/min up to 500-750ml, or until the decelerations abate. Thereafter the maintenance rate is 3ml/min. For prophylaxis the initial rate can be slower: 10ml/min up to 500ml, and then 3ml/min. The rates can be adjusted if there is a large fluid loss with maternal movement. One should guard against the development of polyhydramios and be aware that occasionally a rapid worsening of the FHR pattern may occur. Amnioinfusion has been incriminated in very rare cases of amniotic fluid embolism and abruptio placentae. Generally it takes about 20-30 minutes before the beneficial effects on the FHR are seen.

B. If there is no correctable cause and the ominous pattern persists:

- Individual factors may influence the decision in favour of immediate delivery by caesarean section:
  - Fresh thick meconium.
  - Premium pregnancy
  - Likelihood of several hours until vaginal delivery feasible.
- If vaginal delivery is likely in 1-3 hours then fetal blood pH analysis may allow one to await delivery, or alternatively, confirm the need for immediate delivery.

REFERENCES

1. Thacker SB, Stroup DF, Peterson HB. Efficacy and safety of intrapartum electronic fetal monitoring: an update. Obstet Gynecol 1995;86:613-20.
2. Umstad MP, Permezel M, Pepperell RJ. Litigation and the intrapartum cardiotocograph. Br J Obstet Gynaecol 1995;102:89-91.
3. Haverkamp AD, Orleans M, Langendoerfer S, McFee J, Murphy J. Thompson HE. A controlled trial of the differential effects of intrapartum fetal monitoring. Am J Obstet Gynecol 1979;134:399-412.
4. Kelso IM, Parsons RJ, Lawrence GF et al. An assessment of continuous fetal heart monitoring in labour. Am J Obstet Gynecol 1978;131:526-32.
5. Renou P, Chang A, Anderson I et al. Controlled trial of fetal intensive care. Am J Obstet Gynecol 1976;126:470-6.
6. MacDonald D, Grant A, Sheriden-Pereira MP et al. The Dublin randomised controlled trial of intrapartum fetal heart rate monitoring. Am J Obstet Gynecol 1985;152:524-39.

7. Grant A, Joy MT, O'Brien N et al. Cerebral palsy among children born during the Dublin randomised trial of intrapartum monitoring. Lancet 1989;2:1233-5.
8. Wood C, Renou P, Oats J, Farrell E, Beischer N, Anderson I. A controlled trial of fetal heart monitoring in a low-risk obstetric population. Am J Obstet Gynecol 1982;141:527-34.
9. Leveno KJ. Cunningham FG, Nelson S. A prospective comparison of elective and universal electronic fetal monitoring in 34,995 pregnancies. N Engl J Med 1986;315:615-9.
10. Ingemarsson I, Arulkumaran S, Ingemarsson E. Admission test: a screening test for fetal distress in labor. Obstet Gynecol 1986;68:800-6.
11. Mires G, Williams F, Howie P. Randomised controlled trial of cardiotocography versus Doppler auscultation of fetal heart at admission in labour in low risk obstetric population. BMJ 2001;322:1457-62.
12. Impey L, Reynolds M, MacQuillan K, Gates S, Murphy J, Sheil O. Admission cardiotocography: a randomised controlled trial. Lancet 2003;361:465-70.
13. Hon EH. The Mechanisms of FHR Deceleration Patterns. In: An Atlas of Fetal Heart Rate Patterns. New Haven: Harty Press, 1986.pp. 48-51.
14. Intrapartum surveillance. FIGO Study Group. Int J Gynaecol Obstet 1995;49:213-21.
15. Young P, Hamilton R, Hodgett S et al. Reducing risk by improving standards of intrapartum fetal care. JR Soc Med 2001;94:226-31.
16. Murphy AA, Halamek LP, Lyell DJ, Druzin ML. Training and compentency assessment in electoronic fetal monitoring: a national survey. Obstet Gynecol 2003;101:1243-8.
17. Westgren M, Kruger K, Ek S, et al. Lactate compared with pH analysis at fetal scalp blood sampling: a prospective randomised study. Br J Obstet Gynaecol 1998;105:29-33
18. Lösch A, Kainz C, Kohlberger P et al. Influence of fetal blood pH when adding amniotic fluid: an in vitro model. Br J Obstet Gynaecol 2003;110:453-6.
19. Elimian A, Figueroa R, Tejani N. Intrapartum assessment of fetal well-being: a comparison of scalp stimulation with scalp blood pH sampling. Obstet Gynecol 1997;89:373-6.
20. Skupski DW, Rosenberg CR, Eglinton GS. Intrapartum fetal stimulation tests: a meta-analysis. Obstet Gynecol 2002;99:129-34.
21. Edersheim TG, Hutson JM, Druzin ML et al. Fetal heart response to vibratory acoustic stimulation predicts pH in labor. Am J Obstet Gynecol 1987;157:1557-60.
22. Miyazaki FS, Nevarez F. Saline amniotic infusion for relief of repetitive variable decelerations: a prospective randomized study. Am J Obstet Gynecol 1985;153:301-13.
23. Mohomed K, Mulambo T, Woelk G et al. The collaborative randomised amnioinfusion for meconium (CRAMP): Zimbabwe. Br J Obstet Gynaecol 1998;105:309-13.
24. Pitt C, Ramos LS, Kaunitz AM, Gaudier F. Prophylactic amnio infusion for intrapartum oligohydramnios: A meta-analysis of randomised controlled trial. Obstet Gynecol 2000;96:861-6.

BIBLIOGRAPHY

American College of Obstetricians and Gynecologists. Technical Bulliten 216. Fetal heart rate patterns: monitoring, interpretation and management. Washington DC: ACOG, 1995.

American College of Obstetricians and Gynecologists. Committee Opinion No 258. Fetal pulse oximetry. Washington DC:ACOG, 2001. (Obstet Gynecol 2002;98:523-4).

American College of Obstetricians and Gynaecologists. Neonatal Encephalopathy and Cerebral Palsy. Washington DC: ACOG,2003.

Cowan F, Rutherford M, Groenendaal M et al. Origin and timing of brain lesions in term infants with neonatal encephalopathy. Lancet 2003;361:736-42.

Dildy GA. Fetal pulse oximetry. Obstet Gynecol Surv 2003;58:225-6.

Electronic fetal heart rate monitoring: research guidelines for interpretation. National Institute of Child Health and Human Development Research Planning Workshop. Am J Obstet Gynecol 1997;177:1385-90.

Ellison PH, Foster M, Sheridan-Pereira M et al. Electronic fetal heart monitoring, auscultation, and neonatal outcome. Am J Obstet Gynecol 1991;164:1281-9.

Freeman RK. Problems with intrapartum fetal heart rate monitoring interpretation and patient management. Obstet Gynecol 2002;100:813-26.

Gibb D, Arulkumaran S. Fetal Monitoring in Practice. Oxford: Butterworth-Heinemann Ltd, 1992.

Gimovsky ML, Dolpe JL. Fetal heart rate monitoring in fetuses with congenital anomalies. J Perinatol 1998;18:83-4.

Glantz JC, Letteney DL. Pumps and warmers during amnioinfusion: is either necessary. Obstet Gynecol 1996;87:150-5.

Low JA. Intrapartum fetal asphyxia: definition, diagnosis, and classification. Am J Obstet Gynecol 1997;176:957-9.

MacLennan A. A template for defining causal relation between acute intrapartum events and cerebral palsy: international consensus statement. BMJ 1999;319:1054-9.

Modanlou HD, Freeman RK. Sinusoidal fetal heart rate pattern: its definition and clinical significance. Am J Obstet Gynecol 1982;42:1033-8.

Murphy KW, Russell V, Collins A et al. The prevalence, aetiology, and clinical significance of pseudo-sinusoidal fetal heart rate patterns in labour. Br J Obstet Gynaecol 1991;98:1093-1101.

Noren H, Amer-Wahlin I, Hagberg H et al. Fetal electrocardiography in labor and neonatal outcome: data from the Swedish randomised controlled trial on intrapartum fetal monitoring. Am J Obstet Gynecol 2003;188:183-92.

Ouzounian JG, Paul RH. Clinical role of amnio-infusion. Clin Obstet Gynaecol 1996;10:259-72.

Royal College of Obstetricians and Gynaecologists. Evidence-based Clinical Guideline No 8. The use of electronic fetal monitoring. London: RCOG Press, 2001.

Shy KK, Luthy DA, Bennett FC et al. Effects of electronic fetal heart rate monitoring as compared with periodic auscultation, on the neurologic development of premature infants. N Engl J Med 1990;322:588-93.

Society of Obstetricians and Gynaecologists of Canada. Clinical Practice Guideline No 112. Fetal health surveillance in labour. J Obstet Gynaecol Can 2002;24:250-62.

Tharmaratnam S. Fetal distress. Best Prac Res Clin Obstet Gynaecol 2000;14:155-172.

CHAPTER 17

Uterine rupture

The incidence of this potentially catastrophic complication varies greatly throughout the world: from approximately 1 in 250 deliveries in developing countries to 1 in 3000 in countries with more sophisticated health services. Maternal mortality due to uterine rupture in developed countries is rare but severe morbidity, including emergency hysterectomy is common. In developing countries uterine rupture may contribute up to 15 per cent of maternal deaths.[1]

Because of the increased number of scarred uteri, secondary to the rise in caesarean section rates, the incidence of uterine rupture is not falling.

TYPES

Complete rupture involves the full thickness of the uterine wall.

Incomplete rupture occurs when the visceral peritoneum remains intact and usually occurs in dehiscence of a previous lower segment caesarean scar.

Bleeding may extend into the broad ligament and track into the retroperitoneal space.

Complete rupture is more likely to be lethal to mother and fetus.

CAUSES

A. UTERINE SCAR

1. **Caesarean section:** The classical section scar is much more prone to subsequent rupture than the transverse lower segment scar. This is because the classical scar is in the upper contractile portion of the uterus which may disrupt initial healing during involution, as well as contracting during a subsequent pregnancy and labour. Implantation of the placenta over the site of a previous caesarean section scar can predispose to rupture due to the poor decidual response and subsequent invasion of the scar and adjacent myometrium by the trophoblast. The placenta is obviously more likely to overlie a scar in the upper uterine segment.

2. **Hysterotomy:** Wide experience with pregnancy and labour after hysterotomy is lacking. However, this scar seems to behave in the same treacherous manner as the classical caesarean scar and should be treated in the same way.[2]
3. **Myomectomy:** This type of scar is not encountered frequently in modern obstetrics. If not extensive, and particularly if the uterine cavity was not entered, it seems to withstand subsequent labour quite well.
4. **Uteroplasty.**
5. **Previous perforation** or weakening of the uterine wall by curettage.
6. **Cervical scar:**
   – Cervical amputation or conisation.
   – Deep cervical lacerations.
   – Cervical cerclage.
7. **Salpingectomy with cornual resection.**

B. EXCESSIVE UTERINE ACTION

1. **Oxytocic drugs** used injudiciously are an important, and ideally preventable, cause of uterine rupture.
2. **Neglected obstructed labour** may end with uterine rupture. In this regard the labouring multiparous uterus must be viewed differently from that of the nullipara. The multiparous uterus will often respond to obstruction by increasing the strength of contractions, culminating in rupture. Thus, in non-progressive labour in a multiparous patient any cause for obstructed labour should be carefully sought and oxytocin augmentation of labour used with extreme caution (see Chapter 11).

C. TRAUMA

1. **Internal version and breech extraction** – virtually the only place for this procedure in modern obstetrics is in delivery of the second twin.
2. **Forceps delivery –** more likely with forceps rotation and with the classical application of the anterior blade of Kielland's forceps.
3. **Manual removal of the placenta** – especially if there are accretic areas of placental tissue implanted over a uterine scar.
4. **Fetal destructive operations.**
5. **Shoulder dystocia.**
6. **Excessive fundal pressure** in the second stage of labour.
7. **Termination of early pregnancy.**
8. **Direct trauma,** e.g. car accident.

D. MISCELLANEOUS

1. **Multiparity** is a predisposing factor in all causes of uterine rupture. Repeated labour and delivery may lead to pregressive fibrosis and thinning of the uterine muscle.
2. **Uterine anomalies.**
3. **Placenta increta and percreta.**
4. **Cornual pregnancy.**
5. **Gestational trophoblastic disease.**

CLINICAL FEATURES

The clinical findings may vary from mild and non-specific to an obvious abdominal catastrophe.

The classic signs and symptoms of complete uterine rupture are the sudden onset of tearing abdominal pain, cessation of uterine contractions, vaginal bleeding, recession of the presenting part, absent fetal heart and signs of intra-abdominal haemorrhage associated with hypovolaemic shock. Alternatively, the lower uterine segment may rupture with few such dramatic signs and symptoms. In particular, the thin relatively avascular scar of the lower segment caesarean section may dehisce with no symptoms and labour continue, only for the rupture to manifest itself post partum.

This great variation in the severity of the signs and symptoms means that a constant vigil and awareness must prevail with all patients at risk of uterine rupture.

The following **signs and symptoms of impending or early uterine rupture** are not consistent, but can aid early detection:

1. Persistent lower uterine segment pain and tenderness between contractions. This is quite variable and may occur to a minor degree in normal labour.
2. Swelling and crepitus over the lower uterine segment, particularly if unilateral.
3. Vaginal bleeding.
4. Maternal tachycardia, hypotension, and syncope.
5. Haematuria: The bladder is often adherent to a previous lower segment caesarean scar.
6. Fetal heart rate abnormalities: such as tachycardia; variable, late and prolonged decelerations. **This is the most reliable warning sign**.

MANAGEMENT

1. **Treat hypovolaemia** (see Chapter 24).

2. **Laparotomy:**
   a) **Remove fetus and placenta**
   b) **Secure haemostasis:**
      - Bring the uterus out of the incision. An assistant's hands behind the uterus, pulling it up and with the fingers and thumbs occluding the uterine vessels, may aid the surgeon.
      - Apply Green-Armytage or ring forceps to the bleeding edges of the lacerations.
      - Manual compression of the aorta may be necessary to help see the extent of the lacerations.
      - Uterine and ovarian artery ligation may be of value in reducing blood loss before moving to definitive surgery (see Chapter 25).
      - Internal iliac artery ligation may be required to control bleeding in the base of the broad ligament.

   c) Always carefully check the integrity of the bladder wall, which is often adherent and can be torn in lower segment ruptures. (see Chapter 19).

3. **Surgical options:**
   The choice of operative procedure depends on a number of factors, including the patient's condition, type of rupture, facilities available, and experience of the surgeon.
   3.1. **Total hysterectomy:**
   Provided the surgeon is experienced this is the procedure of choice if the cervix and/or paracolpos are involved in the rupture. It is also indicated if there is infection.
   3.2. **Subtotal hysterectomy:**
   If the patient's general condition demands a short operation, and there is no sepsis or involvment of the cervix or paracolpos, this procedure is chosen. It is simpler, faster, and there is less risk of injury to the bladder and ureters than with total hysterectomy.
   3.3. **Laceration repair and tubal ligation:**
   If the rupture is simple and uninfected this procedure has the merits of speed and simplicity.
   3.4. **Laceration repair alone:**
   This is only considered for simple lacerations when the patient's desire to retain her reproductive potential is strong. A recent report supports this approach in selected cases.[3]

These procedures should be covered with perioperative antibiotics and thromboprophylaxis.

The surgical aspects are covered in Chapter 19.

When uterine rupture occurs a thorough review should be conducted by the unit staff.

REFERENCES

1. Bouvier-Colle MH, Ouedraogo C, Dumont A et al. Maternal mortality in West Africa. Rates, causes and substandard care from a prospective survey. Acta Obstet Gynecol Scand 2001;80:113-5.

2. Clow N, Crompton AC. The wounded uterus: pregnancy after hysterectomy. BMJ 1973;1:21-23.

3. O'Connor RA, Gaughan B. Pregnancy following simple repair of the ruptured gravid uterus. Br J Obstet Gynaecol 1989;96:942-4.

BIBLIOGRAPHY

Aboyeji AP, Ijaiya MDA, Yahaya VR. Ruptured uterus: a study of 100 consecutive cases in Ilorin, Nigeria. J Obstet Gynaecol Res 2001;27:341-8.

Al-Sakka M, Harusho A, Khan L. Rupture of the pregnant uterus: a 21 year review. Int J Gynecol Obstet 1998;63:105-8.

Eden RD, Parker RT, Gall SA. Rupture of the pregnant uterus: a 53 year review. Obstet Gynecol 1986;68:671-3.

Gardeil F, Daly S, Turner MJ. Uterine rupture in pregnancy reviewed. Eur J Obstet Gynecol Reprod Biol 1994;56:107-10.

Kieser KE, Baskett TF. A 10-year population-based study of uterine rupture. Obstet Gynecol 2002;100:749-53.

Miller DA, Goodwin TM, Gherman RB, Paul RH. Intrapartum rupture of the unscared uterus. Obstet Gynecol 1997;89:671-3.

Mokgokong ET, Marivate M. Treatment of the ruptured uterus. S Afr Med J 1976;50:1621-4.

Phelan JP, Korst LM, Settles DK. Uterine activity patterns in uterine rupture: a case –control study. Obstet Gynecol 1998;92:394-7.

Solton MH, Khashoggi T, Adelusi B. Pregnancy following rupture of the pregnant uterus. Int J Gynecol Obstet 1996;52:37-42.

Turner MJ. Uterine rupture. Best Prac Res Clin Obstet Gynaecol 2002;16:69-79.

CHAPTER 18

Vaginal Delivery After Caesarean Section

During the last quarter of the 20th century caesarean rates increased world wide – quadrupling in some countries. Repeat caesarean section accounted for about one-third of this increase. In many developed countries one in 10 pregnant women have previously been delivered by caesarean section. In an attempt to reduce the caesarean section rate many hospitals, particularly in the United States and Canada, that had previously adhered to a policy 'once a always a caesarean always a caesarean' began to promote vaginal birth after caesarean (VBAC). In selected cases, and with widening indications, this became a standard of care in 1980s and 90s. By the late 1990s it was apparent that broadening the indications and the facilities appropriate for VBAC was associated with a small but definite risk of potentially catastrophic uterine rupture.[1] Thus, the 'pendulum syndrome' has occurred and many hospitals are not providing VBAC services or limiting them to strictly selected cases.

Unfortunately the term 'trial of labour 'has been widely adopted to describe labour in patients with a uterine scar. 'Trial of labour' is a well established obstetric term used when labour is undertaken in a case of real or suspected disproportion. Strictly speaking, therefore, a trail of labour is contraindicated in any patient with a uterine scar. In the modern sociological environment the word 'trial' is considered inappropriate as applied to the woman in labour. She is not 'on trial', but, as for a trial of forceps (chapter 11), the word and its clinical and medico-legal connotations remain relevant for the attendants looking after her. The correct term is trial for vaginal delivery.

SELECTION FOR TRIAL OF VAGINAL DELIVERY

It is important that the records of the previous operation and perioperative events be obtained and scrutinised. The following factors need to be considered:

1. **Scar contraindications**
   a) **Classical caesarean section** scars rupture in 3-5 per cent of subsequent pregnancies: about ten times more likely than lower segment scar rupture. Classical scar ruptures are much more likely to occur suddenly and before the onset of labour. These characteristics make them more lethal.
   b) **Low vertical caesarean** sections are usually done in early gestation when the lower uterine segment is not well enough developed to permit a large enough transverse lower segment incision. As a result these vertical incisions usually encroach on the upper uterine segment. From the point of view of subsequent labour they are probably best treated like a classical scar.
   c) **Hysterotomy** scars are treated as a classical scar.
   d) **Extension of a transverse lower segment caesarean incision** requires individual consideration. In general any marked angular or 'T' extensions are best not subjected to labour.
   e) **Myomectomy** incisions if extensive, and particularly if the uterine cavity is entered, are probably best treated by elective caesarean section.
   f) **Previous rupture** of any type of uterine scar is obviously a contraindication to subsequent labour.

2. **Previous vaginal delivery**
   This increases the safety and chances of successful VBAC.[2]

3. **Timing of previous caesarean**
   The woman who had a previous caesarean with no labour, or in the latent phase of labour, will show a nulliparous type of uterine activity in the subsequent pregnancy, requiring greater and longer uterine work to efface and dilate the cervix.[3] Those who had the previous caesarean in active labour are more likely to show the multiparous pattern with less uterine work and less strain in a subsequent labour.

4. **Uterine incision closure**
   There is some, but by no means conclusive, data that suggests that a previous single-layer uterine incision closure may be more likely than double-layer closure to rupture in a subsequent labour.[4]

5. **Post operative infection**
   Post partum endometritis may interfere with adequate healing of the uterine scar.[5] This does not mean that all previous cases with postpartum fever should be denied attempted VBAC, but it may be prudent to select out those cases with severe or obvious intrauterine sepsis for repeat caesarean section.

6. **Inter-pregnancy interval**
An inter-pregnancy interval of less than six months may be associated with an increased risk of scar rupture.[6]

7. **Recurrent indication for caesarean**
A previous caesarean for dystocia or cephalo-pelvic disproportion is not necessarily a recurrent indication and many will subsequently deliver by the vaginal route.

8. **More than one previous caesarean**
There are successful series of women who undertake VBAC after two previous caesarean sections but overall the risk of uterine rupture is probably doubled.[7,8]

9. **Twins**
There are small series showing successful VBAC in twin pregnancy.[9] However, the possible need for interuterine manipulation and over distension of the uterus potentially increases the risk.

10. **Lower uterine segment thickness**
Preliminary work in a number of women suggests that ultrasonographic measurement of the lower uterine segment in the third trimester may help select those women with a very thin lower segment and an increased risk of scar rupture.[10] Further work is required to establish the role of this promising approach.

11. **Individual factors**
A number of 'soft' factors may influence the decision including: maternal age, secondary infertility, previous perinatal morbidity or mortality.

12. **Facilities and personnel**
This is a very real and practical factor. A trial for vaginal delivery can only be contemplated in a hospital with immediately available nursing, anaesthesia and obstetric staff. In addition, appropriate operating and blood transfusion facilities must be present. These have been reviewed in national guidelines.[11,12]

13. **Informed consent:**
Unless the woman understands and accepts the principles involved, a trial for vaginal delivery is inappropriate.

MANAGEMENT OF TRIAL FOR VAGINAL DELIVERY

Antenatal Care

Apart from the careful selection of patients this will be routine.

Induction of Labour

If there is a valid indication and the cervix is favourable, amniotomy is an acceptable method of induction. Intravenous oxytocin can be used with caution if amniotomy alone does not produce progressive labour.

The use of prostaglandins to ripen an unfavourable cervix should only be undertaken with great trepidation, if at all, and only after one has answered the questions: 'Is there a compelling indication for induction?' 'Why am I not doing a repeat caesarean section?' and 'Is this medico-legally prudent?' Misoprostol has an unacceptably high risk of uterine rupture and is contraindicated.[13]

Although there is increasing experience with oxytocin and prostaglandins in women with a previous caesarean section, the fact remains that most cases of uterine rupture are associated with the use of oxytocics.[14] It seems ironic that those who 15 years ago rigidly adhered to the dictum 'once a caesarean, always a caesarean', and would not countenance a physiological contraction in women with a uterine scar, are now willing to impose prostaglandin-induced contractions on a scarred uterus with an unyielding cervix of carrot-like consistency.

Induction of labour with oxytocics, particularly prostaglandins, increases the risk of uterine rupture and the women should be so informed.[15,16]

Labour

- The woman should be advised to come into the **hospital early in labour**. On admission blood should be taken for **group and screen**. The **progress of labour** should be closely watched. Only if labour is normally progressive should the trial be continued.
- A careful watch is kept for the **signs and symptoms of impending uterine rupture** as outlined in Chapter 17. If there is any doubt about scar integrity, or if the progress of labour is slow, **discretion is the better part of valour** with early rather than late recourse to repeat caesarean section.
- The use of **epidural analgesia** in these patients is not contraindicated. The main argument against is the potential masking of the pain and tenderness of early rupture. However, this is not so and epidural analgesia can can be safely used if available and indicated.

- There is increasing data and experience with **oxytocin augmentation of labour**. However, extreme caution is advised and this should be limited to hospitals with on-site obstetric and anaesthetic personnel. If oxytocin augmentation is carried out a smooth progressive response should be expected. If this does not occur a repeat caesarean should be performed.
- Continuous electronic **fetal heart rate monitoring** is preferable. In patients with epidural analgesia and/or oxytocin augmentation, continuous monitoring is essential as fetal heart abnormalities are one of the earliest warnings of scar rupture.
- **The second stage of labour may be shortened**, but only when the head is low in the pelvis and easy assisted vaginal delivery can be accomplished. This reduces the strain on the scar which is greatest at this stage.
- The **third stage of labour** is managed in normal fashion.

The increase in primary caesarean section rates, while most pronounced in North America, is also a world-wide trend. Thus, the management of women previously delivered by caesarean section has assumed increasing importance in modern obstetric practice. Enough experience has now accumulated to show that in many obstetric units up to 50 per cent of those previously delivered by lower segment caesarean section can safely expect to deliver vaginally in a subsequent pregnancy.

As is often the case, however, the pendulum of medical management tends to swing to extremes. Excessive zeal in pursuit of vaginal delivery after previous caesarean section, more often manifest in those with limited experience, will lead to more scar ruptures. Adherence to safe guiding principles allows the majority of women to deliver vaginally with minimal risk. Pushing beyond these safe principles accomplishes few more vaginal deliveries at the cost of a sharply rising risk of scar rupture.

REFERENCES

1. Zinberg S. Vaginal delivery after previous cesarean delivery: a continuing controversy. Clin Obstet Gynecol 2001;44:561-70.
2. Zelop CM, Shipp TD, Repke JT, Cohen A, Lieberman E. Effect of previous vaginal delivery on the risk of uterine rupture during a subsequent trial of labor. Am J Obstet Gynecol 2000;183:1184-6.
3. Arulkumaran S, Gibb DMF, Ingemarson I, Kitchener HS, Ratnam SS. Uterine activity during spontaneous labour after previous lower-segment caesarean section. Br J Obstet Gynaecol 1989;96:933-8.
4. Bujold E, Bujold C, Hamilton EF, Harel R, Gauthier RJ. The impact of single-layer or double-layer closure on uterine rupture. Am J Obstet Gynecol 2002;186:1326-30.
5. Shipp TD, Zelop C, Cohen A, Repke JT, Lieberman E. Post-cesarean delivery fever and uterine rupture in a subsequent trial of labor. Obstet Gynecol 2003;101:136-9.
6. Esposito MA, Menihan CA, Malee MP. Association of interpregnancy interval with uterine scar failure in labor: a case-control study. Am J Obstet Gynecol 2000;183:1180-3.
7. Caughey AB, Shipp TD, Repke JT, Zelop CM, Cohen A, Lieberman E. Rate of uterine rupture during a trial of labor in women with one and two prior cesarean deliveries. Am J Obstet Gynecol 1999;181:872-6.
8. Bretalle F, Cravello L, Shojair R, Roger V, D'ercole C, Blanc B. Vaginal birth after two previous cesarean sections. Eur J Obstet Gynecol Reprod Biol 2001;94:23-6.
9. Delaney T, Young DC. Trial of labor compared to elective caesarean in twin gestations with a previous caesarean delivery. J Obstet Gynaecol Can 2003;25:289-92.
10. Rozenberg P, Goffinet F., Phillippe HJ. Thickness of the lower segment: its influence in the management of patients with previous cesarean sections. Eur J Obstet Gynecol Reprod Biol 1999;87:39-45.
11. Society of Obstetricians and Gynaecologists of Canada. Clinical Practice Guideline No.68. Vaginal birth after previous caesarean birth. J Soc Obstet Gynaecol Can 1997;19:1425-8.
12. American College of Obstetricians and Gynecologists. Practice Bulletin No.5. Vaginal birth after previous cesarean delivery. Washington DC:ACOG,1999.
13. Wing DA, Lovett K, Paul RH. Disruption of prior uterine incision following misoprostol for labor induction in women with previous cesarean delivery. Obstet Gynecol 1998;91:828-30.
14. Confidential Enquiry into Stillbirths and Deaths in Infancy. 5th Annual Report. London: Maternal and Child Health Consortium, 1998.
15. Ravasia DJ, Wood SL, Pollard JK. Uterine rupture during induced trial of labor among women with previous cesarean delivery. Am J Obstet Gynecol 2000;183:176-9.
16. Lydon-Rochelle M, Hoet VL, Easterling TR, Martin DP. Risk of uterine rupture during labor among women with a prior cesarean delivery. N Engl J Med 2001;345:3-8.

BIBLIOGRAPHY

Appleton B, Targett C, Rasmussen M, Readman E, Sale F, Rermezal M. Vaginal birth after caesarean section: an Australian multicentre study. Aust NZ J Obstet Gynaecol 2000;40:87-91.

Beckett VA, Regan L. Vaginal birth after cesarean: the European experience. Clin Obstet Gynecol 2001;44:594-603.

Brill Y, Windrim R. Vaginal birth after caesarean section: review of antenatal predictors of success. J Obstet Gynaecol Can 2002;25:275-86.

Chauhan SP, Magann EF, Wiggs CD, Barrilleaux PS, Martin JN. Pregnancy after classic cesarean delivery. Obstet Gynecol 2002;100:946-50.

Gee H. Trail of scar? In: Sturdee D, Olah K, Keane D.(eds). The Yearbook of Obstetrics and Gynaecology. London: RCOG Press. 2001;9:263-9.

Irvine LM, Shaw RW. Trial of scar or elective repeat caesarean section at maternal request? J Obstet Gynaecol 2001;21:463-7.

Mozurkewich EL, Hutton EK. Elective repeat cesarean delivery versus trial of labor: a meta-analysis of the literature from 1989 to 1999. Am J Obstet Gynecol 2000;183:1187-97.

Patterson LS, O'Connell CM, Baskett TF. Maternal and perinatal morbidity associated with classical and inverted T cesarean sections. Obstet Gynecol 2002;100:633-7.

Smith GCS, Pell JP, Cameron AD, Dobbie R. Risk of perinatal death associated with labor after cesarean delivery in uncomplicated term pregnancies. JAMA 2002;287:2684-90.

Socol ML. VBAC-is it worth the risk? Semin Perinatol 2003;27:105-11.

CHAPTER 19

Emergency Obstetric Hysterectomy

Emergency postpartum hysterectomy represents one of the accepted markers of severe maternal obstetric morbidity. The incidence varies from approximately 1 in 350 to 1 in 7000 deliveries. In most obstetric units the incidence is about 1 in 2000. Maternal mortality ranges from 0 to 25%. The higher incidence and mortality rates tend to occur in developing countries and in hospitals serving obstetric populations with limited resources.

CAUSES

The three main conditions leading to obstetric hysterectomy are:

1. **Abnormal placentation: placenta praevia and/or accreta**. The rising incidence of delivery by caesarean section is followed by higher risk of placenta praevia or placenta praevia accreta in subsequent pregnancies.
2. **Uterine atony**. Despite the improved availability of oxytocic drugs there are still occasions when they are ineffective, particularly in the exhausted infected uterus following prolonged labour.
3. **Uterine rupture and trauma**. Here again the rising incidence of delivery by caesarean section can be followed by greater risk of uterine rupture in subsequent pregnancies.

Other, less common causes, are sepsis and secondary postpartum haemorrhage. Previous caesarean section and caesarean delivery in the current pregnancy are additional risk factors.

Maternal mortality and morbidity are associated with haemorrhage, disseminated intravascular coagulation, transfusion of blood products, damage to bladder and/or ureters and sepsis.

SURGICAL ASPECTS

The choice between total and subtotal hysterectomy is relevant. In many cases, provided the bleeding is coming from the upper uterine segment, subtotal hysterectomy is effective, quicker, easier and less likely to injure the bladder or ureters. If, however, the cervix, lower uterine segment and/or paracolpos are involved total hysterectomy will be required to achieve haemostasis.

The following surgical tips are offered:

- Beware of the very thick, vascular and oedematous pedicles. To avoid haematoma formation double clamp the pedicle, put a free tie proximally and a second transfixing suture distal to the free tie. Smaller pedicles are more likely to be secure.
- Clamp the uterine arteries and thereafter place all other clamps medial to these thereby avoiding the ureter.
- Dissect the bladder down mostly in the midline and less laterally where the bladder pillars are extremely vascular.
- If there is any doubt about the integrity of the bladder, it can be filled with dye or sterile milk intraoperatively via Foley catheter. Be particularly cautious in the case of a ruptured lower segment scar which, due to adherence, may also tear the bladder. If in doubt the best way to establish the integrity of the ureters and bladder is to perform postoperative cystoscopy having given intravenous indigo carmine 10-15 minutes before to highlight the efflux of dye-stained urine from the ureters. If no cystoscope is available a diagnostic laparoscope or hysteroscope can be used.
- It can be hard to distinguish the level of the cervix. This is best done by entering the vagina posteriorly. If may also be helpful to put a finger through the uterine incision and down to the vagina to identify the rim of the cervix.
- Perioperative antibiotics and postoperative thromboprophylaxis should be given.

In many series up to 20-25% of patients requiring emergency obstetric hysterectomy are primiparous. Application of other techniques to deal with severe obstetric haemorrhage may be both life-saving and uterus-preserving. Many of these are covered in Chapter 20 and include techniques of uterine tamponade and the use of compression sutures. In patients with a previous caesarean section and an anterior placenta praevia in the current pregnancy, placenta accreta may be identified or highly suspected before labour and delivery. Where possible these cases should be delivered at hospitals with more sophisticated facilities so that prophylactic and/or emergency uterine artery embolisation may be performed to allow preservation of the uterus (see Chapter 6).

BIBLIOGRAPHY

Bakshi S, Meyer B A. Indications for and outcomes of emergency peripartum hysterectomy. A five-year review. J Reprod Med 2000;45: 733-7.

Baskett TF. Emergency obstetric hysterectomy. J Obstet Gynaecol 2003;23: 353-5.

Castaneda S, Karrison T, Cibils LA. Peripartum hysterectomy. J Perinat Med 2000;28: 472-81.

Chew S, Biswas A. Caesarean and postpartum hysterectomy. Singapore Med J 1998;39: 9-13.

Engelsen IB , Albrechtsen S, Iverson OE. Peripartum hysterectomy – incidence and maternal morbidity. Acta Obstet Gynecol Scand 2001;80: 409-12.

Kastner ES, Figueroa R, Garry D, Maulik B. Emergency peripartum hysterectomy: experience at a community teaching hospital. Obstet Gynecol 2002;99: 971-5.

Lau WC, Fung HY, Rogers MS. Ten years experience of cesarean and postpartum hysterectomy in a teaching hospital in Hong Kong. Eur J Obstet Gynecol Reprod Biol 1997;74: 133-7.

Sebitlone MH, Moodley J. Emergency peripartum hysterectomy. East African Med J 2001;78: 70-4.

Stanco LM, Schrimmer DB, Paul RH, Mishell DR. Emergency peripartum hysterectomy and associated risk factors. Am J Obstet Gynecol 1993;168: 879-83.

Yamamoto H, Sagae S, Nishik WA, Skuto R. Emergency postpartum hysterectomy in obstetric practice. J Obstet Gynecol Res 2000;26: 341-5.

CHAPTER 20

Complications of the third stage of labour

The third stage of labour is that period of time from the birth of the infant until delivery of the placenta and membranes. It will vary in duration: commonly lasting 5-10 minutes and seldom more than 30 minutes. Postpartum haemorrhage remains in the top five causes of direct maternal death in both the developed and developing world. Most of these deaths are ideally preventable. The more remote and unsophisticated the place of delivery, the more important it is to have a clear understanding of the third stage, its potential complications, and the value of consistent prophylaxis.

PHYSIOLOGY

In this stage of labour the uterus continues to contract rhythmically and retract progressively. Retraction is that unique property of uterine muscle whereby the shortened length of the muscle fibre is sustained even after the contraction that produced the decrease in length has passed. This uterine activity causes separation of the placenta and its passage from the upper to the lower segment, through the cervix and into the vagina.

MECHANISM OF PLACENTAL SEPARATION

There are two mechanisms that usually operate together to cause placental separation:

1. **Reduction in size of placental site:** This is by far the most important of the two mechanisms. There is a progressive decrease in the size of the placental site due to the contraction and retraction of the uterine muscle. The decrease in size of the placental bed causes the placenta to buckle and separate completely from the uterine wall. This is best illustrated by the manner in which a postage stamp stuck to an inflated balloon becomes detached when the balloon is deflated.

2. **Retro-placental haematoma formation:** At a weak contraction pressure the decidual veins are compressed but the spiral arterioles continue to pump blood into the intervillous space, resulting in a haematoma that dissects through the decidua spongiosa layer. This usually begins centrally and gradually enlarges until the entire placenta is separated.

MECHANISM OF HAEMOSTASIS

Separation of the placenta leaves a very vascular placental bed with torn arteries and ruptured venous sinuses. Haemorrhage is prevented mainly by the unique architecture of the uterine muscle fibres; the bundles of smooth muscle being arranged in a criss-cross fashion which forms a lattice-work through which the blood vessels pass. After delivery of the placenta these fibres retract, compress, and occlude the torn vessels. This muscle arrangement is often referred to as the **'living ligatures'** or **'physiological sutures'** of the uterus.

CLINICAL SIGNS OF PLACENTAL SEPARATION

1. As the placenta separates and leaves the upper uterine segment, the fundus of the **uterus rises and changes from a discoid to a more globular shape**. In many instances this can be quite difficult to appreciate clinically: the uterus will, however, be felt to contract.
2. **Bleeding:** A gush of blood usually occurs as the placenta separates, but this is not always a reliable sign of complete placental separation.
3. **Cord lengthening:** This is the most reliable clinical sign of placental separation. It is usually about 8-15 cm.

MANAGEMENT

About 30-60 seconds after the baby has been delivered the cord is clamped and cut and cord blood samples taken as indicated. The clamping forceps should then be placed on the cord at the level of the introitus, so that cord lengthening is easily seen. The attendant's hand should then cup the uterine fundus – 'guarding the fundus' – and so aid early detection of an atonic uterus filling with blood, or appreciation of the fundal changes associated with placental separation. This hand should not manipulate or 'fiddle' with the fundus which may cause partial separation, increase blood loss, or possibly stimulate a constriction ring and retention of the placenta. Fundus fiddling is one of the lower forms of third stage activity.

Once the signs of placental separation have occurred the attendant assists delivery of the placenta by controlled cord traction (Figure 20.1). The abdominal hand is placed on the lower part of the uterus

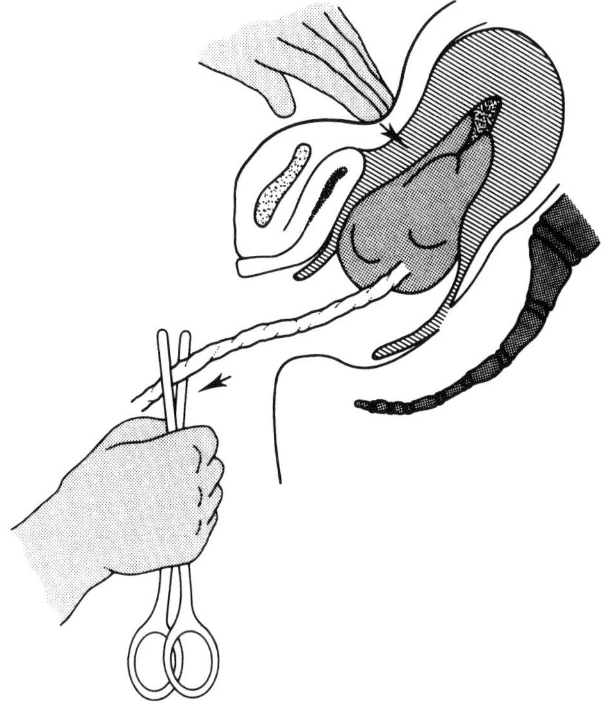

Figure 20.1 Delivery of the placenta by controlled cord traction.

pushing it up and slightly backwards as steady traction with the other hand on the cord clamp, in the axis of the pelvic curve, delivers the placenta through the cervix and out of the vagina. The placenta is then examined to check that it is complete.

There are two schools of thought in the management of the third stage of labour:

The **traditional or physiological management** is to wait for the above events to occur under the influence of normal physiological contractions. The proponents of this school argue that this is less liable to produce a retained placenta and that with careful supervision, and the availability of good oxytocic drugs, a post partum haemorrhage can be promptly and safely managed. The socially and physiologically attractive view that immediate suckling after birth reduces blood loss and post partum haemorrhage is not supported by a randomised controlled trial.[1]

Active management aims to speed up and consistently enlist the factors that normally produce placental separation and haemostasis by inducing a rapid and strong contraction with an oxytocic drug.

Randomised controlled trials have repeatedly shown that active management reduces blood loss, postpartum haemorrhage and the need for blood transfusion – all by about 40%.[2,3] The fear that routine use of an oxytocic drug will increase retained placenta and its manual removal has not been realised – although the longer acting ergometrine may slightly increase this risk.[4] Oxytocin does not and is the drug of choice. Ideally, oxytocin 5 units i.v. or 10 units i.m. should be given after delivery of the anterior shoulder. If this is not feasible it should be given as soon as possible after delivery. The evidence in favour of active management of the third stage is now overwhelming and should be accepted as the basic standard of care. As Ian Donald advocated: '*.... a more active attitude towards the third stage of labour where it is clear that nature often lets us down and masterly inactivity is only acceptable if coupled with really high grade intelligence – an unusual combination*'.[5]

The need for active prophylaxis of post partum haemorrhage continues in the 2 to 3 hours following delivery-sometimes referred to as the fourth stage of labour:

1. For the first 2-3 hours following delivery all patients should be closely observed in a special post partum recovery area. It is very easy for the exhausted, sedated patient to become profoundly shocked as her atonic uterus fills with blood unless she is carefully observed.
2. After delivery of the placenta the uterine fundus should be firmly massaged and all clots expelled. This is very important as the presence of even a few clots will interfere with retraction, and the normal haemostatic mechanism of the uterus. This leads to more oozing of blood into the uterus, more clots, more interference with retraction, and a vicious cycle develops leading to insidious and substantial blood loss.
3. All patients should have an oxytocic drug acting for at least the first two hours following delivery. This may be either 20 units oxytocin in 500 ml i.v. solution, run to keep the fundus firmly contracted, or 0.25mg ergometrine i.m., or 15-methyl prostaglandin F2 alpha 0.25 mg i.m., or misoprostol.
4. The fundus should be frequently checked and massaged to make sure it is not relaxing and that no intrauterine clots are accumulating.
5. A full bladder can also interfere with uterine retraction and this must be kept empty.

The importance of the above points cannot be overemphasized: the more unequipped the place of confinement, the more important is attention to these details. Every place where babies are delivered should have a clear and consistent policy laid down embodying these

principles. None of these routines need interfere with the early attachment of the mother and father with their new baby.
Maternal deaths due to post partum haemorrhage rarely occur within an hour of delivery, though the seeds of disaster may be sown at this time.

They usually occur in the 2-6 hours following delivery because of delayed or inadequate treatment. As Donald said: *'Beware therefore of inertia – not only in the uterus, but in the attendant!'*

OXYTOCIC DRUGS

The properties of the main oxytocic drugs will be outlined here:

Oxytocin produces rapid, strong, rhythmic contractions. Its effect lasts 15-30 minutes. The dose is 10 units intramuscularly (effective in 3-4 minutes) or 5 units intravenously (effective in 30-60 seconds). The main drawback is the short duration of action, so that a prolonged oxytocic effect requires a continuous intravenous infusion: usually 20-30 units in 500 ml crystalloid titrated to the uterine response. In large doses (usually > 200 units) given over a few hours its antidiuretic effect may be enough to cause water intoxication.

Ergometrine (ergonovine) is slightly slower to take effect but produces a more prolonged contraction: up to 60-120 minutes after intramuscular or intravenous injection of 0.25mg. As mentioned above, there is inconclusive data that this may increase the incidence of retained placenta when used in the active management of the third stage. Another potential drawback is the vasopressor effect of this drug in patients with pre-eclampsia or chronic hypertension. Occasionally this effect may be very pronounced and it should not be given to patients who are hypertensive.[6] The larger dose, 0.5 mg, should not be used initially as there is the potential for more side effects without increased efficacy.[7] Ergometrine has a long and noble history in the prevention and management of atonic postpartum haemorrhage. However, it should now be regarded as a second choice to oxytocin for routine use.

The product **Syntometrine** (5 units oxytocin and 0.5 mg ergometrine) combines the rapid onset of oxytocin with the prolonged effect of ergometrine and is used in many countries. The mild vasodilating property of oxytocin may ameliorate the vasopressor effect of ergometrine.

15-methyl prostaglandin F2 alpha: Natural prostaglandins are rapidly metabolised and therefore take high doses to get an oxytocic effect, with a concomitant high incidence of gastro-intestinal and other smooth muscle stimulation side effects. The development of the synthetic 15-methyl analogue of prostaglandin F2 alpha has overcome these drawbacks. This is about ten times as potent as the natural form of prostaglandin and its oxytocic effect lasts 4-6 hours. The dose is

Table 20.1 Oxytocic drugs

Drug	*Dose and route*	*Duration of action*	*Adverse effects*	*Contraindications*
Oxytocin	5 units IV 10 units IM 20 units in	15-30 minutes	Insignificant hypotension and flushing. Water intoxication in high doses (>200 units)	None
Ergometrine	0.2-0.25 mg IV or IM	1-2 hours	Nausea, vomiting, Hypertension. Vasospasm	Pre-eclampsia/ hypertension Cardiovascular disease
Syntometrine (5 units oxytocin 0.5mg ergometrine)	1 ampoule IM	1-2 hours	Nausea, vomiting Hypertension, Vasospasm	Pre-eclampsia/ hypertension Cardiovascular disease
15-methyl PGF2a	0.25 mg IM or IMM 0.25 mg in 500 ml infusion	4-6 hours	Vomiting, Diarrhoea, Flushing, Shivering, Vasospasm. Bronchospasm	Cardiovascular Disease Asthma
Misoprostol	400-600 ug oral 800-1000 ug rectal	1-2 hours	Nausea, Diarrhoea, Shivering, Pyrexia	None
Carbetocin	100 ug IM or IV	1-2 hours	Flushing	None

IM = intramuscular; IMM = intramyometrial; IV = intravenous

Modified from: Baskett TF, Arulkumaran S. Intrapartum Care, London: RCOG Press, 2003. With permission of RCOG Press.

0.25mg intramuscularly or intramyometrially. With this dose, there are no significant cardiovascular side effects and it can be given to hypertensive and preeclamptic patients. It is the most expensive of the oxytocic drugs.

Misoprostol is a prostaglandin E1 analogue. It is the cheapest, most stable and readily available of all the oxytocics. It is usually given orally (400-600ug) or rectally (800-1000ug). It can also be used vaginally or sublingually. Thus, it is the only oxytocic that can be given by the non-parenteral route: a big advantage in areas with limited resources. It is more effective than placebo and as, or slightly less effective than the injectable oxytocics.[8-10] Its side effects are shivering, nausea, diarrhoea and pyrexia; all of which are usually mild and rarely of clinical significance. The application of this drug, which is used off-label in obstetrics, represents a potentially huge advance for areas of the world with limited health services.

Carbetocin is a long-acting synthetic analogue of oxytocin. The dose is 100ug given by intravenous or intramuscular injection. The duration of uterotonic effect is 60-120 minutes. It is more expensive than oxytocin and so far has seen limited use as one-dose alternative to oxytocin infusion for postpartum prophylaxis against uterine atony.[11] Like oxytocin it is relatively free of side effects.

A summary of the oxytocic drugs and their qualities is shown in Table 20.1.

PRIMARY POST PARTUM HAEMORRHAGE

This has been defined as bleeding from the genital tract in excess of 500 ml within 24 hours of delivery. In fact, blood volume studies have shown that the normal parturient loses about 500 ml at delivery. However, clinical estimation of blood loss is usually about half the true blood loss. Therefore, when the clinical estimate of blood loss is 500 ml, the patient has probably lost 1000 ml. Thus, in terms of the need for urgent management the clinical definition is still a practical one to follow. The incidence of primary post partum haemorrhage is approximately 2-5 per cent and is higher in areas where active management of the third stage of labour is not practised.

AETIOLOGY

1. Failure of the uterus to contract and retract (80-90 per cent of cases):
   (a) Uterine atony, which is most often associated with:

   - High parity
   - Multiple pregnancy
   - Polyhydramnios
   - Antepartum haemorrhage
   - Prolonged labour
   - Precipitate labour
   - Deep anaesthesia
   - Full bladder

(b) Mechanical factors preventing retraction:

- Retained placenta or placental fragments
- Uterine fibroids
- Retained blood clots
- Uterine anomalies

2. Genital tract trauma and haematomas:

- Episiotomy
- Lacerations of the uterus, cervix, vagina, and perineum

3. Uterine inversion
4. Coagulation disorders

PROPHYLAXIS

1. Appropriate hospital booking of women who are at increased risk, e.g. those with a previous history of a third stage accident (20-25 per cent chance of recurrence), and those with other known predisposing causes such as grand multiparity. These patients should be delivered in a hospital with adequate anaesthetic and blood transfusion facilities.
2. Active management of the third stage:
   a) Do not 'fundus fiddle' before delivery of the placenta.
   b) Intramuscular or intravenous oxytocin with delivery of the anterior shoulder.
   c) After delivery of the placenta, massage the uterus firmly and expel all clots.
   d) Intravenous infusion of 20 units oxytocin in 500 ml crystalloid solution for at least two hours post partum.
   e) Close surveillance for 2-3 hours following delivery.

MANAGEMENT

1. Contract the uterus by:
   a) Fundal massage.
   b) Intravenous oxytocin 5 units or ergometrine 0.25 mg; these can be repeated within a few minutes if not effective.
   c) Intravenous oxytocin 30 units in 500 ml crystalloid solution run as fast as necessary to keep the uterus firmly contracted.
   d) 15-methyl prostaglandin F2 alpha (0.25 mg) i.m. or injected directly into the myometrium.
   e) Misoprostol 800-1000ug rectally.

The myometrium has different receptors for oxytocin and prostaglandins. Thus, if the uterus is unresponsive to one oxytocic, waste no time in moving to the next. It is usually best to start with oxytocin and if this fails, use ergometrine. If ergometrine is ineffective, or is contraindicated because the patient is hypertensive, then give 15-methyl PGF2 alpha or misoprostol.

2. **Deliver the placenta:** If despite the above treatment the patient continues to bleed, the placenta should be delivered. If it cannot be delivered by controlled cord traction then it should be removed manually. Ideally this should be done under general anaesthesia. If anaesthesia is not available it should be remembered that in most cases the proper application of oxytocic drugs will stem the bleeding enough to allow one to await complete separation and to deliver the placenta by controlled cord traction. If, however, the bleeding persists, manual removal will have to be performed without general anaesthesia (see later).
3. **Seek and suture** lower genital tract lacerations (see later).
4. **Explore the uterus:** If the above measures fail to stop the bleeding, and the uterus has not already been explored during manual removal, one should consider retained placental fragments, uterine rupture or incomplete uterine inversion as possible causes. If general anaesthesia is not available it may be possible to explore the uterus with the aid of inhalation, pudendal and/or paracervical block analgesia. (see Chapter 27).
5. **Treat hypovolaemia** with rapid infusion of crystalloid, colloid and blood as necessary (see Chapter 24).
6. Consider the rare case of coagulation disorder (see Chapter 8).
7. There are extremely rare instances when despite the above measures the uterus fails to contract and retract adequately to control bleeding. In such cases the following may be considered as stop gap measures before more sophisticated supportive and operative treatment:
   a) **Continuous fundal massage:** The value and efficacy of this oxytocic procedure should not be under estimated. The author has seen cases when the administration of oxytocic drugs was still associated with uterine atony which responded to properly applied fundal massage. This can be very exhausting and may require relays of 'masseurs' if it has to be carried out for any length of time. If personnel are sparse the patient herself, or husband, can be instructed how to do it. One of the most proficient the author has seen was an Inuit patient who was taught the technique by a midwife after she had a post partum haemorrhage with her first delivery. She went on to have 12 more children and, after each delivery, immediately rubbed her uterine fundus with great enthusiasm and efficiency!
   b) **Bimanual compression:** The vaginal hand forms a fist in the

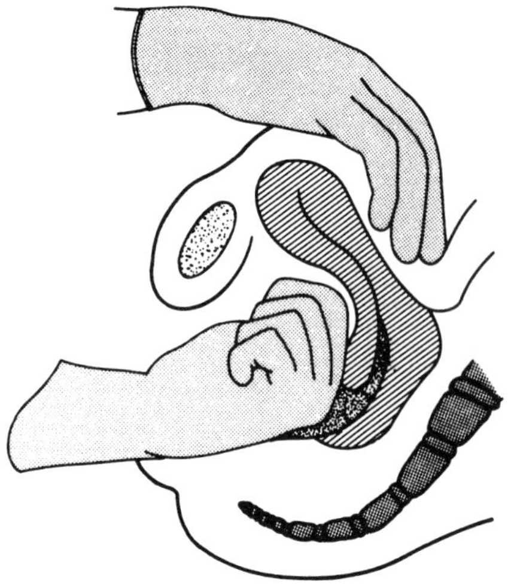

Figure 20.2 Bimanual compression of the uterus.

anterior fornix and pushes the uterus up and out of the pelvis. The abdominal hand is placed on the postero-fundal aspect of the uterus pulling it forward into the anteflexed position (Figure 20.2). In addition to the compression effect, rotary massage of the uterus between the hand and fist may aid contraction.

c) **Aortic compression:** This can be tried in thin patients. With both hands the uterus is lifted up out of the pelvis. The lower hand grips firmly across the lower part of the uterus, as though grasping a fetal head. This serves to attenuate and compress the uterine vessels. The other hand pushes the fundus posteriorly to compress the aorta.

d) **Uterine tamponade:** This can be achieved in a number of ways. Tight packing of the uterus and vagina which largely fell into disrepute in the 1960s, has re-emerged as potentially life and uterus saving in rare cases.[12] It involves very tight packing with several yards of 4-inch gauze in the uterus and vagina. A variety of balloon devices can also be used, including the Sengstaken-Blakemore tube and Rüsch urological balloon, among others.[13-15] A simplified version can be made by tying the cuff of a surgical glove to a straight plastic urinary catheter and using a large syringe to fill the glove. In all balloon applications the device is placed in the uterus and filled with fluid until it can be seen to bulge at the cervix. Observe for a few minutes to see if it has stopped the bleeding, the so-called 'tamponade test',[16] then pack the vagina with guaze and place a Foley catheter in the bladder. Cover with antibiotics and in 12-24 hours slowly deflate and remove the balloon. These procedures may be used in an attempt to save the uterus or to buy time until major vessel ligation/ embolisation or hysterectomy can be performed.

8. **Major vessel embolisation** has been used in cases of uterine atony (see Chapter 25). If hospital facilities are available, stop-gap measures such as continuous fundal massage, bimanual compression and uterine tamponade may sustain the patient until embolisation can be performed.

9. **Laparotomy:** When adequate blood transfusion and surgical facilities are available this may be necessary for those very rare cases refractory to all other measures.
   a) **Uterine and ovarian artery or internal iliac artery ligation** may be performed, and in conjunction with oxytocic drugs allow salvage of the uterus (see Chapter 25).
   b) **Uterine compression suture:** The recently described B-Lynch compression suture aims to compress the myometrium and allow preservation and function of the uterus.[17] Increasing experience with this procedure has confirmed its value, particularly in cases of uterine atony unresponsive to oxytocic drugs.[18] Modifications of the technique have been proposed.[19] Square, through-and-through compression sutures may be useful in dealing with bleeding from the lower segment in cases of placenta praevia.[20] (see Chapter 6).
   c) **Hysterectomy** is the ultimate definitive treatment and should be carried out if other measures fail, and before if child bearing is complete. There always comes a time in cases of relentless haemorrhage when the decision has to be taken to perform a life-saving hysterectomy even when future child bearing is preferred (see Chapter 19).

With the correct application of the full range of oxytocic drugs and the surgical techniques of tamponade, compression sutures and vessel ligation it should be possible to reduce the need for hysterectomy.

Any patient who develops postpartum haemorrhage associated with shock is at risk of partial or complete necrosis of the anterior pituitary **(Sheehan's syndrome)**. This is due to thrombosis and/or spasm of the pituitary portal system, so susceptible to hypovolaemia in the pregnant patient. Since the prolactin-secreting cells are usually the first affected by pituitary ischaemia it is important to note the presence or absence of lactation in the puerperium.

RETAINED PLACENTA

With the correct and active management of the third stage of labour the placenta is usually delivered within 5 to 10 minutes. The longer the placenta is retained the greater the likelihood of post partum haemorrhage. Retained placenta occurs in about 2 per cent of all deliveries and is more likely at earlier gestation.

AETIOLOGY

1. **Retention of separated placenta:**
   (a) Due to uterine atony.
   (b) Due to a constriction ring.
2. **Retention of adherent placenta:**
   (a) Ordinary adherence.
   (b) Pathological adherence due to a deficient decidual reaction. This is more likely in patients whose uterus has been subjected to previous trauma, surgery or infection. There are three degrees: **placenta accreta** is adherent to the myometrium, **placenta increta** invades the myometrium, and **placenta percreta** penetrates to the serosal layer. Placenta praevia is more prone to pathological adherence because of the limited decidual response over the lower uterine segment. Complete pathological adherence of the placenta is extremely rare but areas of partial accreta may be encountered.

MANAGEMENT

1. When the cause is uterine atony, the treatment is as for primary post partum haemorrhage.
2. If at any time the retained placenta is associated with haemorrhage, unresponsive to oxytocic drugs, the treatment is manual removal.
3. In many cases due to ordinary adherence or a constriction ring the bleeding is slight. It is customary to wait approximately 30 minutes and then do a manual removal under general or spinal anaesthesia. If the patient is not bleeding it is reasonable to marshall the staff and equipment required for manual removal under anaesthesia after 30 minutes. This often takes another 30 minutes by which time half of the cases will have resolved. If the patient happened to be delivered under epidural analgesia then this would be done after 10-15 minutes of placental retention.

   However, if anaesthesia is not available a different approach is necessary. Even a successful manual removal under anaesthesia involves increased blood loss. Attempted manual removal without anaesthesia may fail to deliver the placenta and precipitate heavy bleeding by partially separating the placenta which, when completaly adherent, did not bleed. Thus, in remote areas without anaesthesia the 30 minute rule does not apply. Provided the bleeding is minimal, an intravenous mixture of crystalloid and 20 units oxytocin should be infused to keep the uterus contracted and arrangements made to evacuate the patient to a facility where anaesthesia and blood transfusion are available. I have known patients in whom transfer was delayed up to 24 hours, arrive with the placenta still *in situ* and in good condition because the midwife did not panic and applied this treatment.

Obviously this is fraught with the potential for bleeding at any time, but under the circumstances is the best choice. Often times a constriction ring will relax and the placenta deliver normally during the period of waiting to transfer the patient. The situation changes if the patient starts and continues to bleed. The point may then be reached when the attendant will have to decide to proceed with manual removal despite lack of general anaesthesia. In such cases give 1-2 litres of intravenous crystalloid or colloid rapidly and using explanation, pudendal and paracervical block, and inhalation analgesia, proceed to manual removal.

4. Recent work has shown that in some cases of retained placenta the **intra-umbilical cord vein injection of oxytocin** (20 units mixed in 20ml normal saline) will cause separation and delivery of the placenta without elevation of maternal plasma oxytocin levels. The results of this technique are mixed but it is safe and simple and may be useful in cases in which anaesthesia is inadvisable or unavailable.[21,22]
5. In the very rare case of pathological adherence, a piecemeal manual removal may be possible if the adherence is only partial. If the pathological adherence involves the complete placenta then the treatment of choice is hysterectomy. In very rare cases where future child bearing is paramount, the placenta has been left *in situ* to slough off. This is attended by considerable risks of bleeding and infection.

Technique of Manual Removal of the Placenta (Figure 20.3)

1. Put light tension on the cord with the left hand. Place the well lubricated right hand in the vagina and follow the cord up through the cervix.
2. The left hand then firmly cups the fundus and pushes it down.
3. Keeping the fingers and thumb of the right hand extended and together, find the lower margin of the placenta.

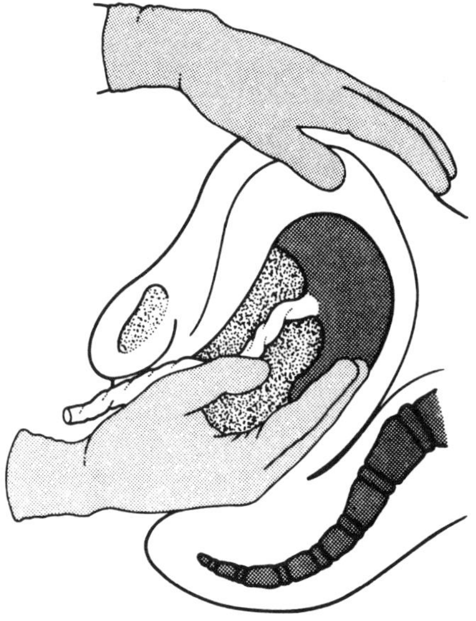

Figure 20.3 Manual removal of the placenta.

4. With side to side sawing movements of the whole hand separate through the decidua spongiosa plane of cleavage.
5. When fully separated, grasp the placenta and slowly withdraw it from the uterus. Too rapid withdrawal risks uterine inversion if any part of the placenta is still adherent.
6. Quickly re-explore the uterus for any placental fragments and integrity of the wall.
7. Run intravenous oxytocin in crystalloid to contract the uterus.
8. Check the cervix and vagina for lacerations.

GENITAL TRACT LACERATIONS AND HAEMATOMAS

LACERATIONS

These often bleed profusely and are the commonest cause of post-partum haemorrhage, except for uterine atony and retained placenta. They should always be sought when the placenta has been delivered, the uterus is firmly contracted, and the patient continues to bleed.

Periurethral and periclitoral lacerations are common. If small (<1cm) and not bleeding they require no treatment. If bleeding, or large, they should be stitched with a continuous suture.

Vaginal lacerations should also be treated with a haemostatic continuous locking suture. On occasions, particularly if one is without assistance, good lighting and retraction facilities, full exposure of higher vaginal lacerations may be impossible. In this case place a suture across the laceration as high as possible and use this as a tractor to pull the apex of the laceration into view. If, under similar circumstances, continuous oozing prevents adequate exposure and there is no arterial bleeding, one may pack the vagina tightly with a gauze pack. This is not ideal but allows time for thought gathering, an intravenous drip, and the muster of equipment and assistance. After about 30 minutes remove the pack: with diminished oozing, better light and retraction, and some assistance, suture of the lacerations should be feasible.

When dealing with higher vaginal lacerations one must have adequate anaesthesia to achieve exposure and haemostasis. If this is not available, suture what you can, clamp bleeding edges with ring forceps, pack the vagina tightly, put in a Foley catheter, run intravenous crystalloid or colloid and transfer to an appropriate facility.

Cervical lacerations: Inspection of the cervix in postpartum haemorrhage is necessary. The anterior lip is easily and painlessly grasped with ring forceps. With a second ring forceps the cervix is grasped beside the first at approximately the 2 o'clock position. The first forceps are removed and 'leap frogged' over the second to the 4 o'clock position. In this way the whole cervix can be inspected. Small lacerations of the cervix are common and usually do not bleed. They most often occur in the lateral (3 and 9 o'clock) positions. If the laceration is small (< 2 cm) and not bleeding, do not suture. You may well regret it if you do, as suturing often provokes bleeding where none existed

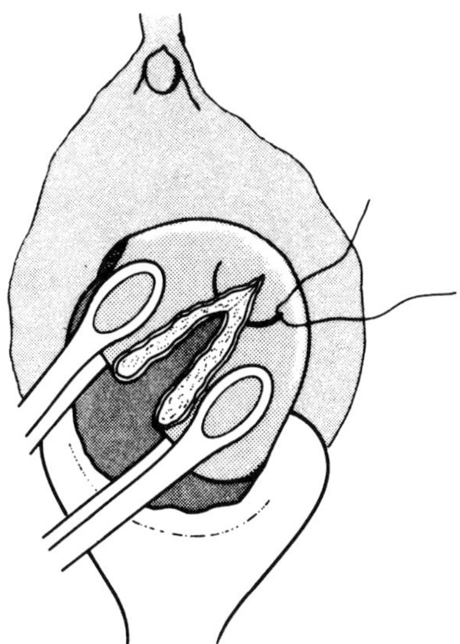

Figure 20.4 Repair of cervical laceration.

before. If the laceration is bleeding or large, use ring forceps on each side of the laceration as tractors (Figure 20.4) and place a continuous haemostatic locking suture. The post partum cervix is often bruised, oedematous, and friable causing sutures to tear out. If, because of this, inadequate exposure, or despite suturing the bleeding continues, apply ring forceps to the bleeding edges and leave them in place for several hours if necessary. This can be done with minimal disruption to the patient.

Uterine rupture (see Chapter 17).

HAEMATOMAS

These may be caused by instrumental delivery, pudendal or paracervical block. In many cases, however, they follow normal delivery, particularly precipitate labour and delivery. Often the vessel causing the haematoma is damaged without laceration of the overlying vaginal skin.

Vulval haematomas present as extremely painful and tender swellings in the area of the labium majus with the overlying skin purple and glistening. They usually manifest themselves shortly after delivery. A vulval haematoma may extend into the paravaginal tissues and ischiorectal fossa.

Paravaginal haematomas are not visible externally. The classical presentation is in the few hours following delivery with pain, restlessness, inability to pass urine, and rectal tenesmus. The condition is diagnosed by this picture plus an examination revealing a tense swelling that may occlude the vagina. The patient may be shocked from the combination of pain and blood loss.

Broad ligament and retroperitoneal haematomas may occur if a vessel ruptures above the pelvic fascia. The bleeding may track between the leaves of the broad ligament or extend retroperitoneally as far as the kidneys. A large broad ligament haematoma can be felt on bimanual examination, may push the uterus to one side and, if large enough, may track up to the pelvic brim and be felt on the lateral abdominal wall. When a broad ligament haematoma occurs one should always consider rupture of the lower uterine segment as a cause. Retroperitoneal haematomas may become very large, rupture into the peritoneal cavity, and be associated with profound hypovolaemia and shock. Ultrasound may help delineate the extent and/or progression of these haematomas.

MANAGEMENT

Vulval and paravaginal haematomas require incision and evacuation. Any bleeding points should be carefully sought and tied off.

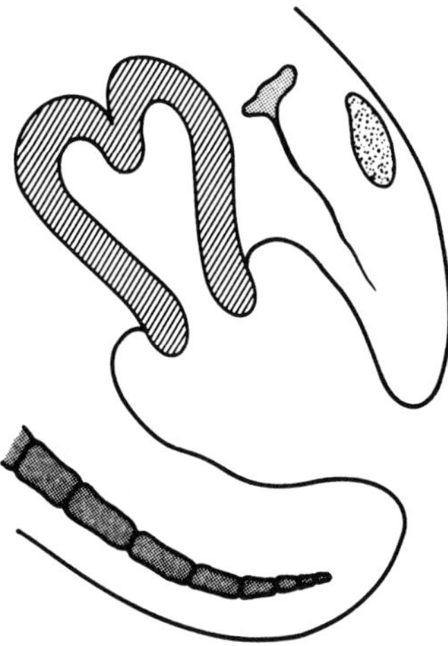

Figure 20.5 Incomplete uterine inversion.

Frequently none is found. Oozing areas may be oversewn. The vagina must be packed tightly with gauze and a Foley catheter inserted. Intravenous crystalloid or colloid should be started and blood cross-matched, in case the haematoma recurs. Both the pack and catheter may be removed in 24 hours. In order to accomplish the above, general or regional anaesthesia is required.

Broad ligament haematomas may be initially treated conservatively with intravenous crystalloid or colloid, blood cross-matched and observation. If there is no progression and the patient's vital signs are good the haematoma may be self-limiting and absorb in the coming weeks. If, however, the haematoma increases in size and the patient becomes shocked, then blood transfusion and intervention are required. At laparotomy the clot is evacuated and any bleeding points secured. An extraperitoneal drain should be inserted. On occasions hysterectomy and/or internal iliac ligation may be necessary to achieve haemostasis. If available, angiographic embolisation of the involved branches of the internal iliac vessels is the treatment of choice. This obviates the need for, and represents an attractive alternative to, surgery (see Chapter 25).[23]

ACUTE UTERINE INVERSION

This is a rare but potentially disastrous complication. The incidence varies from 1 in 2000 to 1 in 50,000 deliveries, depending upon the standard of management of the third stage of labour. There are two

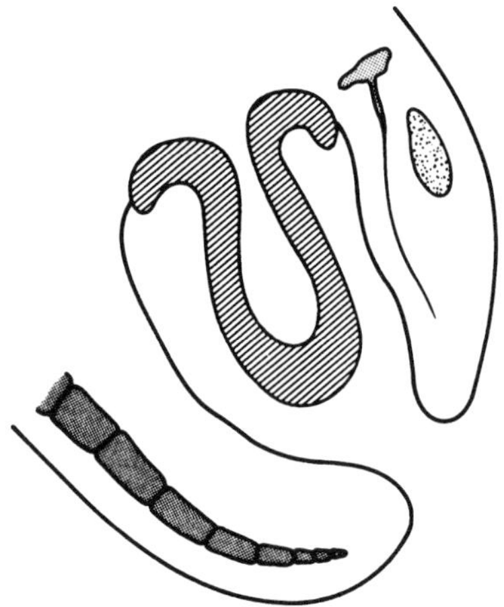

Figure 20.6 Complete uterine inversion.

types, based on the degree to which the uterine fundus turns itself inside out.

Incomplete inversion occurs when the fundus, though inverted, does not herniate through the cervix (Figure 20.5).

Complete inversion occurs when the fundus has passed completely through the cervix and lies within the vagina, or more rarely outside the vulva (Figure 20.6).

AETIOLOGY

1. Mismanagement of the third stage involving fundal pressure and/or cord traction performed before placental separation when the uterus is relaxed. This is a factor in the majority of cases.
2. Sudden rise in intra-abdominal pressure when the uterus is relaxed, e.g. coughing or vomiting.
3. Short cord-either short or shortened by being wrapped around the baby.
4. Fundal insertion of the placenta is probably an important predisposing factor in most of the above causes.
5. Rapid withdrawal of the placenta during manual removal.

DIAGNOSIS

1. Incomplete inversion can be quite deceptive and the dimpling of the uterine fundus may be missed on abdominal palpation. It will only become apparent with vaginal or uterine exploration, usually done because of persistent post partum bleeding. On rare occasions

incomplete inversion may not manifest itself immediately, but progress to complete inversion a few days after delivery.

2. Sudden and profound shock is the most common presentation of complete inversion. This is usually due to both neurogenic and hypovolaemic components. The neurogenic element is due to the traction on the infundibulo-pelvic ligaments, round ligaments, and ovaries. After the initial neurogenic shock, heavy bleeding commonly leads to hypovolaemia.
3. The patient may experience severe lower abdominal pain and a bearing down sensation.

MANAGEMENT

It is wrong to assume that all of the shock is neurogenic in origin, even if the apparent blood loss is not great. Therefore intravenous crystalloid should be rapidly infused and cross-matched blood obtained as soon as possible.

Delay in replacement of the uterus is acccompanied by the formation of the cervical ring and increasing oedema and congestion of the uterus. Thus, the sooner the diagnosis is made, and the earlier attempted correction is carried out, the more likely is an easy and successful replacement of the uterus.

1. As soon as the inversion is recognised try **manual replacement** of the uterus without removing the placenta. If the inversion is diagnosed as soon as it occurs, this may occasionally be achieved without anaesthesia.
2. If a single attempt without anaesthesia does not succeed then do not persist, as you will almost certainly fail and worsen the patient's condition. Instead await the induction of regional or general **anaesthesia** and repeat the attempt at manual replacement. Provided this is done within one hour of inversion it is likely to succeed.
3. The **technique for replacement** is to cup the fundus in the palm of the hand and, with the finger tips at the junction of the corpus and cervix, lift the entire uterus out of the pelvis toward the umbilicus (Figure 20.7). This position may need to be held for 3-5 minutes before correction occurs. On occasions countertraction with ring forceps on the lips of the cervix may help. Once corrected, the placenta, if not previously delivered, is removed manually and withdrawn slowly. An intravenous oxytocin infusion is run and the uterus re-explored to ensure that inversion is not recurring. The oxytocin infusion and fundal checks should be continued for several hours. Alternatively, 15-methyl prostaglandin F2 alpha or misoprostol may be used to reduce the risk of excess oxytocin administration and water intoxication.

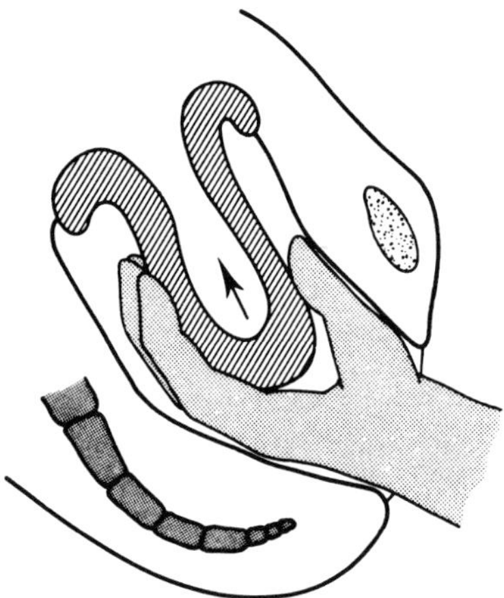

Figure 20.7 Manual replacement of uterine inversion.

4. **Tocolytic agents** may be successful in relaxing the cervical constriction ring enough to allow manual replacement – occasionally without anaesthesia, but more often as an adjunct to a regional anaesthetic. The drug of choice here is intravenous nitroglycerin, given in aliquots of 100-200 ug every 2-3 minutes until relaxation occurs (see Chapter 10).
5. If this fails the **hydrostatic method of O'Sullivan** may work.[24] First ensure that there are no tears in the vagina, cervix or uterus-if there are they should be sutured. One litre bags of warmed saline and an intravenous giving set can be used with a pressure infuser. With one hand in the vagina guide the tubing into the posterior fornix. The other hand seals the labia around the forearm. The saline bag is raised 1-2 metres above the level of the vagina. As the vaginal vault is distended with fluid the fornices are ballooned and stretched, pulling on the constricting cervical ring and allowing replacement of the inversion. The amount of fluid required may be up to 3-5 litres. Alternatively the intravenous set can be attached to a silastic ventouse cup which may help provide a better seal at the introitus.[25]
6. If the inversion is refractory to the above treatment, which is rare, surgical correction will probably be required. At laparotomy, the inversion may be reduced with **Huntington's technique** using tenacula to grasp the inverted uterine fundus in sequential fashion until the entire inversion has been corrected. If the constriction ring is too tight to allow this, the **Haultain technique** of incising the constriction ring posteriorly is required to allow correction of the inversion.
7. If facilities for general anaesthesia are not available, and an attempt to replace the inversion without it is unsuccessful, the situation is

indeed grave. If the placenta is completely attached, do not remove it as this will cause more bleeding. An attempt can be made to lessen the neurogenic component of the shock by replacing the uterus in the vagina and elevating the end of the bed to reduce the tension on the uterine supports. Small doses of intravenous morphia can be given. Intravenous crystalloid and colloid should be run to try and counteract hypovolaemia, with the addition of oxytocin if there is bleeding from uterine atony. Arrangements should be made to evacuate the patient to an appropriate hospital at once. If this is not feasible, or it appears the patient may succumb before she can be transferred, it is worth trying tocolysis with nitroglycerin and/or O'Sullivan's hydrostatic method with the aid of inhalation analgesia and local anaesthetic infiltration.

In hospitals with trained personnel, anaesthesia facilities, and blood transfusion acute uterine inversion is rarely fatal. However, if it occurs without these facilities the risk of maternal death is great. Hence the emphasis on meticulous management of the third stage, and the need for early diagnosis of this condition when immediate replacement without anaesthesia may be feasible.

SECONDARY POST PARTUM HAEMORRHAGE

Although not a complication of the third stage of labour, this condition will be discussed in this section. Abnormal bleeding between 24 hours and 6 weeks post partum occurs in approximately I per cent of cases, with the majority presenting between 5 and 10 days after delivery.

AETIOLOGY

1. Retained placental fragments (found in about 30 per cent).
2. Intrauterine infection (often coexists with the above).
3. Lacerations and haematomas.
4. Submucous fibroid.
5. Trophoblastic disease (a very rare but important cause).
6. Chronic uterine inversion.

MANAGEMENT

One of the main problems in the management of these patients is in the selection of those that require exploration of the uterus with curettage. In some cases the initial bleed may be quite mild and settle, only to be followed hours, or days, later by serious haemorrhage. In general those patients with heavy bleeding and those with evidence of intrauterine sepsis or subinvolution on bimanual examination require immediate exploration as follows:

1. Intravenous crystalloid and blood cross-match.
2. Intravenous antibiotics if any signs of sepsis.
3. Under anaesthesia using the finger and ring forceps seek, loosen and remove any placental tissue. Follow this with cautious curettage. Any tissue should always be sent for histopathological diagnosis – keeping in mind the very rare case of trophoblastic disease.

There are two serious potential complications of exploration of the uterus in these patients. The placental tissue can become quite organized and adherent to the myometrium – indeed the retained placental fragments may represent small isolated areas of placenta accreta. In removing these fragments, strips of myometrium may be torn off. This, plus the curettage disrupting thrombosed vessels, may on occasion lead to severe haemorrhage. The other potential risk is uterine perforation. These cases are unresponsive to oxytocics and may require hysterectomy for control. Occasionally, if future child bearing is paramount, careful and tight uterine and vaginal packing, or balloon tamponade under general anaesthesia may be haemostatic. The pack or balloon is removed in 12-24 hours. Alternatively, if available, angiographic vessel embolisation may avoid laparotomy and hysterectomy (see Chapter 25).

If the bleeding is mild and settles, if there are no signs of sepsis, and if the uterus is firm, not tender and appropriately involuted, then conservative treatment is justified. When available, ultrasound may help consolidate this decision if it shows the uterine cavity to be empty.

REFERENCES

1. Bullough CHW, Msuku RS, Karonde L. Early suckling and postpartum haemorrhage: controlled trial in deliveries by traditional birth attendants. Lancet 1989;2: 522-25.
2. Prendiville W, Elbourne D, Chalmers I. The effects of routine oxytocic administration in the management of the third stage of labour: an overview of the evidence from controlled trials. Br J Obstet Gynaecol 1988; 95: 3-16.
3. Nordstrom L, Fogelstam K, Fridman G, Larsson A, Rydhstroem PH. Routine oxytocin in the third stage of labour: a placebo controlled randomised trial. Br J Obstet Gynaecol. 1997;104:781-6.
4. Hammar M, Bostrom K, Borgvall B. Comparison between the influence of methyergometrine and oxytocin on the incidence of retained placenta in the third stage of labour. Gynecol Obstet Invest 1990;30:91-4.
5. Donald I. In: Practical Obstetric Problems. 3rd ed. London: Lloyd-Luke. 1966 p. ix.
6. Browning DJ. Serious side effects of ergometrine and its use in routine obstetric practice. Med J Aust 1974;1: 957-61.
7. Paull JD, Ratten GJ. Ergometrine and third stage blood loss. Med J Aust 1977;1:178-9.

8. Gühmezoglu AM, Villar J, Ngoc NT et al. WHO multicentre randomised trial of misoprostol in the management of the third stage of labour. Lancet 2001;358:689-95.
9. Caliskan E, Meydanli MM, Dilbaz B, Aykan B, Sönmezer M, Haberal A. Is rectal misoprostol really effective in the treatment of third stage of labor? A randomised controlled trial. Am J Obstet Gynecol 2002;187:1038-45.
10. Sharma S, El-Refaey H. Prostaglandins in the prevention and management of postpartum haemorrhage. Best Prac Res Clin Obstet Gynaecol 2003;17:811-23
11. Boucher M, Horbay GLA, Griffin P et al. Double-blind, randomized comparison of the effect of carbetocin and oxytocin on intraoperative blood loss and uterine tone of patients undergoing cesarean section. J Perinatol 1998;18:202-7.
12. Maier RC. Control of postpartum hemorrhage with uterine packing. Am J Obstet Gynecol 1993;169:17-23.
13. Chan C, Razyi K, Thom KF, Arulkumaran S. The use of a Sengstaken-Blakemore tube to control postpartum haemorrhage. Int J Gynecol Obstet 1997;58:251-2.
14. Johanson R, Kumar M, Obhrai M, Young P. Management of massive postpartum haemorrhage: use of hydrostatic balloon catheter to avoid laparotomy. Br J Obstet Gynaecol 2001;108:420-2.
15. Bakri YN, Amri A, Jabbar FA. Tamponade balloon for obstetrical bleeding. Int J Gynecol Obstet 2001;74:139-42.
16. Condous GS, Arulkumaran S, Symonds I, Chapman R, Suiha A, Razvi K. The "tamponade test" in the management of massive postpartum haemorrhage. Obstet Gynecol 2003;101:767-72.
17. B-Lynch C, Coker A, Lowell AH, Abu J, Cowan MJ. The B-Lynch surgical technique for the control of massive postpartum haemorrhage: an alternative to hysterectomy? Five cases reported. Br J Obstet Gynaecol 1997;104:372-5.
18. Smith KL, Baskett TF. Uterine compression sutures as an alternative to hysterectomy for severe postpartum haemorrhage. J Obstet Gynaecol Can 2003;25:197-200.
19. Hayman RG, Arulkumaran S, Steer PJ. Uterine compression sutures: surgical management of postpartum haemorrhage. Obstet Gynecol 2002;99:502-6.
20. Cho JH, Jun HS, Lee CN. Hemostatic technique for uterine bleeding during cesarean delivery. Obstet Gynecol 2000;96:129-31.
21. Gazvaric MR, Luckas MJM, Drakeley AJ et al. Intraumbilical oxytocin for the management of retained placenta: a randomised controlled trial. Obstet Gynecol 1998;91:203-7.
22. Carroli G, Belizan JM, Grant A et al. Intra-umbilical vein injection and retained placenta: evidence from a collaborative large randomised controlled trial. Br J Obstet Gynaecol 1998;105:179-85.
23. Chin HG, Scott DR, Resnik R et al. Angiographic embolization of intractable puerperal hematomas. Am J Obstet Gynecol 1989; 160: 434-8.
24. O'Sullivan JV. Acute inversion of the uterus. BMJ 1945; 2: 282-4.
25. Ogueh O, Ayida G. Acute uterine inversion: a new technique of hydrostatic replacement. Br J Obstet Gynaecol 1997;104:951-2.

BIBLIOGRAPHY

Baskett TF, Writer DR. Postpartum hemorrhage. In: Datta S (ed). Anesthetic and Obstetric Management of High Risk Pregnancy. New York: Mosby, 1996.pp 110-33.

Baskett TF. A flux of the reds: evolution of active management of the third stage of labour. J R Soc Med 2000;93:489-93.

Baskett TF. Acute uterine inversion: a review of 40 cases. J Obstet Gynaecol Can 2002;24:953-6.

Drife J. Management of primary postpartum haemorrhage. Br J Obstet Gynaecol 1997;104:275-7.

Dombrowski MP, Bottoms SF, Saleh AA et al. Third stage of labor: analysis of duration and clinical practice. Am J Obstet Gynecol 1995;172:1279-84.

El-Refaey H, O'Brien P, Morafa W, Walder J, Rodeck C. Use of oral misoprostol in the prevention of postpartum haemorrhage. Br J Obstet Gynaecol 1997;104:336-9.

Elbourne D, Prendiville W, Chalmers I. Choice of oxytocic preparation for routine use in the management of the third stage of labour: an overview of the evidence from controlled clinical trials. Br J Obstet Gynaecol 1988;95: 17-30.

Granstrom L, Ekinan G, Ulmsten U. Intravenous infusion of 15 methyl prostaglandin F2 alpha in women with heavy post-partum haemorrhage. Acta Obstet Gynecol Scand 1989; 68: 365-7.

Hoveyda F, Mackenzie IZ. Secondary postpartum haemorrhage: incidence, morbidity and current management. Br J Obstet Gynaecol 2001;108:927-30.

Hsu S, Rodgers B, Lele A, Yeh J. Use of packing in obstetric hemorrhage of uterine origin. J Reprod Med 2003;48:67-71.

Mamani AW, Hassan A. Treatment of puerperal uterine inversion by the hydrostatic method: Report of five cases. Eur J Obstet Gynaecol Reprod Biol 1989;32:281-5.

Mousa HA, Walkinshaw S. Major postpartum haemorrhage. Curr Opin Obstet Gynaecol 2001;13:595-603.

Ridgway LE. Puerperal emergency: vaginal and vulvar hematoma. Obstet Gynecol Clin North Am 1995;22:275-82.

Sawhney H, Gopalan S. Home deliveries and third stage complications. Aust NZ J Obstet Gynaecol 1994;34:531-4.

Society of Obstetricians and Gynaecologists of Canada. Clinical Practice Guideline No.88. Prevention and management of postpartum haemorrhage. J Obstet Gynaecol Can 2000,22:271-81.

Skinner J, Turner MJ. Postpartum exploration of the genital tract under general anaesthesia reviewed. J Obstet Gynaecol 1997;17:273.

Soriano D, Dulitzki M, Schiff E, Barkai G, Mashiach S, Seidman DS. A prospective cohort study of oxytocin plus ergometrine compared with oxytocin alone for prevention of postpartum haemorrhage. Br J Obstet Gynaecol 1996;103:1068-73.

Wendel PJ, Cox SM. Emergent obstetric management of uterine inversion. Obstet Gynecol Clin North Am 1995;22:261-74.

CHAPTER 21

Post partum infection

Puerperal sepsis is a major cause of maternal morbidity and remains in the top five causes of maternal death. Post partum pelvic infection occurs in about 1-3 per cent of vaginal deliveries, but is 10 to 20 times more likely in patients delivered by caesarean section. The serious sequelae of septic shock, pelvic abscess and septic pelvic thrombophlebitis occur in < 2 per cent of appropriately treated patients. In only 10 per cent is bacteraemia demonstrable.

PATHOPHYSIOLOGY

The scourge of the pre-antibiotic era – 'childbed fever' – puerperal sepsis due to group A beta-haemolytic streptococci, spread from exogenous sources, is a rare occurrence nowadays – although occasional life-threatening cases still occur.[1] The normal flora of the female lower genital tract contains many potential pathogens. It is this endogenous source that provides the causative organisms for most cases of puerperal pelvic infection.

Certain factors operating in pregnancy help protect against infection: the amniotic fluid is bactericidal and the number and activity of white blood cells increase during labour and the early puerperium. On the other hand the traumatised and necrotic tissues of the genital tract following delivery allow access and provide a culture medium for ascending infection.

Most infections are polymicrobial involving a mixture of aerobic and anaerobic bacteria indigenous to the lower genital tract of the patient. Commonly involved organisms are anaerobic streptococci, *E. coli, Klebsiella, and Bacteroides* species. Other less frequently incriminated organisms are *Clostridia, Staphylococcus aureus* and *Pseudomonas*. Group B beta-haemolytic streptococci are more likely to cause neonatal sepsis but can also cause puerperal pelvic infection.

Predisposing factors to puerperal sepsis include:

1. Caesarean section is the most important predisposing factor. The

suturing and ischaemic necrosis of infected muscle along the uterine incision provide an ideal environment for sepsis.

2. Prolonged labour and ruptured membranes leading to chorioamnionitis.
3. Trauma and tissue necrosis associated with vaginal delivery. The following factors have been incriminated as increasing this risk, though by no means consistently:
   - Forceps delivery.
   - Episiotomy.
   - Manual removal of placenta.
   - Repeated vaginal examinations during labour.
   - Intrauterine manipulation, e.g. internal version.
   - Internal monitoring of fetal heart and uterine contractions.
4. Low socio economic status.

The initial infection is usually confined to the endometrium and myometrium – endomyometritis. If not adequately treated the infection may spread directly or via the lymphatics to cause parametritis, salpingooophoritis, pelvic peritonitis, septic pelvic thrombophlebitis, pelvic abscess, generalised peritonitis, and intra-abdominal abscesses with associated bacteraemia and septicaemia.

CLINICAL FEATURES

Puerperal pelvic infection can present with varying degrees of symptoms and signs. **Mild endometritis** usually presents 2-3 days after delivery with a low grade temperature, lower abdominal pain, and slight uterine tenderness. Cases of **severe endomyometritis** present with a higher temperature (> 38.5°C), general malaise, anorexia, foul lochia, abdominal pain, uterine tenderness, and subinvolution. As the infection spreads beyond the uterus, parametrial tenderness and signs of pelvic and generalised peritonitis may develop.

With appropriate treatment it is rare for a **pelvic abscess** to develop. This should be suspected if the patient is ill with a spiking temperature, vomiting with lower abdominal pain and ileus, and a tender mass in the pelvis. The latter can be hard to feel and ultrasound examination may assist localisation.

Puerperal sepsis due to group A beta-haemolytic streptococci may run a fulminant course with a rapidly progressive pelvic cellulitis, peritonitis, and septicaemia. It should be treated with high dose benzyl penicillin. If group A beta-haemolytic streptococcus is cultured, hospital personnel must be screened to try and identify the source.

DIAGNOSIS

When a recently delivered patient develops a temperature a careful clinical appraisal should consider the following sources of infection:

1. Endomyometritis.
2. Urinary tract.
3. Episiotomy site.
4. Abdominal incision.
5. Pulmonary – particularly if general anaesthesia used.
6. Epidural site.
7. Breast.
8. Thrombophlebitis: legs, pelvis, intravenous site.
9. Others: e.g. influenza.

If the clinical picture suggests endomyometritis the following cultures should be considered:

1. Vaginal/cervical cultures are of limited value only to seek the acquired organisms-chlamydia, gonococci and group A beta-haemolytic streptococci, as well as the endogenous group B beta-haemolytic streptococci.
2. Intrauterine aerobic and anaerobic cultures are the ideal, but hard to get. If the cervix is cleansed, a soft catheter can be passed and uterine contents aspirated with a syringe.
3. Blood, urine, and incision sites may also be cultured if clinically indicated.
4. At the time of caesarean section in high risk cases, it is reasonable to take intrauterine aerobic and anaerobic cultures.

Depending on local experience and economic considerations, an argument can be made for limiting cultures in mild, clinically straightforward cases.

The white cell count and differential are of limited value as they are frequently abnormal in the early puerperium even in uninfected patients.

MANAGEMENT

PREVENTION

Although most of the causative organisms are endogenous this should not be an excuse for slovenly technique. The value of correct aseptic technique, limitation of pelvic examinations during labour, and minimising trauma to tissues during operative delivery should not be underestimated.[2]

Over the last 20 years the use of prophylactic antibiotics at the time of caesarean section, both elective and in labour, has consistently been shown to reduce post-operative febrile morbidity and the duration of hospital stay.[3,4] It is advocated that patients who have a caesarean section be given one dose of a simple broad spectrum antibiotic such as ampicillin or cefazolin when the cord is clamped. However, in patients with prolonged rupture of membranes and labour, plus other high-risk factors, it may be advisable to continue prophylactic antibiotics for 24-48 hours. It may seem illogical that antibiotic prophylaxis effective only against aerobes should be so effective in preventing sepsis known to have anaerobic involvement in the majority of cases. However, it is likely that the reduction of aerobic bacterial infection cuts down the tissue destruction and pus formation that provide the conditions necessary for the anaerobic bacteria to multiply. This allows the normal host defences to cope with the anaerobes.

TREATMENT

Most cases of endomyometritis are caused by mixed infection with both aerobes and anaerobes. The choice of antibiotics will depend on their availability and expense, as well as knowledge of local organisms and their sensitivity. Treatment has to be started before culture results are available and is therefore based on past experience and the probable organisms involved. The development of broad-spectrum cephalosporins and the newer penicillins have made it possible to treat many patients with single-agent therapy which may be less toxic. In practice, the following guidelines are acceptable:

1. Mild cases following vaginal delivery will usually respond to a simple broad-spectrum antibiotic such as ampicillin 1 g i.v. every 4-6 hours.

2. Endomyometritis following caesarean delivery should be given intravenous antibiotics as follows:
   Cefoxitin 2 g every 6 hours
   or
   Aminoglycoside (gentamicin or tobramycin) 5mg/Kg q 24hr plus Clindamycin 600-900 mg every 8 hours.

3. If the temperature persists for 48-72 hours after treatment, then one should suspect wound sepsis or infection with an organism resistant to the chosen antibiotics. If there is no wound infection the antibiotics can be changed on the basis of culture results if available, and if not, on the basis of probabilities. Thus, patients who were initially started on the aminoglycoside/clindamycin combination should have

penicillin added (5 million units every 6 hours) to cover the enterococcus, which is the most likely causative organism resistant to aminoglycoside/clindamycin. Patients who were initially started on cefoxitin should be changed to the clindamycin/aminoglycoside/penicillin combination.

Treatment with intravenous antibiotics should be continued for 48 hours after the patient's fever and symptoms have abated. Continued treatment with oral antibiotics is not necessary.

4. Septic shock can develop and is treated along the lines described in Chapter 3.

The more antibiotics used, the greater the risk of maternal toxic effects, particularly necrotising colitis. For this reason, single and double agent antibiotic therapy is chosen initially and is adequate in the vast majority of cases. It should be stressed, however, that this will depend on local factors and is some large hospitals the experience with certain high-risk groups of patients may dictate the earlier and more frequent use of triple antibiotic therapy.

Antibiotics will appear in breast milk in small amounts. In most instances this is probably of no clinical significance. However, it must be remembered that the neonate with immature enzyme systems may not excrete the antibiotic efficiently and thus get a cumulative effect. With some of the more potentially toxic antibiotics it may be wise to temporarily discontinue breast feeding and maintain lactation by pumping.

A **puerperal pelvic abscess** is most likely to point in the pouch of Douglas, in which case drainage via posterior colpotomy is indicated. On other occasions the abscess may extend above the inguinal ligament where incision and drainage are feasible.

Septic pelvic thrombophlebitis is more likely to be associated with anaerobic sepsis. The incidence of this condition has fallen with earlier recognition and better treatment of anaerobic infections. The diagnosis is usually made in a patient already on adequate antibiotic coverage, without evidence of a pelvic abscess, in whom a high spiking fever persists. On rare occasions there may be septic pulmonary emboli. Usually the diagnosis is impossible to confirm absolutely and is one of exclusion. The treatment is intravenous heparin infusion which reduces the risk of embolisation and also seems to improve the patient's response to the pelvic infection. If the diagnosis is correct the response is usually dramatic with resolution of the fever within 24-72 hours of initiation of heparin treatment.

Episiotomy infection, if recognised early, is usually successfully treated by antiobiotics and sitz baths. If there is any fluctuation or pus, removal of sutures to allow drainage is required. This is usually all that is needed and even quite large gaping areas will granulate and heal well in the ensuing weeks. Early debridement and re-suturing are feasible but must be delayed until all infection is eradicated.[5,6]

Necrotising fasciitis is a very rare but serious condition, with a high mortality that may follow caesarean section,vaginal delivery and episiotomy. The organisms involved are usually mixed aerobes and anaerobes. The clinical picture is one of rapid progression of local inflammation and oedema followed by gangrene and necrosis of the skin and underlying fascia. The patient is toxic and febrile. High dose antibiotics in a manner similar to that for septic shock should be given (see Chapter 3). The most important part of treatment is early and extensive surgical debridement.[7,8]

Puerperal mastitis may occur on a sporadic or epidemic basis. The offending organism is usually *Staphylococcus aureus*, which is often penicillin-resistant. Other organisms less commonly incriminated are *Streptococcus pyogenes, Staphylococcus albus*, and *Escherichia coli*. The source of infection is the baby, the mother or carrier personnel. Nipple fissures, milk stasis, poor hygiene and technique are predisposing factors. The onset is usually between one and three weeks post partum, but can be any time during lactation. The clinical presentation is fever, chills, and pain along with local tenderness, swelling, and redness in the breast: often the upper outer quadrant.

The following treatment is recommended:

1. The breast milk, baby and mother, should be cultured. If hospital carriers are found, appropriate isolation and treatment techniques are followed.
2. While awaiting the culture results the mother should be treated with penicillin G and a penicillinase-resistant penicillin such as methicillin or cloxacillin. Depending on the culture results, one of these can be stopped or another appropriate antibiotic started.
3. It is often advised that breast feeding should be discontinued. In fact the opposite is true; the breast should be thoroughly emptied by feeding and manual expression. The importance of emptying the breasts and avoiding stasis cannot be overemphasised.

The early diagnosis and institution of the above treatment is essential to prevent the progression to abscess formation. Most cases will resolve rapidly with the above treatment, although the antibiotics should be continued for 7-10 days.

If a breast abscess develops it should be drained by a radial incision under general anaesthesia. A finger is inserted through the incision to break down any loculi and the cavity drained or packed with gauze. Antibiotics should also be given as above.

REFERENCES

1. Kent ASH, Haider Z, Beynon JL. Puerperal sepsis: a disease of the past? Br J Obstet Gynaecol 1999;106:1314-5.
2. Iffy L, Kaminetsky HA, Maidman JE. Control of perinatal infection by traditional, preventive measures. Obstet Gynecol, 1979;54: 403-11.
3. Mugford M, Kingston J, Chalmers 1. Reducing the incidence of infection after caesarean section: implications of prophylaxis with antibiotics for hospital resources. BMJ 1989;299: 1003-6.
4. Bagratee, Moodley J, Kleinschmidt I, Zawilski W. A randomised controlled trial of antibiotic prophylaxis in elective caesarean section. Br J Obstet Gynaecol 2001;108:143-8.
5. Hankins GDV, Hauth JC, Gilstrap LC. Early repair of episiotomy dehiscence. Obstet Gynecol 1990;75: 48-51.
6. Arona AJ, Al-Marayati L, Grimes DA et al. Early secondary repair of third and fourth degree perineal lacerations after outpatient wound preparation. Obstet Gynecol 1995;86:294-6.
7. Ammari N N, Hasweh YG, Hassan AA, Karyoute S. Postpartum necrotising fasciitis. Br J Obstet Gynaecol 1986;93: 82-3.
8. Pauzner D, Wolman I, Abramov L. Post cesarean necrotizing fasciitis: report of a case and review of the literature. Gynecol Obstet Invest 1994;37:59-62.

BIBLIOGRAPHY

Baker CJ. Group B streptococcal infections. Clin Perinatol 1997;24:59-70.

Balk RA. Severe sepsis and septic shock: definitions, epidemiology, and clinical manifestations. Crit Care Clin 2000,16:179-92.

Calhoun BC, Brost B. Emergency management of sudden puerperal fever. Obstet Gynecol Clin North Am 1995;22:357-67.

Del Priore G, Stone MJ, Shin EK et al. A comparison of once-daily and 8-hour gentamicin dosing in the treatment of postpartum endometritis. Obstet Gynecol 1996;87:994-1000.

Edwards MS. Antibacterial therapy in pregnancy and neonates. Clin Perinatol 1997;24:251-66.

Faro S. Sepsis in obstetric and gynecology patients. Curr Clin Top Infect Dis 1999;19:60-82.

Goepfert AC, Guinn DA, Andrews WW et al. Necrotizing fasciitis after cesarean delivery. Obstet Gynecol 1997;89:409-12.

Henderson EJ, Love EJ. Incidence of hospital-acquired infections associated with caesarean section. J Hosp Infect 1995;29:245-55.

Noronha S, Yue CT, Sekosan M. Puerperal group A beta-hemolytic streptococcal toxic shock-like syndrome. Obstet Gynecol 1996;87:728.

Summers PR. Surgical aspects of peripartal infection. Clin Obstet Gynecol 1994;37:324-36.

CHAPTER 22

Post partum depression

Pregnancy and childbirth represent a time of increased vulnerability to mental illness, most often exhibited postpartum. The most extreme manifestation of this disorder is evident in the latest United Kingdom review of maternal deaths: 12 per cent of which were associated with psychiatric disorders. In the triennial review, 1997-99, there were 42 psychiatric related maternal deaths, of which 28 were by suicide.[1] Many cases of infanticide and child abuse are linked to post partum mental disorders. At a less dramatic level there may be untold misery for the woman and her husband, as well as a deleterious effect on their attachment to the baby.

For the doctor without specialised training in psychiatry, three main types of post partum mental disturbance should be recognised:

1. 'POST PARTUM BLUES'

This affects 50-60 per cent of normal women on the third to fifth day post partum. The predominant symptoms are lethargy, irritability, weeping, and anxiety over their ability to cope with the baby. The probable basis is a combination of psychological adjustment and profound hormonal and metabolic changes. The rapid physiological withdrawal of steroid hormones, particularly progesterone, has been linked with postpartum blues.[2,3] The only treatment required is explanation, reassurance, and support. The condition resolves within two weeks. A minority of women feel unusually elated-sometimes called the 'post partum pinks'.

2. POST PARTUM DEPRESSION

About 10 per cent of women will need some type of medical support for depression, usually mild and transitory, in the puerperium. Perhaps it should not surprise us that some degree of puerperal depression is so common. When the immediate post partum applause has died down and the congratulatory flowers have withered the woman is left with the harsh reality of looking after an unpredictable and demanding baby.

The emotional and physical strain of meeting the baby's relentless requirements day and night are considerable. She may have ambivalent feelings towards the baby as the cause of a changed relationship with her husband, career interruption, and her altered physical image. These feelings are normal, but all that she reads and hears from society suggests that this should be a time of ultimate joy. A lack of extended family presence and support may cause further feelings of isolation. Overzealous and rigid antenatal classes, extolling the virtues of analgesia-free labour and breast feeding, can backfire on the woman who feels she has failed if she does not achieve these aims.[4]

Prevention

Before discharge home with her baby a discussion should be held about the realities of the early puerperium and the normality of the ambivalent feelings she may experience. Antenatal and postnatal classes may help in this respect. She should be exhorted not to become housebound. Even though it takes extra effort she should get out with her baby and, if possible, for brief outings alone with her husband. Different racial and cultural traditions also need to be taken into account.

Clinical Features

The clinical manifestations of puerperal depression can be obvious or quite subtle. The patient may become progressively lethargic, tearful and withdrawn, be unable to cope with housework or show disinterest in the baby. Other women may repeatedly phone their doctor with vague complaints before the scheduled postnatal visit or seek help later under the guise of complaints of insomnia, dyspareunia, reduced libido, infant feeding problems, etc. Keep in mind that medical conditions, such as thyroiditis, are more common in the six months postpartum and may present as fatigue and depression.

Any patient who expresses, however obliquely, the fear that she may harm herself or her baby should be taken seriously.

Management

Recognition of the condition and explanation with emphasis that she can be treated and expect full recovery is, in itself, therapeutic. Putting aside the time to listen, explain, and reassure the patient is the mainstay of treatment. Explanation to the husband and closely involved family members is required. The husband often feels bewildered, helpless, and rejected.

Practical assistance at home can be mustered from family or social agencies. This should aim at helping the woman regain control of her affairs rather than relieving her of all duties.

The careful, short-term, administration of tranquillisers and hypnotics, such as benzodiazepines may be of value-especially to break the sleep deprivation and fatigue cycle.

More serious cases are best treated with selective serotonin reuptake inhibitors (SSRIs) and psychotherapy under the guidance of a psychiatrist. The most commonly used SSRIs are fluoxitime, sertraline and paroxetine, and appear to be safe in lactating women. A few patients will need hospital admission.

About 30 per cent of these women may have a recurrence in a subsequent pregnancy and prophylactic psychotherapy or antidepressent drugs are recommended by some.

3. POST PARTUM PSYCHOSIS

Approximately 1 in 500-1000 women will experience a severe psychosis in the puerperium. The onset is usually within two weeks but not before the third or fourth day, which coincides with the post partum fall in hormone levels.

The presentation may be acute with confusion, delusions, and hallucinations or mania. In others, the development is more insidious, with anxiety and depression the predominant features. Many of these patients have a past history of, or will develop, schizophrenia or bipolar affective disorder.

It is important to rule out an organic cause such as infection, exhaustion or, later on, the rare case of Sheehan's post partum pituitary necrosis. Drug reactions, for example to scopolamine or barbiturates, should be considered.

These patients need specialist psychiatric care which may include phenothiazines, lithium, tricyclic antidepressants, and electroconvulsive therapy. The details of such treatment are beyond the scope of this book.

Facilities should be provided to admit both mother and baby if hospital care is required.

About 50 per cent of these patients will have a recurrence in a subsequent pregnancy.

REFERENCES

1. Why Mothers Die 1997-1999: The Confidential Enquiries into Maternal Deaths in the United Kingdom. London: RCOG Press, 2001 pp165-187.
2. Harris B, Lovett L, Newcombe RG, Read GF, Walker R, Fahmy D. Maternity blues and major endocrine changes: Cardiff puerperal mood and hormone study. BMJ 1994;308:949-53.
3. Nappi RE, Petraglia F, Luisi S, Polatti F, Forina C, Genazzini AR. Serum allopregnanolone in women with postpartum "blues". Obstet Gynecol 2001;97:77-80.
4. Stewart DE. Psychiatric symptoms following attempted natural childbirth. Can Med Assoc J 1982;127:713-7.

BIBLIOGRAPHY

Appleby L. Suicide during pregnancy and in the first postnatal year. BMJ 1991;302:137-40.

Cox JL, Connor Y, Kendell RE. Prospective study of the psychiatric disorders of childbirth. Br J Psychiatry 1982;140: 111-7.

Forman DN, Videbech P, Hedegaard M, Salvig JD, Secher NJ. Post partum depression: identification of women at risk. Br J Obstet Gynaecol 2000;107:1210-17.

Hendrick V, Altschuler L. Management of major depression during pregnancy. Am J Psychiatry 2002;159:1667-73.

Henshaw CA. Maternal suicide. In: Sturdee D, Olah K, Keane D(eds). The Yearbook of Obstetrics and Gynaecology. London:RCOG Press. 2001;9:270-6.

Josefsson A, Angelsioo L, Berg G et al. Obstetric, somatic and demographic risk factors for postpartum depressive symptoms. Obstet Gynecol 2002;99:223-8.

Lumley J, Austin MP. What interventions may reduce postpartum depression. Curr Opin Obstet Gynecol 2001;13:6-5-11.

O'Hara MW, Swain AM. Rates and risk of postpartum depression – a meta-analysis. Int Rev Psychiatry 1996;8:37-54.

Pop VJ, Wijnen HA, van Montfort M et al. Blues and depression during early pueperium: home versus hospital deliveries. Br J Obstet Gynaecol 1995;102:701-6.

Stocky A, Lynch J. Acute psychiatric disturbance in pregnancy and the puerperium. Best Prac Res Clin Obstet Gynaecol 2000;14:73-87.

CHAPTER 23

Amniotic fluid embolism

This is a rare but devastating complication. The incidence is about 1 in 50,000 deliveries. The mortality rate is very high (50-90 per cent), although a recent report suggests improvement is possible.[1] Despite its rarity, the high mortality rate means that amniotic fluid embolism accounts for 5-10 per cent of all maternal deaths.

PREDISPOSING FACTORS

The amniotic fluid may gain entry to the maternal circulation through a trivial injury to the endocervical veins, such as often occurs during labour or amniotomy, or through a more dramatic uterine wound such as caesarean section or uterine rupture. It can occur with first and second trimester pregnancy termination.

The classic profile of the women with amniotic fluid embolism was felt to be the multipara with tumultous labour and strong uterine contractions. However, a recent review of cases from a national registry has shown that there is no typical picture of the woman who suffers amniotic fluid embolism.[2] There are associations with operative delivery, abruptio placentae, minor manipulations such as intrauterine pressure catheter insertion, amnio-infusion and amniotomy. However, it may occur during the course of normal labour and up to four hours postpartum.

PATHOPHYSIOLOGY

It has been known for some time that amniotic fluid commonly enters the maternal circulation without ill effect. It seems that it is the presence of fetal cells within the amniotic fluid that may trigger the syndrome known as amniotic fluid embolism in certain susceptible women. This initiates a complex pathophysiological cascade involving complement activation similar to that seen with anaphylaxis and septic shock.[3] An acute inflammatory response develops which disrupts the pulmonary capillary endothelium and alveoli. The main features are:

1. Initially the combined effects of the amniotic particulate manner and prostaglandins on the pulmonary circulation may cause acute pulmonary vascular obstruction and hypertension leading to cor pulmonale. Recent work suggests that this pulmonary hypertension is transient and is soon superceded by left atrial and ventricular failure leading to profound hypotension and shock.[4]
2. Ventilation-perfusion imbalance causing severe hypoxia, cyanosis, convulsions and/or coma.
3. About half the patients that survive for more than one hour develop disseminated intravascular coagulation. This is due to the amniotic fluid and fetal cells activating coagulation factors, and may be compounded by the profound shock.

DIAGNOSIS

The definitive diagnosis can only be made by confirming the presence of amniotic fluid debris in the maternal circulation. This may be achieved as follows:

1. Post mortem examination showing amniotic fluid debris in the pulmonary pre-capillary arterioles. This may require serial lung sections and special fat stains. Newer immunohistochemical techniques to identify fetal isoantigens are available.[5]
2. In the patient who survives, the diagnosis is suspect. Some of these cases have been confirmed by special staining of blood obtained from the right side of the heart via a central venous pressure line or from fetal squames obtained in sputum, although it has been shown that fetal squamous cells may be present in the maternal pulmonary circulation in pregnancies without the clinical syndrome of amniotic fluid embolism.[6]

CLINICAL FEATURES

The clinical diagnosis is based on all, or some, of the following presenting features in a patient in labour or just delivered:
1. Respiratory distress and cyanosis.
2. Cardiovascular collapse.
3. Convulsions and/or coma.
4. Haemorrhage and coagulation failure may be the presenting sign but usually this only develops after one hour, if the patient survives.
5. Pulmonary oedema often develops. Bronchospasm can occur but is unusual.

Obviously other acute catastrophes can present with similar features, e.g. thrombotic pulmonary embolism, eclampsia, acid aspiration, drug reaction, etc. Careful assessment of the clinical details should differentiate between these conditions.

The key to diagnosis is to suspect amniotic fluid embolism when a previously normal patient develops cardio-respiratory distress in labour or soon after delivery. There is no time for confirmatory tests as 25-50 per cent of these patients die within the first hour.

MANAGEMENT

1. Cardiopulmonary resuscitation.
2. Oxygenation by intermittent positive pressure ventilation.
3. Circulatory support:
   (a) Intravenous dopamine infusion as necessary to maintain adequate cardiac output.
   (b) Intravenous hydrocortisone 500mg and repeat 6 hourly.
4. Treat metabolic acidosis with intravenous sodium bicarbonate.
5. Treat haemorrhage and coagulopathy (see Chapter 8).

If the patient survives the initial insult time may permit more sophisticated monitoring and manipulation of the cardio-respiratory systems by central venous pressure, systemic and pulmonary arterial lines, along with coagulation profile assessment. Treatment can then be guided by experts.

It may then be feasible to take a sample of blood from the right side of the heart using the central venous pressure line, to try and confirm the diagnosis by seeking amniotic fluid debris. Newer immunohistochemical technique to identify isoantigens may be helpful in establishing the diagnosis. Unfortunately the hypoxic insult is so great that many of the survivors have permanent neurological damage.

If undelivered at the time of diagnosis, the outlook for the fetus is also grave. The rapid cardio-respiratory collapse of the mother has the obvious detrimental effect on fetal oxygenation. Unless rapid delivery can be effected the perinatal mortality and asphyctic morbidity is high.

REFERENCES

1. Gilbert WM, Danielson B. Amniotic fluid embolism: decreased mortality in a population-based study. Obstet Gynecol 1999;93:973-7.
2. Clark SL, Hawkins GDV, Dudley DA, Dildy GA, Porter TF. Amniotic fluid embolism: analysis of the national registry. Am J Obstet Gynecol 1995;172:1158-69.
3. Benson MD, Kobayashi H, Silver RK, Oi H, Greenberger PA, Terao T. Immunologic studies in presumed amniotic fluid embolism. Obstet Gynecol 2001;97:510-4.
4. Clark SL, Cotton DB, Gonik B, Greenspoon J, Phelan JP. Central hemodynamic alterations in amniotic fluid embolism. Am J Obstet Gynecol 1988;158:1124-6.
5. Kobayashi H, Oi H, Hayakawa H. Histological diagnosis of amniotic fluid embolism by monoclonal antibody TKH-2 that recognizes Neu Ac 2-6 Gal NAc epitope. Hum Pathol 1997;28:428-33.
6. Clark SL, Pavlova Z, Greenspoon J, Horenstein J, Phelan JP. Squamous cells in the maternal pulmonary circulation. Am J Obstet Gynecol 1986;154:104-6.

BIBLIOGRAPHY

Burrows A, Khoo SK. The amniotic fluid embolism syndrome: 10 year's experience at a major teaching hospital. Aust NZ J Obstet Gynaecol 1995;35:245-50.

Clark SL. New concepts of amniotic fluid embolism: a review. Obstet Gynecol Surv 1990; 45: 360-8.

Fletcher SJ, Parr MJA. Amniotic fluid embolism: a case report and review. Resuscitation 2000;43:141-6.

Girard P, Mal H, Laine JF. Left heart failure in amniotic fluid embolism. Anesthesiology 1986;64:262-5.

Khang TY. Expression of endothelin-1 in amniotic fluid embolism and possible pathophysiological mechanism. Br J Obstet Gynaecol 1998;105:802-4.

Maher JE, Wenstrom KD, Hauth JC, Meis PJ. Amniotic fluid embolism after saline amnioinfusion: two cases and review of the literature. Obstet Gynecol 1994;83:851-4.

Morgan M. Amniotic fluid embolism. Anaesthesia 1979; 34: 20-32.

Ratten,GJ. Amniotic fluid embolism-two case reports and a review of maternal deaths from this cause in Australia. Aust NZ J Obstet Gynaecol 1988; 28: 33-5.

Yong W, Zhou N, Zhou L, Li Y. Study of the diagnosis and management of amniotic fluid embolism: 38 cases of analysis. Obstet Gynecol 2000;95(4 Suppl):38S.

CHAPTER 24

Haemorrhagic (hypovolaemic) shock

As referred to throughout this book there are many complications of pregnancy in which hypovolaemic shock associated with obstetric haemorrhage threatens the life of the mother and/or fetus. An outline of the principles involved and the management will be presented here.

PATHOPHYSIOLOGY

The physiological adaptation to pregnancy includes an increase in blood volume of about 40-50 per cent, so that in some ways the pregnant woman is better prepared to withstand haemorrhage. Thus, the average blood loss of about 500 ml and 1000 ml associated with vaginal delivery and caesarean section respectively, are tolerated with relative impunity. This is not the case with all pregnant women. Those with anaemia, prolonged labour and dehydration, or with a reduced blood volume and contracted intravascular space associated with pre-eclampsia, may not tolerate even limited blood loss. This is especially likely if the blood loss is rapid, as it so frequently is with obstetric haemorrhage.

In response to severe haemorrhage with hypotension there is increased catecholamine release and stimulation of the baroreceptors leading to increased sympathetic tone which results in:

1. Increase in the rate and force of myocardial contraction.
2. Selective peripheral arteriolar constriction reducing blood flow to all organs except the heart and brain.
3. Venous constriction causing, in effect, an autotransfusion from these capacitance vessels and increasing the return of blood to the right side of the heart.
4. The consequent reduction of hydrostatic pressure in the capillaries causes them to imbibe extracellular fluid to augment the intravascular volume.
5. An increase in the release of aldosterone and antidiuretic hormone cause greater retention of sodium and water by the kidneys.

All of the above mechanisms are an attempt to improve cardiac output, sustain blood pressure, maintain tissue perfusion, and restore the intravascular volume. Appropriate treatment at this stage will reverse the shock and restore full circulation to all organs.

- If the blood loss continues, these mechanisms will fail to sustain adequate circulation resulting in tissue hypoxia, metabolic acidosis, and cell damage. In response to the hypoxic tissue metabolites, the capillaries dilate leading to pooling and stagnation of blood, further reducing the circulating blood volume.
- More volume is lost from the intravascular space as fluid leaks through the damaged capillary walls into the tissues.
- The extensive hypoxic tissue damage may initiate disseminated intravascular coagulation.
- As the diastolic pressure falls, coronary artery perfusion is reduced leading to myocardial hypoxia and cardiac failure.
- Sustained reduction of organ perfusion may lead to varying degrees of damage; the most vulnerable organs being the lung ('shock lung', adult respiratory distress syndrome), the kidney (acute tubular and cortical necrosis), and the pituitary (Sheehan's syndrome).

In the initially healthy patient haemorrhagic shock is reversible until quite late in the above sequence, so that vigorous resuscitative efforts should be made even in the apparently exsanguinated patient. A stage is reached, however, when the changes are irreversible and all treatment fails.

CLINICAL FEATURES

The above pathophysiological mechanisms produce the changes that bring about the clinical features of hypovolaemic shock:

- Tachycardia
- Hypotension
- Tachypnoea and air hunger
- Skin changes-sweating, cold, pallor, and cyanosis
- Dry mouth and thirst
- Oliguria/anuria
- Restlessness, anxiety, confusion, and coma

It should be remembered that in the early phase of compensated blood loss the peripheral arteriolar constriction may sustain a normal blood pressure but still cause a critical reduction in utero-placental perfusion, so that the fetus is jeopardised before the mother. Thus, a normal fetal heart rate recording is reassuring for both mother and fetus.

In addition to the cardiovascular and respiratory responses assessed by the vital signs, it can be useful to think of the skin, brain and kidney as the most sensitive end-organs to reduced perfusion and hypoxia, leading to clinically detectable manifestations of hypovolaemia. These include, respectively, skin: pallor, cold, shivering and prolonged capillary refill time*; brain: restlessness, anxiety, confusion and coma; kidney: oliguria and anuria.

Another rough working clinical sign is if the radial pulse is impalpable the systolic blood pressure is <70mmHg – at which level perfusion to the heart, brain and kidney is critically reduced.

MANAGEMENT

The basic aims of management are the maintenance or restoration of the circulation in order to sustain tissue perfusion and oxygenation. At the same time specific measures are taken to stop the blood loss.

The guiding "rule of 30s" may be clinically helpful in both diagnostic and management terms: The patient may lose up to 30 percent of her blood volume without major haemodynamic changes, and aim to keep the haematocrit above 30 per cent and the urinary output above 30ml/hour.

1. **POSITION**

Raise the legs to aid venous return.

2. **OXYGEN**

By face mask.

3. **INTRAVENOUS FLUIDS**

In the absence of blood there are two types of fluids available:

- Crystalloids-Ringer's lactate and normal saline.
- Colloids-5 percent albumin,plasma protein fraction(plasmanate), hydroxyethyl starches (pentaspan) the dextrans (macrodex, rheomacrodex), and the gelatins (gelofusine).

Crystalloids have the advantage of being safe, cheap, and easily available. If transfused rapidly, at a volume approximately two to three

*Capillary refill time is easily assessed by compressing a fingernail for five seconds. The time is normal if the colour returns within two seconds).

times the estimated blood loss, they can provide short-term expansion of the intravascular space being soon excreted by the kidneys and rapidly distributed to the extracellular fluid. This too is of benefit, as the extracellular fluid is also depleted in haemorrhagic shock. In the lung crystalloid is readily reabsorbed from the interstitium whereas colloid will persist and occasionally may exacerbate pulmonary oedema by drawing further fluid into the extracellular tissues. The drawback of crystalloids is their rapid loss from the intravascular space, such that 80 per cent is lost to the circulation. The combination of pre-eclampsia and hypovolaemic shock is a circumstance of special pathophysiology. The combination of vasospasm and reduced intravascular capacity, hypoproteinaemia, and increased capillary permeability make these patients very susceptible to overload with crystalloid leading to pulmonary and generalised oedema (see chapter 7).

Remember that crystalloid has no powers of coagulation or of oxygenation, and is merely a short-term volume expander.

The natural colloids, 5 per cent albumin and plasmanate, have the advantage of remaining longer in the intravascular space but are expensive and in limited supply. The dextrans and starches may cause clotting defects and interfere with blood cross-matching unless the haematologist is given prior warning of their presence. The synthetic gelatins do not have this disadvantage and on balance are superior to the dextrans. All artificial colloids carry a small risk of an allergic reaction.

The controversy is unresolved over which fluid is superior – crystalloid or colloid. The final decision must take into account the availability, expense, and safety of each fluid, the speed with which blood can be obtained and the degree of shock. Overall, crystalloid is the safest choice and as effective as colloid, provided there is not undue delay in obtaining blood. The fluid should be warmed.

- Whatever fluid is chosen the key is **rapid** infusion and restoration of the blood volume through wide bore intravenous cannulae. Crystalloid can be infused twice as fast through a 14 guage, compared to an 18 guage cannula.
- In the previously healthy pregnant woman a blood loss of up to 1500 ml can usually be safely managed by rapid infusion of crystalloid alone, provided the source of bleeding is arrested.
- In patients with a blood loss >2000 ml, and readily available blood for transfusion, the initial management is rapid crystalloid infusion followed by packed red blood cells.
- In patients with massive blood loss, profound shock and/or delay in getting blood, both crystalloid and colloid infusion are indicated. If available, albumin is the colloid of choice. It is very viscous and is best drawn up with a wide bore needle and added to saline so it can be infused rapidly.

The above guidelines are based on the non-pregnant physiological formula: blood volume (litres) = weight (kg) ÷14. Thus, a 70kg woman would have a blood volume of 5 litres, in contrast to 3.5 litres in a 50kg woman. The importance of taking maternal weight into account when estimating blood loss and its management is obvious.

4. BLOOD TRANSFUSION

In massive haemorrhage, as well as restoration of the intravascular volume, the oxygen-carrying capacity of blood is essential. The main drawbacks to blood transfusion are:

- Availability and expense.
- Hepatitis, HIV and other transmittable infectious diseases.
- Transfusion reaction.
- Development of antibodies to atypical blood group antigens. These may not represent an immediate problem, but can pose a threat to the fetus with isoimmunisation in a subsequent pregnancy.
- It is unacceptable to a small number of women for religious or other beliefs.

Blood transfusion practices have changed drastically over the past decade. Each unit of this scarce resource is now split into its separate components, with specific indications for transfusion.

Whole blood is rarely used, and now largely unavailable.

Packed red blood cells have a haematocrit of 70-80 per cent and are used to restore the oxygen carrying capacity, while simultaneously transfused crystalloid or colloid provides the volume. With such a high viscosity packed cells cannot be rapidly transfused. This can be overcome by adding about 50-100 ml normal saline to each unit. Ringer's lactate should not be used for this purpose as its calcium content may cause clotting.

Practical Aspects of Blood Transfusion:

(a) Blood Type/Antibody Screen/Cross-match

The universal blood donor is Type O, Rh negative which, lacking both the A and B antigens, cannot be haemolysed by anti-A or anti-B antibodies in the recipient's blood. However O Rh negative donors may have anti-A and anti-B antibodies in their plasma that react with A or B cells of a non-Type O recipient. Therefore, if two or more units of O Rh negative blood are transfused, the amount of anti-A and anti-B antibodies mean, that if more units are needed, only O Rh negative blood can be given. Thus, even the universal donor blood type is not without dangers and it should only be used in dire emergencies.

If the patient's ABO and Rh type are ascertained (10 minutes) and type-specific blood given without cross-match, about 1 in 100 patients will develop irregular antibodies. However, the potential for a serious reaction is only about 1 in 1000, in patients not previously transfused. If the patient's blood is typed and screened for irregular antibodies and a short (20 minute) saline cross-match performed, the chance of a transfusion reaction is reduced to about 1 in 10,000.

Thus, any patient in whom haemorrhage is a risk should be typed and screened ahead of time. This ensures that safe blood can be rapidly made available.

(b) Temperature

The rapid transfusion of cold blood is dangerous. Blood <30°C can cause ventricular fibrillation and cardiac arrest. At a less dramatic level, cold blood will cause shivering which increases oxygen consumption; obviously an undesirable extra stress in the shocked patient. In addition, although the quantity of coagulation factors does not fall due to hypothermia, the enzyme systems necessary for their action are depressed, resulting in reduced coagulation activity, Other physical functions adversely affected by hypothermia are citrate and lactate metabolism, increased intracellular potassium release, and an unfavourable shift of the oxygen-haemoglobin dissociation curve to the left. The metabolism of drugs is also adversely affected by hypothermia.

Ideally, the blood transfusion line should be conducted through an electric blood warmer with a thermostat maintaining body temperature. A recently introduced device working on the current principle allows high flow, constant temperature, transfusion through an 8FG intravenous cannula placed in the antecubital, internal or external jugular vein. If this is not available, the blood is passed through a coil placed in an electrically heated water bath or simply a basin of water warmed to 37-40°C. The water should not exceed this temperature because of the risk of haemolysis. The water temperature in the simple basin is monitored by a thermometer and warm water has to be added frequently as the heat loss from the cold blood is considerable. In an emergency, if a thermometer is not available, the water temperature can be safely assessed by the elbow, in the same way as one tests the bath water for a baby.

(c) Blood pH

Stored blood has a pH of about 6.8-6.9 and it has been recommended that sodium bicarbonate should be given empirically with massive blood transfusion. However, the citrate in stored blood provides a source for the body to generate bicarbonate and, in fact, it is not uncommon to get a metabolic alkalosis, especially if Ringer's lactate is also infused in large amounts. Thus, bicarbonate should be given only if a metabolic acidosis is demonstrated by arterial blood gases.

(d) Hyperkalaemia

Stored red blood cells lose potassium into the plasma so that large transfusions may involve a significant increase in serum potassium. Provided renal perfusion and function is maintained, this is rarely a serious threat. Indeed, some patients may become hypokalaemic.

(e) Citrate Intoxication

The storage anticoagulant citrate binds calcium so that theoretically massive blood transfusion could deplete circulating calcium, which may need to be replaced with calcium chloride or gluconate. To get significant changes of either calcium or potassium, massive transfusions at rates of a unit every 5-10 minutes are required.

(f) Dilutional Coagulopathy

With massive blood loss, and its replacement with fluids deficient in clotting factors and platelets, a critical deficiency of coagulation factors may develop and lead to a dilutional coagulopathy. Factors 5 and 8, particularly the latter, are unstable in stored blood. Packed or resuspended red blood cells have fewer clotting factors than whole blood. As a working rule therefore, one unit of fresh frozen plasma should be transfused for every five units of packed cells.

Most of the platelets in stored blood are not viable after 24-48 hours. With transfusion of 15 units, or more, of stored blood the platelet count often falls below 100,000. Therefore, after 20-25 units of blood, 5 units of platelets should be given. Each unit will raise the platelet count about 10,000/mm^3.

The need for fresh frozen plasma and platelets to augment red cell transfusion is variable and depends on the volume and speed of transfused blood. If possible, guidance from a haematologist is advisable.

5. AUTOTRANSFUSION

In certain types of haemorrhage this may have a role (see Chapter 4).

6. MEDICAL (MILITARY) ANTISHOCK TROUSERS (MAST)

Antishock trousers are composed of three separate inflatable compartments, one for each leg and one for the abdomen. When all compartments are inflated, in the patient with hypovolaemic shock, the effect is an autotransfusion of 500-1000 ml of blood. This can be lifesaving as a part of pre-hospital or emergency room care before adequate replacement of blood volume with intravenous fluids. They have not been widely used in pregnancy but can have a place in the initial management of hypovolaemic shock secondary to abortion and ectopic pregnancy. In haemorrhage of later pregnancy only the leg compartments would be used.

Great care must be taken before the suit is deflated as the intravascular space will be suddenly increased and the blood pressure will fall dramatically unless sufficient volume has been transfused. Deflation should only occur when all facilities for intervention to arrest the haemorrhage are available.

7. DISSEMINATED INTRAVASCULAR COAGULATION

The larger and more severe the haemorrhagic insult, the more likely is the release of thromboplastins from hypoxic, acidotic tissues leading to disseminated intravascular coagulation (see Chapter 8).

8. VASOACTIVE DRUGS

The role of vasoactive drugs is not well established and requires expert guidance. They tend to be used as a last resort when the patient is close to irreversible shock:

- Purely vasoconstrictor drugs are contraindicated, though dopamine or dobutamine may be used in myocardial failure (as indicated by hypotension and rising central venous pressure) or oliguria associated with hypotension. No more than 10 ug/kg/min should be infused.
- Phenoxybenzamine and chlorpromazine can help relax the vasoconstriction and may aid tissue perfusion, although they may be associated with a profound fall in blood pressure and reduction in forward flow to the extent of jeopardising tissue oxygen supply. A less dramatic effect may be achieved with small incremental doses of opiates given intravenously.

The use of vasodilator drugs should always be associated with active transfusion, efforts to arrest bleeding, and careful monitoring of the arterial and central venous pressure.

9. STOP THE BLEEDING

Unless the origin of the blood loss is stopped the replacement of blood volume and peripheral circulation may increase bleeding from the haemorrhagic site. Obviously at the same time as the hypovolaemia is being treated specific measures are taken to stop the source of the bleeding. These will depend on the cause of bleeding and are covered in the appropriate sections of this book.

10. MONITORING PROGRESS

As a guide to the above management and depending on the severity of blood loss and the facilities available, some or all of the following monitoring is carried out:

- Arterial blood pressure, pulse, and respiration.
- Indwelling catheter to measure urinary output. If the hourly urinary output is at least 30 ml there is probably adequate renal perfusion.
- Frequent auscultation of the lung bases.
- Haemoglobin and haematocrit, although it must be remembered these do not reflect acute changes.
- Platelets and coagulation profile.
- Electrolytes.
- Arterial blood gases, with artificial ventilation if respiratory failure occurs.
- Central venous pressure gives a guide to right atrial pressure and should be interpreted in the light of the arterial pressure readings. A low central venous pressure reading (< 10 cm H_2O) with a low arterial pressure indicates the need for further transfusion. A high central venous pressure with a low arterial pressure suggests myocardial failure.
- A Swan-Ganz catheter measures pulmonary artery wedge pressure and provides an indication of left atrial pressure. When compared with the central venous (right atrial) pressure an appraisal and comparison of right and left ventricular performance can be made. This is rarely indicated or used, except in patients with haemorrhage and severe pre-eclampsia.

BIBLIOGRAPHY

American Society of Anesthesiologists Task Force on Blood Component Therapy. Practice guidelines for blood component therapy. Anesthesiology 1996;84:732-47.

American College of Obstetricians and Gynaecologists. Educational Bulletin No 235. Haemorrhagic shock. Washington DC:ACOG,1997

Contreras M, DeSilva M. Preventing incompatible transfusions. BMJ 1994;308:1180-1.

Grady K, Cox C. Shock. In: Johanson R, Cox C, Grady K. Howell C (eds). Managing Obstetric Emergencies and Trauma. London: RCOG Press, 2003 pp81-90.

Greaves I, Porter KM, Revell MP. Fluid resuscitation in pre-hospital trauma care: a consensus view. J R Coll Surg Edinb 2002;47:451-7.

Grimes DA. A simplified device for intra-operative autotransfusion. Obstet Gynecol 1988;72: 947-50.

Guidelines for red blood cell and plasma transfusion for adults and children. Can Med Assoc J 1997;156(Suppl) S1-24.

Hess J. Blood substitutes. Semin Hematol 1996;33:369-78.

Hofmeyr CJ, Mohala BKF. Hypovolaemic shock. Best Prac Res Clin Obstet Gynaecol 2001;15:645-62.

Nolan TE, Gallup DG. Massive transfusion: a current review. Obstet Gynecol Surv 1991;46:289-95.

Practice parameter for the use of fresh-frozen plasma, cryopreciptate and platelets. Development Task Force of the College of American Pathologists. JAMA 1994;271:777-81.

Rees GAD, Willis BA. Resuscitation in late pregnancy. Anaesthesia 1998;43:347-9.

Sandberg EC, Pellegra R. The medical antigravity suit for management of surgically uncontrollable bleeding associated with abdominal pregnancy. Am J Obstet Gynecol 1983;146: 519-23.

Santoso JT, Lin DW, Miller DS. Transfusion medicine in obstetrics and gynaecology. Obstet Gynecol Surv 1995;50:470-81.

Schierhout G, Roberts I. Fluid resuscitation with colloid or crystalloid solutions in critically ill patients: a systematic review of randomised trials. BMJ 1998;16:975-6.

Shevell T, Malone FD. Management of obstetric hemorrhage. Semin Perinatol 2003;27:86-104.

Society of Obstetricians and Gynaecologists of Canada. Clinical Practice Guidelines No 115. Haemorrhagic Shock. J Obstet Gynaecol Can 2002;24:504-11.

Spahn DR, Leone BJ, Reves JG et al. Cardiovascular and coronary physiology of acute isovolaemic hemodilution: a review of nonoxygen-carrying and oxygen-carrying solutions. Anesth Analg 1994;78:1000-21.

CHAPTER 25

Obstetric haemorrhage: major vessel ligation and embolisation

Uncontrolled obstetric haemorrhage is one of the most frightening and testing of all medical emergencies. Sometimes the bleeding is so heavy as to be audible, promoting the valid fear that the woman may exsanguinate within minutes. Such fear can lead to hasty and ill-considered action. In other sections of this book, specific measures to deal with haemorrhage from different causes have been outlined. Here we are concerned with the role of major vessel ligation or embolisation when the usual measures to control bleeding have failed. It is emphasised, however, that careful application of the principles of treatment will promptly deal with most cases of obstetric haemorrhage without recourse to major vessel ligation or embolisation. It is further emphasised that where feasible, the proper measures to prevent obstetric haemorrhage have been outlined and should be diligently applied. It is in the shadow of the omission of prophylaxis that the seeds of disaster proliferate.

GENERAL PRINCIPLES

- Apart from uterine atony, virtually all intra-operative bleeding can be temporarily controlled by pressure, allowing time for the surgeon to regain equanimity and summon adequate assistance, instruments, lighting and blood transfusion.
- Apply pressure for 4-5 minutes. In the case of venous haemorrhage, it is often surprising how formerly brisk bleeding will be stopped completely or reduced to oozing from identifiable points that can be precisely clamped and sutured. It is necessary to ligate both sides of a venous tear as there are no valves in the pelvic veins and blood may flow both ways.
- Beware of venous bleeding that stops completely with pressure however, as this may only be temporary. Careful observation without pressure for several minutes is required to rule out a return of bleeding or haematoma formation.

- Do not apply clamps and sutures blindly.

INDICATIONS

The main indications for consideration of major vessel ligation or embolisation are bleeding of uterine origin in which preservation of the uterus is desirable, and in vaginal and pelvic trauma when local measures fail to achieve haemostasis:

- Abortion
  - cases in which there is associated trauma to the uterus.
  - missed abortion unresponsive to curettage and oxytocics.
- Ectopic pregnancy
  - This may have to be considered in some of the rarer types, such as interstitial, ligamentary and cervical.
- Antepartum haemorrhage
  - placenta praevia, placenta accreta and abruptio placentae.
- Post partum haemorrhage
  - in the rare case of uterine atony that is unresponsive to oxytocics.
  - extensive cervical and vaginal lacerations.
- Uterine rupture.
- Caesarean section
  - associated with extension of the uterine incision into the broad ligament or vagina.
  - uterine flbroids interfering with normal haemostatic mechanisms.

UTERINE ARTERY LIGATION

This is only effective for uterine haemorrhage and is the logical first step in such cases as the uterine artery carries the vast majority of the blood supply to the uterus. It is the simplest major vessel ligation and usually the most effective for uterine haemorrhage. The method described here involves ligation of the ascending branch of the uterine artery.

Method

Grasp and elevate the uterus with one hand, tilting the fundus away from the side to be ligated. Using a large curved needle and absorbable suture, pass the needle through the myometrium about 2 cm medial to the uterine vessels and encircle the vessels bringing the needle back through an avascular portion of the broad ligament. Tie the suture but do not divide the vessels. Repeat on the other side. It is important to include a good amount of adjacent uterine muscle in the suture which serves to catch any branches of the uterine artery in the myometrium and to stabilise the ligature. At the time of caesarean section, the placement of the suture is approximately 3 cm below the level of the transverse incision in the uterus. Ensure that the bladder is well down to avoid ureteric and bladder injury. The vessels usually recanalise and subsequent menstrual and reproductive function is unaffected.

The success of uterine artery ligation in cases of post partum haemorrhage associated with caesarean section, unresponsive to oxytocics, was reported to be 95 per cent by O'Leary.[1] Fahmy recorded an 80 per cent success rate in cases of intractable post partum haemorrhage unresponsive to other measures.[2]

OVARIAN ARTERY LIGATION

The ovarian artery arises directly from the aorta and travels in the infundibulo-pelvic ligament to the mesovarium and mesosalpinx. It passes superior to the ovary, providing branches to the ovary and tube and contributes to the uterine blood supply by anastomosing with the ascending uterine artery in the region of the uterine attachment of the utero-ovarian ligament. It is in this site that an encircling stitch of absorbable suture can be placed to ligate the vessel. The suture is placed just below the ovarian ligament in a similar manner to that for uterine artery ligation. Ligation at this point will not jeopardize the

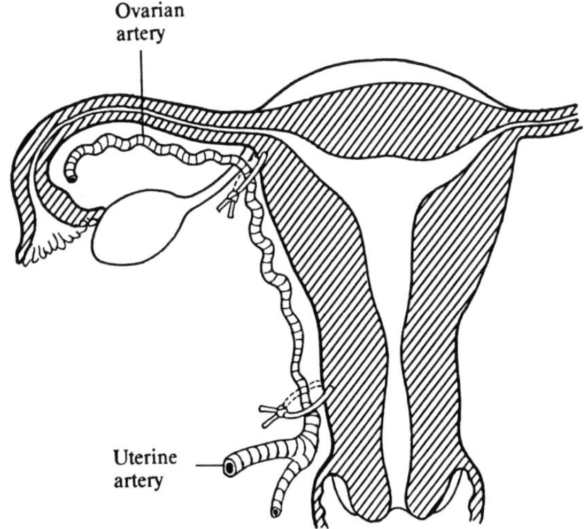

Figure 25.1 Sites for uterine and ovarian artery ligation.

blood supply to the tube or ovary. This can be done following uterine artery ligation and should further reduce blood flow to the uterus (Figure 25.1).

INTERNAL ILIAC ARTERY LIGATION

Uterine and ovarian artery ligation will not reduce flow through the descending cervical branch of the uterine artery or the vaginal arteries, which arise directly from the internal iliac artery. Thus, for haemorrhage originating from the cervix, vagina and broad ligament areas, internal iliac artery ligation may be required.

Anatomy

The internal iliac artery arises from the bifurcation of the common iliac artery, at the level of the lumbo-sacral junction in front of the sacro-iliac joint. The ureter runs antero-lateral to the internal iliac artery, behind which lie the internal iliac veins. The internal iliac artery is 4-5cm long and divides into anterior and posterior divisions. The posterior division divides into three: the ilio-lumbar and lateral sacral arteries and leaves the pelvis through the greater sciatic foramen as the superior gluteal artery to supply the muscles of the buttock. The anterior division usually has eight branches: the superior and inferior vesical, obturator, middle haemorrhoidal, uterine, vaginal and the terminal, internal pudendal and inferior gluteal branches.

Haemodynamics

The haemodynamics of internal iliac artery ligation have been outlined by Burchell.[3] He showed that unilateral ligation reduced the pulse pressure by about 77 per cent on the same side and, with bilateral ligation, the reduction was 85 per cent. The mean arterial pressure is only reduced by 25 but the blood flow is reduced by about 50 per cent. In essence, bilateral ligation almost reduces the pulse pressure to that of a venous system, allowing clotting to take place. Ligation of the internal iliac arteries does not completely stop blood flow due to the presence of three main collateral anastomoses:

1. The lumbar artery arises from the aorta and anastomoses with the ilio-lumbar artery.
2. The middle sacral artery, also arising from the aorta, joins with the lateral sacral artery.
3. The superior haemorrhoidal artery, which is the terminal branch of the inferior mesenteric artery, anastomoses with the middle haemorrhoidal artery.

Additional collaterals may link the aorta with the uterine artery via the ovarian artery, the femoral artery with the internal pudendal artery via the profunda femoris and femoral circumflex vessels, and the common iliac with the superior gluteal via the circumflex iliac arteries.

Immediately after ligation of the internal iliac artery, these collateral channels open and flow is reversed so that all the branches of the internal iliac artery are again filled and flowing blood-but with the reduced pressures already noted. This collateral system is virtually limited to each side with very few crossing the midline. The full capacity of this collateral system is available immediately and does not increase subsequently. The efficiency of this collateral system is such that bilateral internal iliac ligation does not cause tissue necrosis or interfere with subsequent menstrual or reproductive function.

Method

Divide the round ligament between two clamps well out from its uterine attachment. This allows avascular entry of the retroperitoneal space and clear identification of its contained blood vessels and ureter. Identify the ureter and reflect it medially with the attached peritoneum. Find the external iliac artery on the pelvic side wall and trace it proximally to the bifurcation of the common iliac artery. Locate and clear the areolar tissue from the internal iliac artery for 3-4 cm. Pass a right-angle clamp beneath the artery and doubly ligate the artery with absorbable suture. Do not divide the vessel. Also check the femoral pulse before and after, in case of inadvertent ligation of the external iliac artery. It is said to be safer to pass the clamp from lateral to medial to lessen the risk of trauma to the external iliac vein. The main point is to be aware of the risk of trauma to both the underlying internal iliac veins and the laterally placed external iliac vein. Gentle elevation of the artery with a Babcock clamp and passing the right-angle clamp very close to the internal iliac artery should reduce the risk of venous trauma. Burchell felt that bleeding was less if the artery was ligated distal to the posterior division as he found one of the anastomotic channels (superior-middle haemorrhoidal) only functioned when the posterior division was also ligated. This also lessens the risk of subsequent ischaemic buttock pain, by avoiding the posterior division and it's terminal superior gluteal artery. However, location of the posterior division is not always easy and inexperienced attempts to do so add risk of trauma to the underlying internal iliac veins, which can bleed frighteningly. If one ligates the internal iliac artery 2.5-3.0 cm from its origin, it is likely to include only the anterior division.

Clark *et al.*[4] found internal iliac artery ligation to be only 42 per cent effective in controlling intractable post partum haemorrhage in cases in which medical treatment and uterine artery ligation had failed. Evans and McShane had an identical failure rate.[5]

PELVIC VESSEL EMBOLISATION

An increasing number of reports over the past 20 years have confirmed the value of angiographic embolisation of pelvic vessels in the control of obstetrical and gynaecological haemorrhage. The success is high (>95 per cent) because of the accessibility of the internal iliac artery to angiographic catheterisation.

The procedure can be done under local anaesthesia with mild sedation. Via a femoral artery puncture, and under angiographic control, the catheter is guided to the aortic bifurcation. An aortogram then outlines the pelvic vessels and the bleeding sites can be seen from the extravasation of contrast material. The catheter is then advanced to the specific bleeding vessel, which is embolised by the injection of gelfoam particles. Post-embolisation arteriograms demonstrate success, or the need for further embolisation in this or other vessels. If necessary, the internal iliac artery can be embolised, as well as any collateral vessels that are shown to be bleeding. It is this ability to seek and embolise bleeding collateral vessels after internal iliac artery embolisation that makes this method superior to surgical ligation of the internal iliac artery. In addition, surgical ligation makes subsequent pelvic vessel embolisation difficult and, in some cases, impossible. Whereas, if embolisation is tried first and fails, surgical options are still available.

SUMMARY

Obstetricians need to be familiar with both surgical and embolisation techniques for control of haemorrhage. Each method has the potential to save the patient her life and her uterus. The method chosen will depend on the clinical circumstances, surgical skill, facilities and availability of angiographic services. In cases in which one is dealing directly with uterine haemorrhage following caesarean section or uterine rupture, the use of uterine and ovarian artery ligation has much to recommend them. Indeed, these can be simply and rapidly performed before repair of the uterus and while making the final decision about conservation of the uterus. It should not be forgotten that in cases of uterine haemorrhage, hysterectomy should be curative and this option must be constantly balanced with the need to preserve the uterus for future reproduction.

In cases with cervical and vaginal lacerations and haematomas, if direct suturing and packing fail, it is better to proceed to embolisation which saves a laparotomy and is likely to be more successful than internal iliac ligation.

The big advantage with uterine and ovarian artery ligation is the simplicity, speed, and safety of the procedure and that it is within the realm of any general obstetrician. The problem with internal iliac artery ligation is that it is more difficult, the dissection is not commonly performed by the general obstetrician, it is often ineffective, and denies access to subsequent embolisation techniques.

REFERENCES

1. O'Leary JA. Uterine artery ligation for hemorrhage. In: Gynecologic Surgery. Sanz LE (ed). New Jersey: Medical Economics Books, 1988. pp. 385-90.
2. Fahmy K. Uterine artery ligation to control postpartum hemorrhage. Int J Gynecol Obstet 1987;25: 363-7.
3. Burchell RC. Physiology of internal iliac artery ligation. J Obstet Gynaecol Br Commonw 1968;75:642-51.
4. Clark SL, Phelan JP, Bruce SR, Paul RH. Hypogastric artery ligation for obstetric hemorrhage. Obstet Gynecol 1985;66:353-6.
5. Evans S, McShane P. The efficacy of internal iliac ligation. Surg Gynecol Obstet 1985;160:250-3.

BIBLIOGRAPHY

Allahbadia G. Hypogastric artery ligation: a new perspective. J Gynaecol Surg 1993;9:35-7.

Corr P. Arterial embolization for haemorrhage in the obstetric patient. Best Prac Res Clin Obstet Gynaecol 2001;15:557-61.

Chattopadhyay SK, Deb RB, Edrees YB. Surgical control of obstetric hemorrhage: hypogastric artery ligation or hysterectomy. Int J Gynecol Obstet 1990;32:345-51.

Fehrman H. Surgical management of life-threatening obstetric and gynecologic hemorrhage. Acta Obstet Gynecol Scand 1988;67: 125-8.

Hansch E, Chitkara V, McAlpine J et al. Pelvic arterial embolization for control of obstetric haemorrhage: a five-year experience. Am J Obstet Gynecol 1999;180:1454-60.

Mitty HA, Sterling KM, Alvarez M et al. Obstetric hemorrhage: prophylactic and emergency arterial catherization and embolotherapy. Radiology 1993;188:183-7.

Nandanwar YS, Jhalam L, Mayadeo N, Guttal DR. Ligation of internal iliac arteries for control of pelvic haemorrhage. J Postgrad Med 1993;39:194-5.

O'Leary JA. Uterine artery ligation in the control of post-cesarean hemorrhage. J Reprod Med 1995;40:189-93.

Stanacato-Pasik A, Mitty HA, Richard HA, Eskhar N. Obstetric embolotherapy; effect on menses and pregnancy. Radiology 1997;204:791-3.

Thavarasah AS, Sivolingam N, Almohdzar SA. Internal iliac and ovarian artery ligation in the control of pelvic haemorrhage. Aust NZ J Obstet Gynaecol 1989;29: 22-5.

Vedantham S, Goodwin SC, McLucas B et al. Uterine artery embolization: an underused method of controlling pelvic hemorrhage. Am J Obstet Gynecol 1997;176:938-48.

Wells I. Internal iliac artery embolization in the management of pelvic bleeding. Clin Radiol 1996;51:825-7.

Yamashita Y, Takahashi M, Ito M et al. Transcatheter arterial embolization in the management of postpartum haemorrhage due to genital tract injury. Obstet Gynecol 1991;77: 160-3.

CHAPTER 26

Trauma in pregnancy

Accidental injury occurs in approximately five percent of all pregnant women and is the leading cause of non-obstetrical deaths, accounting for 20% in this category.[1-5] The perinatal mortality is much higher, with the ratio of fetal to maternal deaths ranging from 3:1 to 9:1. Abdominal trauma requiring admission to hospital occurs in 0.4-0.6 percent of pregnant women. Of these 35-60 percent are caused by motor vehicle accidents, 25-40 percent by falls, and 15-25 percent from assault.[3,5-6]

Medical and nursing personnel who look after trauma patients rarely look after pregnant women and *vice versa* with obstetrics. However, both specialties require clear decisive action.

GENERAL PRINCIPLES

- What is best for the mother is best for the fetus: A sure cause of fetal death is maternal death.
- Treatment principles are the same as for the non-pregnant trauma victim, with some modifications to account for the anatomical and physiological changes of pregnancy. In general the risk of fetal injury is related to the extent of maternal trauma. However, in rare cases there may be serious fetal injury with trivial injury to the mother.
- In almost all cases fetal compromise is manifest within four hours of injury.
- Radiographic studies, including CT scan, should not be withheld. For some of the studies the uterus can be protected with lead abdominal shields.
- Tetanus prophylaxis is unaltered by pregnancy.
- Antibiotic administration is unchanged: but avoid tetracyclines, sulphas and chloramphenicol.

ANATOMICAL AND PHYSIOLOGICAL CHANGES IN PREGNANCY

During the first trimester of pregnancy the uterus is protected by the bony pelvis and there are only mild physiological changes. However, by the second trimester there are increasing and significant changes in maternal anatomy and physiology that may alter clinical signs and laboratory data.

Anatomical:

- Uterus: By the second and third trimester the uterus is increasingly vulnerable to blunt and penetrating trauma of the abdomen.
- Bladder: From the second trimester the bladder becomes, at least partially, an abdominal organ. It is therefore more vulnerable to abdominal trauma and may be crushed between the pelvic bones and fetal head in cases of fractured pelvis in later pregnancy. The bladder is more vascular and therefore, if traumatised, more likely to bleed heavily.
- The diaphragm rises approximately four centimetres, with compensatory flaring of the ribs. This may be relevant in the evaluation of penetrating thoracic or abdominal wounds and the placement of thoracostomy tubes.
- The small bowel tends to be pushed into the upper abdomen by the uterus and therefore may avoid penetrating trauma to the lower abdomen. However, penetration of the upper abdomen may injure several loops of tightly crowded small intestine.
- The distension of the abdominal wall may reduce the peritoneal response to irritation, potentially masking significant clinical signs of intra-abdominal organ injury.
- Gastric emptying is delayed and decreased, which increases the risk of acid aspiration during trauma, unconsciousness, and general anaesthesia.
- From the second trimester, bilateral ureteral dilatatoin and incomplete bladder emptying may be physiological and should be considered when interpreting intravenous pyelography.
- Supine hypotension syndrome: In the second half of pregnancy the gravid uterus may occlude both the inferior vena cava and aorta when the pregnant woman lies in the supine position. This may dramatically reduce the cardiac output and, in patients with bleeding and hypovolaemia, critically interfere with venous return to the heart. However, in many patients there are adequate collateral channels so that the brachial blood pressure may be normal despite aorta-caval compression by the gravid uterus. It is important to remember that in such cases the aortic compression may critically reduce the utero-placental circulation to the fetus despite

a normal brachial blood pressure in the mother. *Thus, the supine position should be avoided in the pregnant woman from 20 weeks gestation.*

Physiological:

- Cardiac output increased by 30-40 percent from 10 weeks gestation.
- Blood volume increased 30-50 percent by 28 weeks gestation.
- Heart rate increased 10-15 beats per minute.
- Blood pressure, both systolic and diastolic, falls 10-15 mmHg in the second trimester but returns to normal in the third.
- Maternal tidal volume increases by 40 per cent in late pregnancy and residual volume decreases by 25 per cent. The PO_2 is unchanged but the PCO_2 is decreased to 30 mmHg. There is a compensatory decrease in serum bicarbonate with a reduced buffering capacity of the blood, making the development of metabolic acidosis more rapid after trauma.
- Moderate leukocytosis: 18,000 in second and third trimesters and up to 25,000 during labour.
- Plasma volume increases more than the red cell mass, resulting in a physiological dilutional anaemia with average haematocrits of 30-34 percent by 30-34 week's gestation.
- Coagulation factors increase, including factors 7, 8, 9, and 10. However, platelet count, bleeding time, prothrombin time (PT), and partial thromboplastin time (PTT) remain unchanged. Fibrinogen levels may double during pregnancy and reach 400-500 mg/dl by term. Thus, at term, levels below 150 mg/dl should be considered abnormal in the pregnant woman and may indicate disseminated intravascular coagulation.
- The hypercoagulable state of the pregnant woman may increase the risk of thromboembolism during periods of immobility following trauma.
- Electrocardiograph changes are not specific and represent the left axis deviation due to elevation of the diaphragm. Q waves in lead III and premature atrial contractions may be seen.

RISKS TO THE FETUS

A major cause of fetal death is death of the mother. The next biggest risk is abruptio placentae.

Indirect:

- **Maternal hypovolaemia and hypoxaemia:** The mother will maintain homeostasis at the expense of the fetus. Because of her additional blood volume the mother withstands initial haemorrhage quite well. Thus, the pregnant woman may have a normal heart rate and blood pressure with 20% (~1500 ml) acute blood loss and up to 35% gradual blood loss. However, before clinical evidence of maternal shock occurs, uterine artery vasoconstriction may reduce uterine and, therefore, fetal perfusion by 10-20%.

- **Supine Hypotension:** This may reduce utero-placental circulation even without the obvious clinical manifestation of reduced brachial blood pressure in the mother.

Direct:

Fractured skull: If the maternal pelvis is fractured and the fetus presents as a vertex. It is also possible for there to be acceleration-deceleration forces on the fetal brain even in breech presentation and without apparent major maternal or fetal trauma. Such cases occur but are fairly rare.[7]

Penetrating Trauma (eg. stab or bullet wound): The uterus and its contents may slow and arrest the progress of a bullet, depending on the type and velocity. Thus, the fetus has a much higher injury and mortality level and the mother is relatively protected compared to the non-pregnant state.

Abruptio Placentae: The placenta does not contain elastic tissue but the uterus does and therefore it changes shape in response to acceleration-deceleration forces. Hence the tendency for shearing and the inelastic placental edge to separate. Thus, there does not have to be much direct trauma to the abdomen to cause abruptio placentae. The manifestations of abruptio placentae usually occur within a few hours of the injury. There have been a number of isolated reports suggesting delayed abruptio placentae up to five days following trauma. This is a dubious entity (see later).

Feto-maternal haemorrhage: Recent studies have shown that the incidence and volume of feto-maternal haemorrhage following injury is five times greater than in uninjured pregnant women. This may cause subsequent isoimmunisation in Rh negative women. Or, if big enough, the bleed may present the direct threat of fetal exsanguination.[8,9]

Uterine rupture is not common, occurring in approximately 1 in 200 episodes of trauma during pregnancy.[10] The presentation may vary from fairly subtle findings with mild uterine tenderness and fetal heart rate abnormalities (tachycardia and late decelerations), up to an obvious abdominal catastrophe associated with fetal and maternal death.

Premature labour may be associated with abruptio placentae or possibly prostaglandin release from bruising of the myometrium.

Premature rupture of the membranes: which may lead to premature labour, chorioamnionitis or chronic oligohydramnios.

RISKS TO THE MOTHER

In addition to the usual effects of trauma, which are unrelated and unchanged by pregnancy, the following aspects may alter the risks to the mother:

- Uterine rupture.
- Bladder trauma due to the intra-abdominal position and increased vascularity.
- Retroperitoneal haemorrhage due to increased vascularity, particularly in the pelvis.
- Rupture of the spleen has been shown in some series to be more common in pregnancy.
- Acid aspiration (Mendelson's) syndrome: If general anaesthesia is required or if there is reduced level of consciousness.
- Supine hypotension due to compression of the inferior vena cava by the gravid uterus, which may reduce maternal cardiac output by up to 30 percent.
- Amniotic fluid embolism associated with uterine rupture.
- Disseminated intravascular coagulation (DIC) which may be associated with uterine rupture, amniotic fluid embolism and/or severe haemorrhage.
- The incidence of spousal and partner physical abuse against pregnant women has been under-reported and only recently acknowledged. When the cause of injury is not obvious this should be considered and the woman asked gently but directly about this possibility. She should be made aware that help is available and put in contact with the appropriate resources.[11,12]

MANAGEMENT

- The trauma victim who is obviously pregnant will often precipitate diagnostic and therapeutic paralysis in emergency department personnel. It cannot be over emphasised that the interests of the fetus are best served by the prompt and appropriate treatment of the mother.
- If the injury is severe and life-threatening, treat the mother first and worry about the pregnancy later.

- Initial management includes a quick primary appraisal of injury and the ABC's – Airway, Breathing, and Circulation (see below for CPR in the pregnant woman).
- Place a sandbag under the right hip to displace the uterus and avoid aorta-caval compression. If the patient is on a spinal board, the whole board can be tilted at least 15 degrees to the left. When safe and feasible nurse the patient in the left lateral position.
- Establish intravenous access and take appropriate bloods including Kleihauer test for feto-maternal bleed.
- If a Medical Anti-Shock Suit is to be used, inflate only the leg compartments.
- Radiographic studies should be carried out as for the non-pregnant woman,with shielding of the uterus when feasible.
- The presence of a pelvic fracture should warn of possible damage to the greatly dilated pelvic veins with subsequent massive retroperitoneal haemorrhage.
- Peritoneal lavage is not contraindicated in pregnancy. The indications are the same as for the non-pregnant. A site just above the uterine fundus is chosen or through an intraumbilical incision. The procedure and interpretation are the same as in the non-pregnant.[13]

OBSTETRICAL CONSIDERATIONS

- The conscious injured pregnant woman is usually as, or more, worried about damage to her fetus as she is about herself. Within the limits imposed by her injuries and the need for maternal resuscitation, early attempts should be made to confirm the well being of her fetus – this reassurance can be of great therapeutic value.
- Establish the gestational age, either from history or a clinical assessment of uterine size. It is important to do this as early as possible in case rapid decisions have to be made regarding fetal viability, should laparotomy be necessary.
- If maternal transfer is required after stabilisation, consider the choice of hospital vis a vis adjacent obstetrical and neonatal services.
- Clinical assessment of the uterus and fetus involve seeking signs of abruptio placentae and fetal distress or death. If available and feasible, an external doppler fetal heart monitor may show signs of fetal distress (bradycardia, tachycardia, loss of baseline variability, late decelerations). In early gestation (≥7 weeks) ultrasound may confirm fetal heart activity.
- Ultrasound is unreliable in detecting the presence or absence of retroplacental clot in many cases. The diagnosis of abruptio placentae is therefore based on the clinical picture of uterine irritability, contractions and tenderness, allied to vaginal bleeding

(the latter may be absent in concealed abruptio). Fetal heart abnormalities may also presage the full clinical picture of abruptio placentae, which may not become manifest for 24 hours. Isolated cases of so-called delayed (up to five days following trauma) abruptio placentae have been reported but usually without the early fetal heart monitoring. This is a dubious entity and in the vast majority of cases with significant abruptio the clinical picture, or at least fetal heart rate changes, is manifest within 24 hours and usually, if life threatening to the fetus, within four hours. Thus, in a woman with minor trauma who does not require hospital admission, and in whom there is no uterine tenderness or bleeding, normal fetal heart rate monitoring and no regular uterine contractions after four hours should provide adequate reassurance. If there is uterine tenderness, vaginal bleeding, regular uterine contractions or a nonreassuring fetal heart rate pattern more prolonged fetal monitoring is needed.

- Delivery of the fetus by caesarean section may be required for uterine rupture or abruptio placentae with a live, viable fetus. In some instances laparotomy may be required for maternal injuries and caesarean section be necessary to empty the uterus and allow room to deal with the maternal trauma. Hence the need to establish gestational age and potential fetal viability early on so that obstetrical and neonatal resources can be marshalled if required.
- If the patient is Rh negative and the Kleihauer test is positive, Rh immune globulin (300 micrograms) should be given. Prolonged fetal heart monitoring, up to 24 hours, may assist in detecting cases of slow fetal exsanguination (usually manifest initially by fetal tachycardia followed by loss of baseline variability and late decelerations).
- It is, of course, easy to say monitor the fetal heart rate continuously for 24 hours to detect early signs of abruptio placentae, fetal exsanguination and fetal distress. However, this may be quite difficult and impractical in some trauma victims. Therefore the guiding principle should be to do ones best and at least intermittently monitor the fetus for 15 to 30 minutes every one to two hours. Again, the practical requirements for maternal treatment should dominate the decisions.
- Formula to calculate the amount of Rh immune globulin required to prevent isoimmunisation in Rh negative women:

$$\underset{\text{(estimated maternal blood volume)}}{5000} \times \frac{\text{\% fetal cells}}{100}$$

eg. Kleihauer of 0.5% (= 5 fetal cells per thousand RBC's)

$$5000 \times \frac{0.5}{100} = 25 \text{ ml}$$

10ug of Rh Immune globulin (RhIg) covers one ml fetal blood. Thus, a standard dose of 300ug RhIg covers up to 30 ml. Therefore if the Kleihauer is 0.5% or less, the standard dose of 300ug will be adequate.

If no Kleihauer result is available, or if the quantitative result is delayed, in cases of abdominal trauma give 300ug RhIg within 72 hours. One can then send the quantitative Kleihauer as soon as feasible.

CARDIOPULMONARY RESUSCITATION (CPR) IN THE PREGNANT WOMAN

The objectives of CPR are the same in the pregnant as the non-pregnant woman – the re-establishment of adequate oxygenation and cardiac output. The previously noted anatomical and physiological changes of pregnancy necessitate modification of some of the practical aspects of CPR:

- The reduction of lung residual volume added to elevation of the diaphragm by the pregnant uterus, which may be further aggravated by the Trendelenburg position, makes ventilation more difficult and the development of hypoxia and acidosis more rapid. This, plus the propensity to gastric acid regurgitation and aspiration, make the early placement of an endotracheal tube essential.
- Ensure adequate venous return by avoiding the supine position and vena caval compression. This requires a left lateral tilt of at least 15 degrees. Soft wedges are unsuitable for external chest compression. Thus, sand bags or a special wooden wedge with a non-slip covering long enough to support the patients hips and thoracic spine should be used to achieve this tilt.
- External chest compressions should then be performed so the line of force is at 15 degrees to the vertical.
- To accommodate the elevated diaphragm and the marginally higher and more horizontal position of the heart, the hands should be placed slightly higher, at mid-sternum, to clear the uterine fundus during compression.

POST MORTEM CAESAREAN SECTION

- Post mortem caesarean section is replete with a long history and rich mythology. It is extremely rare for this procedure to be necessary, feasible, or appropriate. Personnel and resources should not be diverted from maternal resuscitation unless additional skilled personnel and equipment are available to perform the caesarean section, resuscitate, and look after the infant (which is often premature).

- It has been suggested that emptying the pregnant uterus may assist in the resuscitation of the mother by removing aorta-caval compression and improving ventilation. This may be so in isolated cases, but should rarely be necessary if the principles of CPR in the pregnant woman are followed properly.
- Nonetheless there are rare cases in which post mortem caesarean section may be considered. Gestational age is crucial and the decision to perform postmortem caesarean section will depend on the facilities immediately available for managing the infant if it is premature. If there is a full neonatal intensive care unit immediately available, postmortem caesarean section as early as 26-28 weeks gestation may be considered. If not, one has to tailor the gestational age to the ability to look after the infant.
- With no perfusion irreversible brain damage occurs within 4-6 minutes. The literature shows that most intact fetal survivors are delivered within five minutes of maternal cardiac arrest. It is very rare to get survival of a normal fetus if delivered ≥10 minutes following maternal cardiac arrest.

REFERENCES

1. Newfeld JDG, Moore EE, Marx JA.Trauma in pregnancy. Emerg Med Clin North Am 1987;5:623-30.
2. Patterson RM. Trauma in pregnancy. Clin Obstet Gynaecol 1984;27:32-8.
3. Why Mothers Die 1977-1999:The Confidential Enquiry into Maternal Deaths in the United Kingdom, London: RCOG Press,2001 pp241-51.
4. Pearlman MD, Tintinalli JE, Lovern RP. Blunt trauma during pregnancy. N Engl J Med 1990;323:1609-13.
5. Williams JK, McClain L, Rosemurgy AS. Evaluation of blunt abdominal trauma in the third trimester of pregnancy - maternal and fetal considerations. Obstet Gynecol 1990;75:33-7.
6. Lavin JP, Polsky SS. Abdominal trauma during pregnancy. Clin Perinatol 1983;10:423-38.
7. Sokal MM, Katz M, Lell ME.Neonatal survival after traumatic fetal subdural hematoma. J Reprod Med 1980;24:131-3.
8. Pearlman MD, Tintinalli JE, Lorenz RP. A prospective controlled study of outcome after trauma during pregnancy. Am J Obstet Gynecol 1990;162:1502-10.
9. Goodwin TM, Breen M, Kelly JV. Pregnancy outcome and feto maternal haemorrhage after non-catastrophic trauma. Am J Obstet Gynecol 1990;126:665-71.
10. Rothenberger D, Quattlebaum FW, Perry JF. Blunt maternal trauma: a review of 103 cases. J Trauma 1978;18:173-9.
11. Heltan AS, McFarlane J, Anderson ET. Battered and pregnant: a prevalence study. Am J Public Health 1987;77:1337-9.
12. Cokkinides VE, Coker AL, Sanderson M, Addy C, Bethea L. Physical violence during pregnancy: maternal complications and birth outcomes. Obstet Gynecol 1999;93:661-6.
13. Rothenberger DA, Quattlebaum FW, Zabel J. Diagnostic peritoneal lavage for blunt trauma in pregnant women. Am J Obstet Gynecol 1977;129:479-81

BIBLIOGRAPHY

American College of Obstetricians and Gynaecologists. Obstetric aspects of trauma. Educational Bulletin No.251 Washington DC:ACOG,1998.

Awwad JT, Azar GB, Seoud MA. High-velocity penetrating wounds of the gravid uterus: review of 16 years of civil war. Obstet Gynecol 1994;83:259-64.

Dildy GA, Clark SL. Cardiac arrest during pregnancy. Obstet Gynecol Clin North Am 1995;22:303-14.:

Fries MH, Hawkins GAV. Motor vehicle accidents associated with minimal maternal trauma but subsequent fetal demise. Ann Emerg Med 1989;18:301-4.

Goodwin H, Holmes JF, Wisner DH. Abdominal ultrasound examination in pregnant blunt trauma patients. J Trauma 2001;50:689-93.

Higgins SD, Garite TJ. Late abruptio placentae in trauma patients: implications for monitoring. Obstet Gynecol 1984;63:105.

Hyde LK, Cook LJ, Olson LM, Weiss HB, Dean JM. Effect of motor vehicle crashes on adverse fetal outcomes. Obstet Gynecol 2003;102: 279-86.

Katz VL, Dotters DJ, Droegemueller W. Perimortem cesarean delivery. Obstet Gynecol 1986;68:571-6.

Mayer L, Liebschultz J. Domestic violence in the pregnant patient: obstetric and behavioural interventions. Obstet Gynecol Surv 1998;53:627-35.

Muhajarine N, D'Arcy C. Physical abuse during pregnancy: prevalence and risk factors. Can Med Assoc J 1999;160:1007-11.

Oates S, Williams GL, Rees GAD. Cardiopulmonary resuscitation in late pregnancy. BMJ 1988;297:404-5.

Parker J, Balis N, Chester S. Cardiopulmonary arrest in pregnancy. Aust NZ J Obstet Gynaecol 1996;36:207-10.

Pearlman MD, Phillips ME. Safety belt use during pregnancy. Obstet Gynecol 1996;88:1026-9.

Polko LE, McMahon MJ. Burns in pregnancy. Obstet Gynecol Surv 1998;53:50-6.

Reis PM, Sander CM, Pearlman MD. Abruptio placentae after auto accidents. J Reprod Med 2000;45:6-10.

Sakala EP, Kort DD. Management of stab sounds to the pregnant uterus: a case report and review of the literature. Obstet Gynecol Surv 1988;43:319-24.

Stone IK. Trauma in the obstetric patient. Obstet Gynecol Clin North Am 1999;26:459-67.

Van Hook JW. Trauma in pregnancy. Clin Obstet Gynecol 2002;45:414-24.

Weiss HB, Songer TJ, Fabio A. Fetal deaths related to maternal injury. JAMA 2001;286:1863-8.

Whitten M, Irvine LM. Post mortem and perimortem caesarean section: what are the indications? J R Soc Med 2000;93:6-9.

CHAPTER 27

Analgesia for emergency obstetric procedures

The purpose of this chapter is to cover the simpler methods of analgesia available in all hospitals. These may be chosen for safety reasons in preference to general anaesthesia or the major regional blocks (spinal and epidural). It is particularly aimed at those working in hospitals, with limited specialist anaesthetic services, where these techniques may be all that is available. Skilfully combined and carefully applied, much can be achieved with these simple procedures.

INHALATION ANALGESIA

This method of analgesia is simple, safe, and, within limits, effective. In obstetrics the most commonly used gases are nitrous oxide and oxygen.

Advantages

1. Limited training and skill are required to administer this form of analgesia, although attention to simple practical points is essential for maximum effectiveness.
2. It can be self-administered by the woman which has a beneficial psychological effect as it gives her some control over events.
3. The woman remains conscious, has full motor power and intact protective reflexes.
4. There is no effect on uterine activity.
5. There is no significant accumulation of the gas and it is very safe for the mother and infant.

Indications

1. Analgesia is the late first and second stages of labour. It is particularly appropriate for the multiparous woman – the majority of whom first request pain relief within one hour of full dilatation or delivery.

2. As an adjunct to local anaesthetic blocks (pudendal and paracervical) for procedures such as: forceps delivery, assisted breech and twin delivery, suture of genital tract lacerations, etc.

Technique

- There is a variety of equipment for self-administration of these gases. The most practical for nitrous oxide is a pre-mixed gas cylinder of 50 per cent nitrous oxide and 50 per cent oxygen (Entonox). Others utilise a blender apparatus that produces the appropriate 50/50 concentration from separate cylinders or hospital pipelines (Nitronox, Midogas).
- There is a latent period from when the woman starts inhalation until there is sufficient gas tension in the central nervous system to produce analgesia. In the first stage of labour, uterine contractions are palpable about 20 seconds before the woman feels pain. Thus, once the contraction is palpable the woman is told to start inhaling the gas so that she is beginning to get some effect by the time the contraction becomes painful. The knowledge and application of this simple point is essential if full benefit is to be obtained. In the late first and second stages of labour the gap between palpation of the contraction and pain perception is shorter and therefore the inhalation is started on the basis of the time interval between contractions. The aim being to start inhalation about 30 seconds before the expected contraction begins.
- When used as an adjunct to local anaesthetic blocks for painful procedures the inhalation is continued until satisfactory analgesia is achieved.
- As long as the gas is self-administered the woman is not in danger, for once she becomes drowsy, and well before the loss of protective reflexes, her grip on the mask relaxes breaking the airtight seal. This seal is necessary to transmit the negative pressure required to activate the demand valve which allows the gas to flow. For women who dislike masks a mouthpiece is available.

NARCOTIC ANALGESIA

This is a long-established method of analgesia in labour, although its main effect is probably sedative. The most commonly used narcotic in obstetrics is meperidine (demerol, pethidine), as some studies suggest it does not pass across the blood-brain barrier of infants as easily as other narcotic drugs. However, it does affect the neurobehaviour of the neonate. It is commonly used in the first stage of labour, as well as an adjunct to other methods of analgesia for painful procedures.

- By subcutaneous injection the dose is 50-150 mg, the effect is maximal 45-60 minutes later and lasts about 3-4 hours.
- Given intravenously in 20-25 mg increments the effect starts in 30 seconds, is maximal in 2-5 minutes and lasts about 1-2 hours. There is much to be said for choosing the intravenous route which provides a more precise and predictable effect. One is also more likely to get maximum analgesic effect with less drug transfer to the fetus. The drug is given in 20-25 mg increments with 3-5 minutes between each dose to assess the effect and guard against hypotension. Satisfactory analgesia is usually achieved with a dose of 40-50 mg. The injection should be given just as a contraction is starting, which in theory reduces the transfer of drug to the fetus due to the diminution in utero-placental blood flow during the contraction and the rapid protein binding in maternal plasma.
- The intravenous route is useful for the woman in labour who is unconsolably or uncontrolably distressed by her pain. It provides quick relief, reassures her that pain control is available and effective, and allows more considered decisions about long term analgesia.
- Fentanyl can be used in a similar manner to meperidine. It has some advantages that have led many to favour its use over meperidine. It has a shorter half-life, causes less nausea and vomiting, and less neonatal neurobehavioural effects. It is usually given intravenously as 50-100ug hourly.
- Both fentanyl and meperidine can be given intravenously via patient-controlled systems. This is no more effective, but does reduce the total dose given and allows the woman an element of control.
- The main potential drawback is respiratory depression in the newborn. This is most likely if delivery occurs 1-4 hours following administration. While this is a real and potentially serious complication one need not be completely intimidated provided one has the equipment and ability to apply assisted ventilation and administer naloxone, which effectively reverses the depressant effect (see Chapter 28). There is no benefit from maternal administration of naloxone just before delivery, as it provides uncertain or incomplete reversal of the narcotic effect. Narcotic analgesia may also impair the establishment of breast feeding.

LOCAL ANAESTHESIA

The use of local anaesthesia is the method of choice for minor obstetric operative procedures. Local infiltration of the perineum and vagina is adequate for the performance and repair of an episiotomy and the suture of vaginal lacerations. More extensive analgesia is provided by paracervical and pudendal blocks.

Local Anaesthetic Toxicity

If local anaesthetics are to be used it is important to be able to deal with their potential toxicity. This is due to inadvertent intravascular injection, exceeding dose guidelines, or injection into a very vascular space allowing rapid absorption (e.g. the paracervical space).

The recommended dose guidelines for the most commonly used local anaesthetic, lidocaine (lignocaine), are 3-4 mg/kg plain solution and 7-8 mg/kg with added epinephrine (adrenaline). A one per cent solution contains 10 mg/ml. Therefore in a 70 kg patient the dose should not exceed 250 mg, or 25 ml, of a one per cent plain solution.

Clinical Features

- In mild cases of local anaesthetic toxicity the patient may have a dry mouth, numbness of the tongue, tinnitus, light headedness, apprehension, excitement, and muscle twitching.
- In severe cases convulsions occur. Respiratory and cardiac depression may follow due to a direct effect of the local anaesthetic and/or secondary to the hypoxia induced by the convulsions.

Management

Convulsions are associated with enormous utilisation of oxygen so that hypoxia develops rapidly. The aim of treatment therefore is to stop the convulsions and ventilate with oxygen without delay:

1. Maintain airway and give 100 per cent oxygen.
2. Protect the patient from injuring herself. Place the patient on her side with slight Trendelenburg to protect the airway and avoid aorto-caval compression.
3. Stop the convulsions with either:
   - Diazepam 5-10 mg i.v. and, if necessary, further increments of 2.5-5 mg, or
   - Thiopentone 50-100 mg i.v. and further increments of 50 mg if required.
4. On rare occasions, the convulsions persist and have to be controlled by paralysis with succinyl choline, endotracheal intubation and intermittent positive pressure ventilation. Diazepam or thiopentone should be given as well to suppress the convulsions at source and to prevent awareness at recovery.

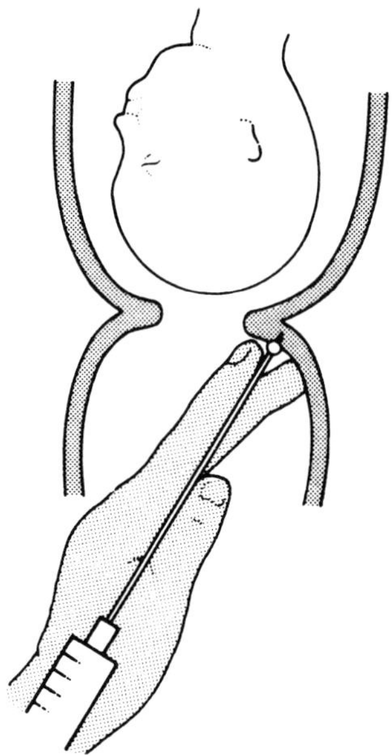

Figure 27.1 Paracervical block.

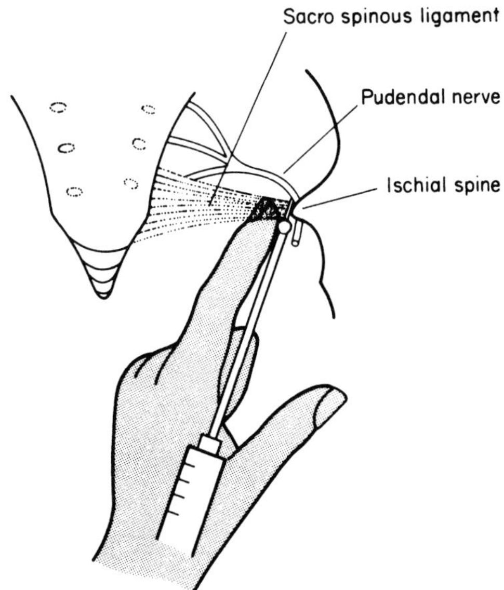

Figure 27.2 Pudendal block.

5. The blood pressure should be monitored throughout, because in severe intoxication myocardial depression may occur which will require treatment with inotropic drugs and other appropriate resuscitative measures.

PARACERVICAL BLOCK

This is a simple and effective method of pain relief in labour when conventional methods of analgesia fail and epidural anaesthesia is unavailable. However, its use in labour is limited by concerns for fetal safety (see later). Paracervical block is also a very useful technique to allow evacuation of the uterus in incomplete abortion. It can also be used in cases when manual removal of the placenta is required but general anaesthesia is not available.

Technique

A specially designed needle and guard are required so that the needle protrudes only 2-3 mm. Using this guard 5-10 ml of local anaesthetic is injected into each lateral fornix between the 3 and 4 o'clock and 8 and 9 o'clock positions (Figure 27.1). Care must be taken to aspirate before, and intermittently during injection as the paracervical space is very vascular.

Complications

Although this technique is very simple to perform, and safe from the maternal aspect the potential fetal side effects cast considerable doubt on the wisdom of using paracervical block in labour. Fetal bradycardia is not uncommon following paracervical block and several cases of intrauterine death related to the block have been recorded. It is felt that in some cases rapid absorption and even transarterial diffusion of the local anaesthetic may cause high fetal levels leading to myocardial and central nervous system depression. In most cases with a bad outcome the fetus was already compromised before the block and high doses of local anaesthetic were used. However, unless modified techniques, with lower doses and less toxic local anaesthetics are developed and shown to be safe, paracervical block cannot be recommended in labour without a strong cautionary note about fetal safety.

PUDENDAL BLOCK

This technique is safe and very useful for low forceps/vacuum and assisted breech delivery. It must be accepted, however, that many pudendal blocks, even in experienced hands, are only partially successful. Therefore augmentation with inhalational analgesia is often appropriate.

Pudendal block can be performed by two methods:

Transvaginal Pudendal Block

This is the method of choice as it is simple, less painful than the transperineal route, and more likely to be successful. Using two fingers in the vagina the ischial spine is identified. The special needle guard is then guided so the end lies just medial and below the ischial spine (Figure 27.2). The needle is then advanced through the vaginal skin and sacrospinous ligament. If the needle is still in the ligament it will not be possible to inject the local anaesthetic. After initial aspiration 7-10 ml of one per cent lidocaine (lignocaine) is injected to block the pudendal nerve.

Transperineal Pudendal Block

This method is used only if the presenting part is so low as to preclude the transvaginal technique. The skin is infiltrated with local anaesthetic halfway between the anus and the ischial tuberosity. With an index finger in the vagina palpating the ischial spine a 10 cm needle is thrust through the infiltrated skin and guided towards the ischial spine and sacro-spinous ligament. The pudendal nerve is blocked in the same manner as the transvaginal technique.

BIBLIOGRAPHY

American College of Obstetricians and Gynecologists. Obstetric analgesia and anesthesia. ACOG Practice Bulliten No 36.Obstet Gynecol 2002;100:177-91.

Bricker L, Lavender T. Parenteral opiods for labor pain relief: a systemic review. Am J Obstet Gynecol 2002;186:S94-109.

Eggleson ST, Lush LW. Understanding allergic reactions to local anesthetics. Ann Pharmacother 1996;30:851-7.

Gall H, Kauffman R, Kalverman CM. Adverse reactions to local anaesthetics: analysis of 197 cases. J Allergy Clin Immuniol 1996;97:933-9.

Halpern SH, Leighton BL, Ohlsson A, Barrett JF, Rice A. Effect of epidural vs. parenteral opiod analgesia on the progress of labor: a meta-analysis. JAMA 1998;280:2105-10.

Kaita TM, Nikkola EM, Rantala MI, Ekblad UU, Salonen MA. Fetal oxygen saturation during epidural and paracervical analgesia. Acta Obstet Gynecol Scand 2000;79:336-40.

Olofsson C, Ekblom A, Ekman-Ordeberg G, Hjelm A, Irestedt L. Lack of analgesic effect of systemically administered morphine or pethidine in labour pain. Br J Obstet Gynaecol 1996;103:968-72.

Rayburn WF, Smith CV, Parriot JE, Wood RE. Randomized comparison of meperidine and fentanyl during labor. Obstet Gynecol 1989;74:604-6.

Rosen MA. Nitrous oxide for relief of labor pain: a systematic review. Am J Obstet Gynecol 2002;186: S110-26.

Rosen MA. Paracervical block for labor analgesia: a brief historic review. Am J Obstet Gynecol 2002;186:S127-30.

Scott DB,. Toxicity caused by local anaesthetic drugs. Br J Anaesth 1984;53:553-4.

Scrimshire JA. Safe use of lignocaine. BMJ 1989;298:1494.

CHAPTER 28

Immediate care of the newborn

The details of neonatal intensive care are beyond the scope of this book. This chapter covers the delivery room care of the normal newborn and the basic principles of neonatal resuscitation.

MANAGEMENT OF THE NORMAL NEWBORN

More than 90 per cent of all newborn infants are mature and vigorous at birth and require only the following routine care:

1. **Airway clearance:** Once the infant's head is delivered the anterior nares and mouth can be gently cleared with a gauze wipe. In the normal infant suction is usually not necessary and vigorous suction is contraindicated as it may induce apnoea, laryngeal spasm and bradycardia.
2. **Avoid heat loss:** The wet newborn with a large surface area in relation to body mass, can suffer enormous heat loss by evaporation within a few minutes. The infant's attempts to sustain its temperature involve greatly increased oxygen consumption, which is undesirable in any newbom and especially in those requiring resuscitation. Therefore a warm towel should be available to thoroughly dry the infant immediately after birth. The infant is then wrapped in a warm blanket to prevent further heat loss. This is one of the simplest and most important aspects of immediate care of the newborn.
3. **Cord clamping:** Immediate cord clamping deprives the infant of about 30 ml blood. If cord clamping is delayed and the infant held below the level of the introitus an increase in blood volume and polycythaemia can result. If the infant is held above the level of the placenta hypovolaemia can ensue. A reasonable compromise is to keep the infant at the level of the introitus and spend about 30 seconds ensuring airway clearance and drying the infant. The cord is then clamped and the infant handed off to be wrapped in a warm blanket. If the infant is depressed at birth there should be no delay in clamping the cord and initiating resuscitation.

Table 28.1 **The Apgar Score**

Sign	0	1	2
Colour	Pale or blue	Body pink: extremities blue	Pink all over
Heart rate	Absent	< 100	>100
Respiration	Absent	Slow, irregular	Vigorous cry
Reflex irritability	No response	Grimace	Cry
Muscle tone	Limp	Some flexion	Well flexed, active motion

The colour and respiration are a visual assessment. The heart rate is recorded from the cord pulsations or by auscultation. Reflex irritability is the response to suction of nares or to flicking the sole of the foot. Muscle tone assessed by manipulating the limbs.

4. **Apgar score:** Performance of this neonatal assessment score should be carried out one and five minutes after delivery (Table 28.1). It ensures a systemic appraisal of the newborn infant, is an indication of its adaptation to extrauterine life, and gives a guide to the need for resuscitation. In the very small pre-term infant the score may be low on the basis of immaturity leading to reduced reflex irritability and muscle tone.

RESUSCITATION OF THE NEWBORN

RESUSCITATION EQUIPMENT

The level of sophistication of facilities for neonatal resuscitation will obviously depend on the size of the hospital. The following is the minimum equipment that should be immediately available in any delivery room-no matter how small the hospital. All personnel should be familiar with the equipment and it should be checked regularly. There is a lot to be said for regular practice drills of neonatal resuscitation using a mannequin.

1. Resuscitation table with the capacity to tilt and an overhead radiant heater.
2. Suction-Wall suction catheter (pressure 50-80 mmHg)
   – DeLee suction trap.
   – Bulb suction.
3. Self-inflating bag and facemasks (assorted sizes).
4. Stethoscope.
5. Oxygen source.
6. Oropharyngeal airways. (Sizes 00 and 0)
7. Laryngoscope with size 0 (preterm) and 1 (term) straight blades.
8. Endotracheal tubes (2.5, 3.0 and 3.5 mm) plus malleable stylets.

7. Umbilical catherisation tray with 3.5 and 5.0 French umbilical catheters.
8. Drugs and syringes:
   Naloxone (0.4 mg/ml).
   Sodium bicarbonate 4.2 (.5mmol/ml)
   Epinephrine (adrenaline) 1 in 10,000.
   Heparin, 1000 u/ml.
   Albumin 4.5%
   10 per cent glucose/water.
   Normal saline.
9. Prominent wall chart with list of drugs, doses for birthweight categories, and route(s) of administration.
10. Wall clock.

ASSESSMENT OF THE INFANT

About 10 per cent of all newborn infants have some degree of cardiorespiratory depression. The main causes are:

1. Asphyxia: Many of the high risk factors for perinatal asphyxia are identifiable in the antepartum or intrapartum periods, for example:

   - Hypertensive disorders
   - Antepartum haemorrhage
   - Diabetes mellitus
   - Rh isoimmunisation
   - Intrauterine growth restriction
   - Chorioamnionitis
   - Preterm delivery
   - Prolonged labour
   - Fetal distress in labour
   - Meconium staining in labour
   - Operative delivery
   - Twin delivery

2. **Drug depression:** Analgesic and anaesthetic drugs cross the placenta and can cause respiratory depression in the newborn.
3. **Fetal haemorrhage:** Fetal blood loss from one twin, a torn vessel in the cord, or vasa praevia may lead to a hypovolaemic and hypoxic newborn.
4. **Congenital anomalies:** Certain anomalies may present with early cardiorespiratory depression; for example diaphragmatic hernia.

Many of the above factors are identifiable in advance of delivery and thus the probable need for resuscitation can be anticipated. In such instances extra personnel can be mustered and the equipment laid out to hand. However, as there is always the possibility of delivery of an asphyxiated infant one must be prepared to initiate resuscitation at any delivery.

In most instances it is not appropriate to wait one minute to perform the formal Apgar score. Rather the elements of the Apgar score are

assessed in a few seconds and the need for, and urgency of, resuscitation based on this evaluation.
Moderate asphyxia (Apgar score 4-6): These infants are usually blue (asphyxia livida), have slow, irregular respiration, heart rate < 100 b.p.m., poor response to stimulation, and decreased muscle tone.
Severe asphyxia (Apgar score 0-3): These infants are pale (asphyxia pallida), have severe bradycardia, absent or slow gasping respiration and are limp and unresponsive. Such infants are in danger of suffering hypoxic brain damage and the resuscitation must proceed apace.

The word 'asphyxia' can have serious social and medico-legal connotations and really should only be applied to the newborn if substantiated by cord gases reflecting acidosis.

MANAGEMENT OF THE RESUSCITATION

1. **Airway clearance:** This is the first move and is carried out with wall, bulb or DeLee suction. This aspect of treatment is covered in detail in the section on meconium aspiration (see later).
2. **Ventilation and oxygenation:**
   (a) **Bag and mask ventilation:** This is a very effective method of applying intermittent positive pressure ventilation provided the practical details are followed. It is appropriate for all cases of moderate asphyxia and some severely asphyxiated infants:
   - The infant's neck should be slightly extended. If there is a lot of caput and moulding of the head it may be necessary to put a rolled towel under the infant's shoulders to facilitate this extension.
   - The face mask must fit tightly over the mouth and nose to avoid leaks. The nose must not be obstructed as it is the route of ventilation. The left index finger and thumb hold the mask over the mouth and nose and the other fingers support the chin and mandible.
   - The 100 per cent oxygen source should flow at 4-6 l/min. There is growing evidence that room air may be as effective as 100 oxygen and possibly less risky in preterm infants.[1]
   - In the first instance the right hand squeezes the bag at a rate of approximately 100 per minute. Initially lung compliance may be quite high because of lung fluid. As the pulmonary circulation is established, the lung stiffness diminishes and less pressure is needed for ventilation. After the initial rapid rate the bag can be squeezed at 30-40 per minute.
   - The adequacy of ventilation is assessed by gauging the movement of the chest wall (the lower sternum should lift by 1-2cm), auscultation of breath sounds, rise in the heart rate, and pinking of the infant.

- Most infants will respond to airway clearance and adequate bag and mask ventilation.

(b) **Endotracheal intubation:** This method is used in severely asphyxiated infants, either initially, or if about 30 seconds bag and mask ventilation fails to achieve a good response. It may also be used in some infants with meconium aspiration.

- The infant's neck should be neutral or in slight extension (the 'sniff 'position). The larynx of an infant is more anterior than that of an adult, so that hyperextension of the neck displaces the larynx even further anteriorly hindering intubation.
- The laryngoscope is grasped between the thumb and index finger of the left hand with the middle and ring fingers supporting the infant's chin. This leaves the little finger resting on the larynx where it can apply pressure to bring the vocal cords posteriorly and into view (Figure 28.1).

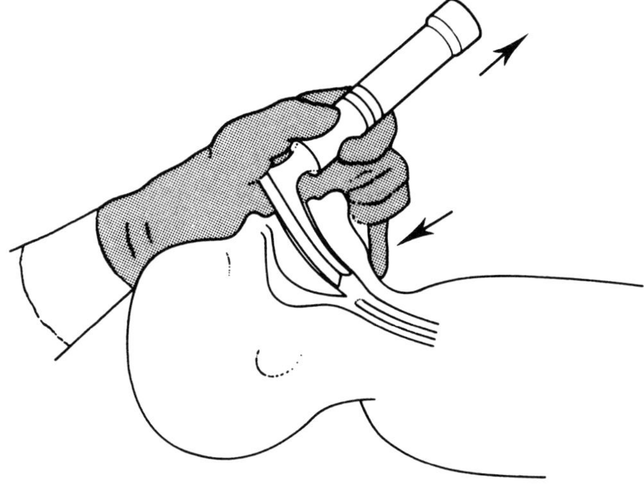

Figure 28.1 Neonatal intubation. Little finger pressed gently on larynx to bring cords into view.

- The laryngoscope is inserted into the right side of the infant's mouth and then rotated to the midline, moving the tongue to the left. Advance the laryngoscope blade into the oesophagus and then slowly withdraw until the vocal cords pop into view.

- The endotracheal tube is inserted from the right side of the mouth 1-2 cm below the cords. The size of tube depends on the estimated weight of the infant:

<1000 g	2.5 mm
1000-2500 g	3.0 mm
>2500 g	3.5 mm

- The bag is attached to the tube and the same principles of ventilation applied.
- Check for correct positioning of tube by: bilateral chest movement, bilateral breath sounds on auscultation and absent breath sounds over the stomach.
- The tube is removed when the infant becomes vigorous and there is sustained regular respiration.

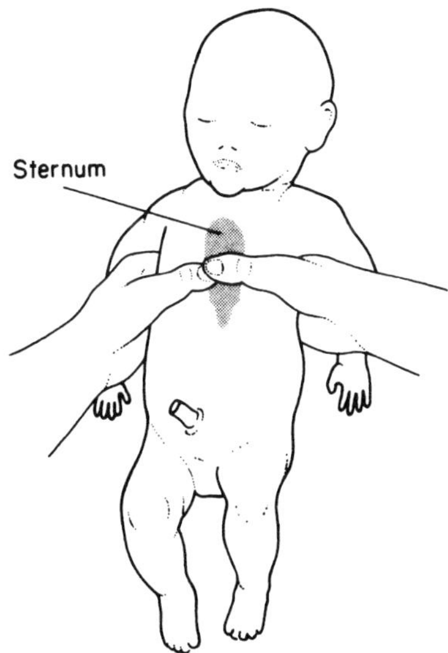

Figure 28.2 Neonatal external chest compression (cardiac massage).

3. **External chest compression (cardiac massage):** This is indicated if the heart beat is absent or if, despite apparently adequate ventilation, a severe bradycardia (< 60 b.p.m.) persists.
   - The hands encircle the infant's chest so that the fingers support the back. The thumbs, one on top of the other, are placed on the middle third of the sternum (Figure 28.2). Placement lower on the sternum may lacerate the liver. It is important that the encircling hands are not placed so tightly around the chest as to interfere with the assisted ventilation.

- The sternum is depressed one-quarter of the antero-posterior diameter of the chest, at a rate of about 120 per minute. The coordination of chest compression and ventilation should be 3:1, with three chest compressions followed by one ventilation. Thus, over one minute there would be 90 chest compressions and 30 ventilations.
- Properly carried out external chest compression (cardiac massage) should maintain enough cerebral and coronary artery perfusion to prevent hypoxic damage.

4. **Umbilical vein catheterisation:** This is necessary if one has to give drugs or intravenous fluids to the infant.

   Access to the umbilical vein can be achieved by dissecting it free of Wharton's jelly and making a nick in the vein with a scalpel close to the abdominal wall. A 3.5 or 5.0 French umbilical catheter is threaded in 5-10 centimetres until blood can be drawn back. The catheter is retained in the same manner as a cutdown intravenous line.
5. **Narcotic antagonist:** The drug of choice is naloxone in a dose of 0.1mg/kg. This can be given intravenously, directly down the endotracheal tube or, if the infant's peripheral circulation is good, by intramuscular injection. This drug is only given after appropriate resuscitation if depression by narcotic drugs is suspected. Should not be given if the mother is opiate dependent.
6. **Epinephrine (adrenaline):** If, despite adequate basic resuscitation, the infant remains severely bradycardiac or without detectable cardiac activity, epinephrine 1 in 10000 solution in a dose of 0.1 to 0.3ml/kg (0.01 to 0.03mg/kg) can be infused through the umbilical vein catheter or directly down the endotracheal tube. When using the endotracheal route one should lean toward the higher dose. This dose can be repeated twice every 3-5 minutes if there is no response.
7. **Correction of acidosis:**
   - If, despite several minutes of appropriate resuscitation, the infant remains unresponsive, pale and bradycardiac, steps should be taken to correct the metabolic acidosis that will by now exist.
   - Sodium bicarbonate is very hyperosmolar and may cause vasodilatation and hypotension if given undiluted and rapidly.
   - When sodium bicarbonate is given the ventilation rate should be increased to eliminate the increased production of carbon dioxide produced as the hydrogen ions react with the bicarbonate.
   - The sodium bicarbonate is infused slowly through an umbilical catheter, at a rate of I mmol/minute to a dose of 1-2 mmol/Kg.It is very irritant if given extravascularly. Flush the catheter with normal saline after adminstration.
8. **10 per cent glucose/water:** This infusion, at an initial rate of 4 ml/kg/ hour, will provide metabolic substrate and a vehicle for drug

administration. The maintenance rate is about 2 ml/kg/hour.

The newborn infant that does not respond to the above resuscitation within 10-15 minutes has a bad prognosis. If spontaneous respiration and a sustained heart rate are not present after 20 minutes, it is almost always appropriate to stop resuscitative efforts.

CONGENITAL ANOMALIES

Certain anomalies are more likely to present in the delivery room with early problems of respiration and ventilation:

Diaphragmatic hernia occurs in about 1 in every 3000 deliveries. The infant presents with immediate respiratory distress, a scaphoid abdomen and heart sounds shifted to the right. The initial management is immediate intubation and ventilation, followed by passage of a naso-gastric tube and decompression of the stomach. The aim is to sustain the infant until paediatric surgery is available.

Choanal atresia is a rare malformation with blocked nasal passages. The infant is initially vigorous and well. Respiratory distress occurs when the infant stops mouth breathing. A nasal catheter cannot be passed. There is chest retraction but no nasal flaring. The initial treatment is an oropharyngeal airway.

Tracheo-oesophageal fistula and oseophageal atresia occur in about 1 in 3000 deliveries. The clue is the inability to pass a nasogastric tube. If respiratory distress occurs, intubation and ventilation may be necessary until surgery can be considered.

Pierre Robin syndrome (micrognathia and glossoptosis): In this condition the tongue may fall back and obstruct the hypopharynx. If possible an oropharyngeal airway should be inserted and this may be facilitated by passing a nasal catheter to help dislodge the tongue forward. The infant should be placed prone.

HYPOVOLAEMIA

This possibility should be considered in twins, abruptio placentae, and placenta praevia. In other suspicious cases inspection of the placenta, cord, and membranes may reveal a torn vessel or vasa praevia as the source of fetal blood loss. The infant presents with pallor, hypotension, and tachycardia. In advanced cases it may be hard to differentiate from asphyxia pallida. A degree of hypovolaemia also occurs in the asphyxiated infant due to the vasoconstriction associated with hypoxia in utero and is compounded by the necessity for immediate cord clamping in these cases.

Management

The initial treatment consists of giving, via the umbilical venous catheter, 10-20 ml/kg over 5 to 10 minutes, one of the following:

- Normal saline/Ringers lactate.
- 4.5 per cent albumin in normal saline.
- Emergency 0 negative blood.

MECONIUM ASPIRATION

The aspiration of thick particulate meconium into the distal airways causes pneumonitis and also acts as a culture medium for secondary infection. Plugs of meconium can lodge in small bronchioles causing complete obstruction and distal collapse of alveoli. A partial ballvalve type obstruction may cause distal alveolar rupture leading to interstitial escape of air and the potential for pneumothorax, pneumomediastinum, and subcutaneous emphysema.

Management

1. As soon as the infant's head is born, and while the thorax is still in the birth canal inhibiting inspiratory efforts which might distribute meconium to the peripheral airways, the nares and oropharynx should be thoroughly cleared of meconium by suction. Use of a catheter via DeLee or wall suction is more effective than bulb suction. Intrauterine fetal gasping associated with hypoxia may have caused some peripheral distribution of meconium prior to delivery. In such cases it is still worth while using careful suction to cut down the total amount of meconium aspirated. There is evidence that amnioinfusion with normal saline during labour complicated by meconium staining reduces the sequelae of meconium aspiration.[2,3]
2. Once delivered, if the infant is crying and vigorous, just apply gentle suction to the oropharynx: laryngoscopy is not required.[4]
3. If the infant is depressed, immediate laryngoscopy should be performed and any visible meconium sucked out. An endotracheal tube is then passed, and suction applied to the tube as it is withdrawn. Special adapters between the endotracheal tube and suction tubing are available. Once removed, blow out the contents. If there is no meconium, leave the tube out and ventilate with oxygen by bag and mask. If there is meconium in the tube blow it out, reinsert the tube, and repeat until the meconium is cleared.
4. It is essential to clear the infant's airway as quickly as possible before established respiration distributes the meconium to the small

airways. However, even if the infant has begun breathing, aspiration of the trachea is still worthwhile in the presence of thick meconium. The other reason for speedy clearance of the airway is to initiate oxygenation as soon as possible.

5. When the infant is stable pass a nasogastric tube and suction the stomach. Infants born through meconium often swallow it and may regurgitate and aspirate later on.

6. The full routine outlined above need not apply to thin watery meconium. In these cases the nares and oropharynx are sucked out but, provided the infant is vigorous, endotracheal intubation is not required. Indeed, persistent attempts to intubate a vigorous, crying infant can be traumatic, as well as unsuccessful.

It is emphasized that the above principles of management for newborn resuscitation are proposed for those working in hospitals without sophisticated neonatal intensive care. By far the most important aspects are clearance and establishment of an airway, ventilation, circulatory support and the avoidance of hypothermia. If one gets to the stage of having to use drugs, other than narcotic antagonists, the chances of successful resuscitation are small.

These clinical skills are easily learned and the equipment is readily obtained. In clinical practice the main reason for failure is a lack of organisation so that equipment is not to hand when an unanticipated resuscitation is required. All personnel should be familiar with the equipment and practice the routines of resuscitation.

REFERENCES

1. Lundstrom KE, Pryds O, Greisen G. Oxygen at birth and prolonged cerebral vasoconstriction in preterm infants. Arch Dis Child 1995;73:F81-6.
2. Mahomed K, Mulambo T, Woelk G et al. The collaborative randomised amnioinfusion for meconium project (CRAMP): 2. Zimbabwe. Br J Obstet Gynaecol 1998;105:309-13.
3. Pierce J, Gaudier FL, Sanchez-Ramos L. Intrapartum amnioinfusion for meconium-stained fluid: meta-analysis of prospective clinical trials. Obstet Gynecol 2000;95:1051-6.
4, Wiswell TE, Gannon CM, Jacob J et al. Delivery room management of the apparently vigorous meconium-stained neonate:results of the multicenter, international collaborative trial. Pediatrics 2000;105:1-7.

BIBLIOGRAPHY

Advanced Life Support Group. Advanced Paediatric Life Support. 3rd ed. London: BMJ Publishing Group, 2000.

American Academy of Pediatrics Advanced Life Support. Elk Grove, Ill: AAP: 1997.

American College of Obstetricians and Gynecologists. Use and abuse of the Apgar score. Committee opinion No.174. Washington DC: ACOG,1996.

Letsky E A. Fetal and neonatal transfusion. BMJ 1990;300: 862-6.

McIntyre J. Neonatal resuscitation. In: Intrapartum Care. Baskett TF, Arulkumaran S. London:RCOG Press, 2002.p 175-84.

Milner AD. Resuscitation of the newborn. Arch Dis Child 1991;66:66-9.

Resuscitation of Babies at Birth. London: BMJ Publishing Group, 1997.

Sims DG, Heal CA, Bartle SM. Use of adrenaline and atropine in neonatal resuscitation. Arch Dis Child 1994;70:F3-10.

Walker DE, Balvert L. A practical program to maintain neonatal resuscitation skills. Can Med Assoc J 1994;151:299-304.

INDEX

Notes

Notes

Notes